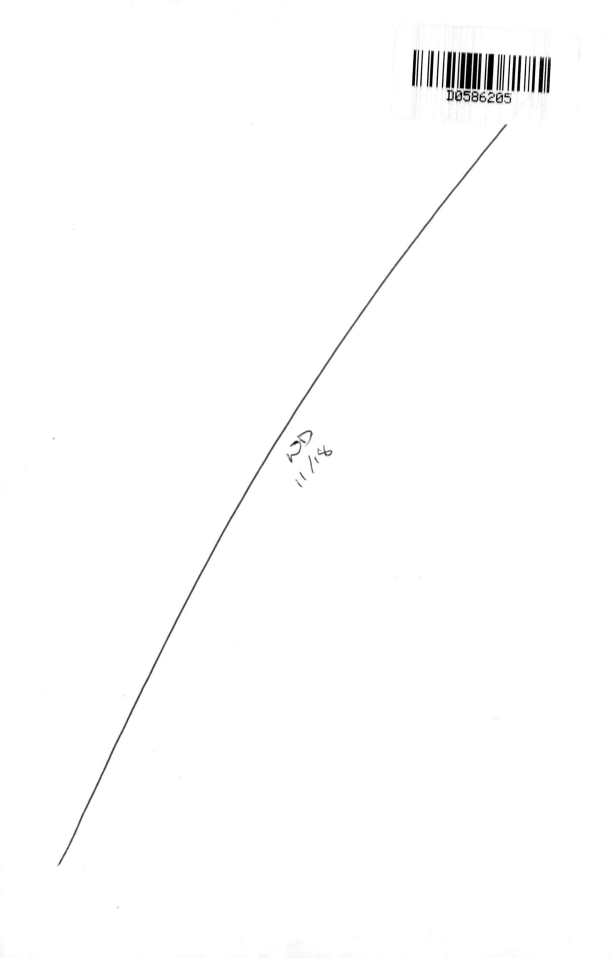

RD
11/18

theclinics.com

BURTON P. DRAYER, MD, Consulting Editor

NEUROIMAGING
CLINICS of North America

Stroke II: Imaging Techniques and Future Directions

MICHAEL H. LEV, MD
Guest Editor

August 2005 • Volume 15 • Number 3

SAUNDERS

An Imprint of Elsevier, Inc.
PHILADELPHIA   LONDON   TORONTO   MONTREAL   SYDNEY   TOKYO

W.B. SAUNDERS COMPANY
A Division of Elsevier Inc.

1600 John F. Kennedy Boulevard • Suite 1800 • Philadelphia, Pennsylvania 19103-2899

http://www.theclinics.com

NEUROIMAGING CLINICS OF NORTH AMERICA	**Volume 15, Number 3**
August 2005	**ISSN 1052-5149**
Editor: Barton Dudlick	**ISBN 1-4160-2734-3**

Neuroimaging Clinics of North America (ISSN 1052-5149) is published quarterly by Elsevier Inc. Corporate and editorial offices: 1600 John F. Kennedy Boulevard, Suite 1800, Pennsylvania, PA 19103-2899. Accounting and circulation offices: 6277 Sea Harbor Drive, Orlando, FL 32887-4800. Periodicals postage paid at Orlando, FL 32862, and additional mailing offices. Subscription prices are USD 190 per year for US individuals, USD 290 per year for US institutions, USD 95 per year for US students and residents, USD 214 per year for Canadian individuals, USD 352 per year for Canadian institutions, USD 255 per year for international individuals, USD 352 per year for international institutions and USD 128 per year for Canadian and foreign students/residents. To receive student/resident rate, orders must be accompanied by name of affiliated institution, date of term and the *signature* of program/residency coordinator on institution letterhead. Orders will be billed at individual rate until proof of status is received. Foreign air speed delivery is included in all *Clinics* subscription prices. All prices are subject to change without notice. POSTMASTER: Send address changes to *Neuroimaging Clinics of North America*, W.B. Saunders Company, Periodicals Fulfillment, Orlando, FL 32887-4800. **Customer Service: 800-654-2452 (US). From outside of the US, call (+1) 407-345-4000. E-mail: hhspcs@harcourt.com.**

Reprints. For copies of 100 or more, of articles in this publication, please contact the Commercial Reprints Department, Elsevier Inc., 360 Park Avenue South, New York, New York 10010-1710. Tel.: (+1) 212-633-3813; Fax: (+1) 212-462-1935; E-mail: reprints@elsevier.com.

Neuroimaging Clinics of North America is covered by *Excerpta Medica/EMBASE,* the RSNA Index of Imaging Literature, Index Medicus, MEDLINE/MEDLARS, SciSearch, Research Alert, and Neuroscience Citation Index.

Printed in the United States of America.

GOAL STATEMENT

The goal of *Neuroimaging Clinics of North America* is to keep practicing radiologists and radiology residents up to date with current clinical practice in radiology by providing timely articles reviewing the state-of-the-art in patient care.

ACCREDITATION

The *Neuroimaging Clinics of North America* is planned and implemented in accordance with the Essential Areas and Policies of the Accreditation Council for Continuing Medical Education (ACCME) through the joint sponsorship of the University of Virginia School of Medicine and Elsevier. The University of Virginia School of Medicine is accredited by the ACCME to provide continuing medical education for physicians.

The University of Virginia School of Medicine designates this educational activity for a maximum of 60 category 1 credits per year, 15 category 1 credits per issue, toward the AMA Physician's Recognition Award. Each physician should claim only those credits that he/she actually spent in the activity.

The American Medical Association has determined that physicians not licensed in the US who participate in this CME activity are eligible for AMA PRA category 1 credit.

Category 1 credit can be earned by reading the text material, taking the CME examination online at *http://www.theclinics.com/home/cme*, and completing the evaluation. After taking the test, you will be required to review any and all incorrect answers. Following completion of the test and evaluation, your credit will be awarded and you may print your certificate.

FACULTY DISCLOSURE/CONFLICT OF INTEREST

The University of Virginia School of Medicine, as an ACCME accredited provider, endorses and strives to comply with the Accreditation Council for Continuing Medical Education (ACCME) Standards of Commercial Support, Commonwealth of Virginia statutes, University of Virginia policies and procedures, and associated federal and private regulations and guidelines on the need for disclosure and monitoring of proprietary and financial interests that may affect the scientific integrity and balance of content delivered in continuing medical education activities under our auspices.

The University of Virginia School of Medicine requires that all CME activities accredited through this institution be developed independently and be scientifically rigorous, balanced and objective in the presentation/discussion of its content, theories and practices.

All authors/editors participating in an accredited CME activity are expected to disclose to the readers relevant financial relationships with commercial entities occurring within the past 12 months (such as grants or research support, employee, consultant, stock holder, member of speakers bureau, etc.). The University of Virginia School of Medicine will employ appropriate mechanisms to resolve potential conflicts of interest to maintain the standards of fair and balanced education to the reader. Questions about specific strategies can be directed to the Office of Continuing Medical Education, University of Virginia School of Medicine, Charlottesville, Virginia.

The authors/editors listed below have identified no professional/financial affiliations for themselves or their spouse/partner:
Brad R. Brobeck, MD; John W. Chen, MD, PhD; Andrew Demchuck, MD, FRCPC; Barton Dudlick, Acquisitions Editor; P. Ellen Grant, MD; David S. Liebeskind, MD; Eng H. Lo, PhD; Michael A. Moskowitz, MD; Pratik Mukherjee, MD, PhD; Leif Østergaard, MD, PhD; Maher Saqqur, MD, FRCPC; Sanjay K. Shetty, MD; Aneesh B. Singhal, MD; James Snyder, MD; Bruce A. Wasserman, MD; Ona Wu, PhD; and, William T.C. Yuh, MD, MSEE.

The authors listed below have identified the following professional/financial affiliations for themselves or their spouse/partner:
Steven C. Cramer, MD is a consultant and on the advisory board for GlaxoSmithKline, EBEWE Pharma, and WL Gore and Associates; is a consultant, on the advisory board, and a stockholder in Stem Cell Therapeutics; and is a consultant for Northstar Neuroscience, AGY Therapeutics, and Biotrofix.
Michael H. Lev, MD has educational grants and is on the speakers' bureau for GE Medical Systems and Bracco Diagnostics.
Howard A. Rowley, MD is a consultant for Forest Labs and Paion Corp., and is a consultant, on the speakers' bureau and the advisory board for GE Healthcare.
Keith R. Thulborn, MD, PhD is a contractor for GE and the owner of Thulborn Associates, Inc, both in the area of MRI.

The authors listed below have not provided disclosure for themselves or their spouse/partner:
Adrei V. Alexandrov, MD; William A. Copen, MD; Turgay Dalkara, MD, PhD; Denise Davis, BS; Andrew Demchuk, MD; Lucy Der Yeghiaian, MA, OTR/L; R. Gilberto Gonzalez, MD, PhD; Rishi Gupta, MD; Tudor G. Jovin, MD; Amin Kassam, MD; Michael H. Lev, MD; David J. Mikulis, MD; Pamela W. Schaefer, MD; A. Gregory Sorenson, MD; Craig D. Takahashi, PhD; Toshihiro Ueda, MD, PhD; and Howard Yonas, MD.

Disclosure of Discussion of non-FDA approved uses for pharmaceutical products and/or medical devices.
The University of Virginia School of Medicine, as an ACCME provider, requires that all authors/editors identify and disclose any "off label" uses for pharmaceutical products and/or for medical devices. The University of Virginia School of Medicine recommends that each reader fully review all the available data on new products or procedures prior to instituting them with patients.

TO ENROLL

To enroll in the Neuroimaging Clinics of North America Continuing Medical Education program, call customer service at 1-800-654-2452 or sign up online at *http://www.theclinics.com/home/cme*. The CME program is available to subscribers for an additional annual fee of USD 156.

FORTHCOMING ISSUES

RECENT ISSUES

CONSULTING EDITOR

BURTON P. DRAYER, MD, Dr. Charles M. and Marilyn Professor and Chairman, Department of Radiology, Mount Sinai Medical Center, New York, New York

GUEST EDITOR

MICHAEL H. LEV, MD, Director, Emergency Neuroradiology and Neurovascular Laboratory, Department of Radiology, Massachusetts General Hospital; and Associate Professor (Radiology), Harvard Medical School, Boston, Massachusetts

CONTRIBUTORS

ANDREI V. ALEXANDROV, MD, Director, Neurosonology Program and Stroke Research, Barrow Neurological Institute, Phoenix, Arizona

BRAD R. BROBECK, MD, Division of Neuroradiology, Massachusetts General Hospital, Boston, Massachusetts

JOHN W. CHEN, MD, PhD, Division of Neuroradiology, Department of Radiology, Massachusetts General Hospital, Boston, Massachusetts

WILIAM A. COPEN, MD, Clinical Assistant (Radiology), Massachusetts General Hospital, Boston, Massachusetts

STEVEN C. CRAMER, MD, Associate Professor, Departments of Neurology and Anatomy and Neurobiology, University of California at Irvine, Irvine, California

TURGAY DALKARA, MD, PhD, Professor (Neurology), Faculty of Medicine, Hacettepe University, Ankara, Turkey

DENISE DAVIS, BS, Instructor (Radiology), Department of Radiology, University of Pittsburgh Medical Center, Pittsburgh, Pennsylvania

ANDREW M. DEMCHUK, MD, FRCPC, Associate Professor (Neurology), Department of Clinical Neurosciences, University of Calgary, Calgary, Alberta, Canada

LUCY DER YEGHIAIAN, MA, OTR/L, Department of Occupational Therapy, University of California at Irvine, Irvine, California

R. GILBERTO GONZALEZ, MD, PhD, Director, Massachusetts General Hospital; and Professor (Radiology), Harvard Medical School, Boston, Massachusetts

P. ELLEN GRANT, MD, Chief, Division of Pediatric Radiology, Massachusetts General Hospital, Boston, Massachusetts

RISHI GUPTA, MD, Clinical Fellow (Vascular Neurology and Neurovascular Surgery), Department of Neurology, Stroke Institute, University of Pittsburgh Medical Center, Pittsburgh, Pennsylvania

TUDOR G. JOVIN, MD, Assistant Professor (Neurology), Department of Neurology, Stroke Institute, University of Pittsburgh Medical Center; and Veterans Affairs Pittsburgh Health Care System, Pittsburgh, Pennsylvania

AMIN KASSAM, MD, Associate Professor, Department of Neurological Surgery, University of Pittsburgh Medical Center, Pittsburgh, Pennsylvania

MICHAEL H. LEV, MD, Director, Emergency Neuroradiology and Neurovascular Laboratory, Department of Radiology, Massachusetts General Hospital,; and Associate Professor (Radiology), Harvard Medical School, Boston, Massachusetts

DAVID S. LIEBESKIND, MD, Assistant Professor (Neurology); Neurology Director, Stroke Imaging; and Associate Neurology Director, University of California at Los Angeles Stroke Center, University of California at Los Angeles Medical Center, Los Angeles, California

ENG H. LO, PhD, Associate Professor (Radiology), Harvard Medical School, Boston; and Neuroprotection Research Laboratory, Department of Radiology, Massachusetts General Hospital, Charlestown, Massachusetts

DAVID J. MIKULIS, MD, Director, Functional MR Imaging Research; Associate Professor, Division of Neuroradiology, Department of Medical Imaging, Toronto Western Hospital of the University Health Network and University of Toronto; and Senior Scientist, Toronto Western Hospital Research Institute and Institute of Medical Science, University of Toronto, Toronto, Ontario, Canada

MICHAEL A. MOSKOWITZ, MD, Professor (Neurology), Harvard Medical School, Boston; and Stroke and Neurovascular Regulation Laboratory, Neuroscience Center, Departments of Radiology and Neurology, Massachusetts General Hospital, Charlestown, Massachusetts

PRATIK MUKHERJEE, MD, PhD, Assistant Professor (Radiology and Bioengineering), Neuroradiology Section, Department of Radiology, University of California at San Francisco, San Francisco, California

LEIF ØSTERGAARD, MD, PhD, Director, Center of Functionally Integrative Neuroscience, Department of Neuroradiology, Århus University Hospital, Århus, Denmark

HOWARD A. ROWLEY, MD, Sackett Professor of Radiology; and Chief (Neuroradiology), Department of Radiology, University of Wisconsin, Madison, Wisconsin

MAHER SAQQUR, MD, FRCPC, Clinical Assistant Professor (Neurology), Division of Neurology, Department of Medicine, University of Alberta, Edmonton, Alberta, Canada

PAMELA W. SCHAEFER, MD, Associate Director (Neuroradiology); Director (MRI), Massachusetts General Hospital; and Associate Professor (Radiology), Harvard Medical School, Boston, Massachusetts

SANJAY K. SHETTY, MD, Clinical Fellow, Division of Neuroradiology, Department of Radiology, Massachusetts General Hospital, Boston, Massachusetts

ANEESH B. SINGHAL, MD, Assistant Professor (Neurology), Harvard Medical School; and Stroke Service, Department of Neurology, Massachusetts General Hospital, Boston, Massachusetts

JAMES SNYDER, MD, Professor, Department of Anesthesiology/Critical Care Medicine, University of Pittsburgh Medical Center, Pittsburgh, Pennsylvania

A. GREGORY SORENSEN, MD, Co-Director, MGH/MIT/HMS Athinoula A. Martinos Center for Biomedical Imaging, Charlestown, Massachusetts

CRAIG D. TAKAHASHI, PhD, Department of Neurology, University of California at Irvine, Irvine, California

KEITH R. THULBORN, MD, PhD, Professor (Radiology, Physiology, and Biophysics), Center for Magnetic Resonance Research, University of Illinois at Chicago, Chicago, Illinois

TOSHIHIRO UEDA, MD, PhD, Director, Division of Stroke Diagnostics and Therapeutics, Yokohama Stroke and Brain Center, Yokohama, Japan

BRUCE A. WASSERMAN, MD, Neuroradiology Division, Russell H. Morgan Department of Radiology and Radiological Science, Johns Hopkins Medical Institutions, Baltimore, Maryland

ONA WU, PhD, Instructor (Computer Science), MGH Department of Radiology, MGH/MIT/HMS Athinoula A. Martinos Center for Biomedical Imaging, Charlestown, Massachusetts

HOWARD YONAS, MD, Chairman; and Professor (Neurosurgery), Department of Neurosurgery, University of New Mexico Health Sciences Center, Albuquerque, New Mexico

WILLIAM T.C. YUH, MD, MSEE, Professor and Vice Chairman, Department of Radiology, Ohio State University Medical Center, Columbus, Ohio

CONTENTS

of disease processes, including ischemic stroke. The changes that occur in acute infarction enable DWI to detect very early ischemia. Also, because predictable progression of diffusion findings occurs during the evolution of ischemia, DWI enables more precise estimation of the time of stroke onset than does conventional imaging.

Acute stroke therapy is evolving rapidly as research moves toward extending the time window for treatment so that more patients can benefit. As physiology-based imaging increasingly is used in patient selection, it is becoming evident that rigid time windows are not applicable to individual patients. Xenon CT has an important role in acute stroke therapeutic intervention as a quantitative, reproducible, rapid, and safe modality, which can provide valuable physiologic data that can optimize patient triage and aid in management.

Single-photon emission CT (SPECT) is an underused noninvasive imaging tool for the management of patients who have acute or chronic ischemia. SPECT was introduced in the late 1970s and is a proven, cost-effective means for the evaluation of regional cerebral blood flow and cerebrovascular reserve. Evaluation of cerebral blood flow using SPECT has become more accessible with the commercial availability of tracers that cross the blood–brain barrier and are retained by cells of the central nervous system.

Collateral circulation is a fundamental determinant of stroke pathophysiology. Distal arterial embolism and hypoperfusion resulting from severe proximal arterial stenosis may be offset by collateral flow. Collaterals influence whether or not infarction results. The detection and characterization of arterial deoxygenation and other consequences of collateral perfusion depend on neuroimaging techniques. Imaging advances will further the understanding of clinical correlates, including collateral sustenance and collateral failure, and possibly promote the development of collateral therapeutics. Refinements of perfusion imaging protocols may quantify the delay and dispersion of collateral flow more accurately. This review explores the role of collateral flow in acute ischemic stroke and describes the imaging modalities used to investigate phenomena "beyond the clot."

Data from intravenous tissue plasminogen activator studies have shown rapidly diminishing clinical benefit beyond 3 hours when noncontrast CT is used for treatment triage. Newer trials, such as the Desmoteplase in Acute Ischemic Stroke trial, have now successfully pushed the time window out to 9 hours using the concept of penumbral imaging and treatment of the perfusion-diffusion mismatch. Advanced imaging with CT or MR imaging protocols is providing a means for rational physiologic selection and outcomes assessment in stroke treatment.

projection pulse sequence with extremely short echo time values. This twisted projection imaging provides high signal-to-noise images at adequate resolution ($5 \times 5 \times 5$ mm^3) in less than 10 minutes at 3.0 T. The images are quantified as tissue sodium concentration (TSC) maps that can be interpreted directly in terms of tissue viability. With infarction, baseline TSC values of less than 45 mmol/L increase at variable rates to approximately 70 mmol/L, allowing monitoring of the progression of stroke pathophysiology.

provides an overview of the major mechanisms of neuronal injury and the status of neuroprotective drug trials and reviews emerging strategies for treatment of acute ischemic stroke. Advances in the fields of stem cell transplantation, stroke recovery, molecular neuroimaging, genomics, and proteomics will provide new therapeutic avenues in the near future. These and other developments over the past decade raise expectations that successful stroke neuroprotection is imminent.

NEUROIMAGING
CLINICS OF
NORTH AMERICA

Neuroimag Clin N Am 15 (2005) xv – xvi

Preface

Stroke II: Imaging Techniques and Future Directions

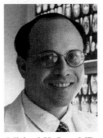

Michael H. Lev, MD
Guest Editor

...all the most acute, most powerful, and most deadly diseases, and those which are most difficult to be understood by the inexperienced, fall upon the brain.

—Hippocrates (circa 400 BC)

"What am I supposed to do? No one can restore a brain!"

—Dr. Leonard "Bones" McCoy
(*Star Trek* Episode #56: "Spock's Brain")

Advances in stroke neuroimaging and therapeutics since the start of the "Decade of the Brain" in 1990 have exceeded the imaginings of science fiction. Technologic developments such as diffusion/perfusion-weighted imaging, multidetector row CT angiography, and endovascular clot dissolution/retrieval strategies have occurred at a staggering pace. Improved understanding of underlying stroke pathophysiology continues to make these advances increasingly clinically relevant.

These two issues of the *Neuroimaging Clinics of North America* attempt to capture the excitement of this evolving field, making it accessible to experts and novices alike. Stroke I provides an overview of differing approaches to stroke prevention and management throughout the world, dealing primarily with the interface between imaging and intervention. Stroke II explores the technical aspects of various neuroimaging modalities in greater detail, with special attention to their physiological underpinnings and future potential. Important differences between adult and childhood stroke are highlighted.

Certain recurrent themes emerge from the outset: diffusion imaging is the most sensitive method for the detection of infarct *core* (tissue likely—but not certain—to die despite early complete reperfusion of ischemic brain), although source images from the CT angiography dataset, like MR diffusion-weighted imaging, can also define core; CT angiography is more accurate than MR angiography for depicting large vessel thrombus; susceptibility MR is more sensitive than CT for detecting chronic microbleeds (the clinical relevance of which for thrombolysis exclusion, however, is unclear); and the ratio between core and salvageable *penumbra* (ischemic tissue that may survive with early reperfusion) might be used to extend the current limited time window for thrombolytic treatment.

The authors have done a wonderful job; they run the spectrum from "up and coming" to established leaders in their respective areas of expertise. There is some overlap—and even occasional disagreement—between authors as they review related topics from different perspectives. Such controversy befits a field undergoing such rapid evolution as stroke neuroimaging.

Acknowledgments

There are several individuals without whom these two issues would not exist. I cannot overstate the foresight of R. Gilberto Gonzalez, MD, Chief of Neuroradiology, and Walter J. Koroshetz, MD, Chief of Stroke Neurology, in both advancing novel MR/CT imaging techniques as clinical tools for patient triage at the Massachusetts General Hospital and in supporting my career goals. Dr. Robert H. Ackerman, director emeritus of the Massachusetts General Hospital Neurovascular Laboratory, has served as a valued mentor for over 15 years. My sincere thanks go to Dr. Burton Drayer for inviting me to participate in this *Clinics* series, and I would also like to acknowledge my research assistants Jonathan Fine, Sarah Gottfried, and Erin Murphy for their editing help. Finally, my heartfelt thanks to my wife, Julie M.

Goodman, PhD, not only for her detailed neuroscience editorial expertise, but also for all else that has made this work possible.

Dedication

These issues are dedicated to Marilyn Lev (1935–2003).

Michael H. Lev, MD

Director
Emergency Neuroradiology and
Neurovascular Laboratory
Department of Radiology
Massachusetts General Hospital
Boston, MA, USA

Associate Professor (Radiology)
Harvard Medical School
Boston, MA, USA

NEUROIMAGING
CLINICS OF
NORTH AMERICA

Neuroimag Clin N Am 15 (2005) 473–480

Transcranial Doppler in Acute Stroke

Andrew M. Demchuk, MD, FRCPC[a],*, Maher Saqqur, MD, FRCPC[b], Andrei V. Alexandrov, MD[c]

[a]Department of Clinical Neurosciences, University of Calgary, Calgary, AB, Canada
[b]Division of Neurology, Department of Medicine, University of Alberta, Edmonton, AB, Canada
[c]Neurosonology Program and Stroke Research, Barrow Neurological Institute, Phoenix, AZ, USA

Neurovascular imaging has revolutionized the understanding of acute stroke and guides the development of reperfusion strategies. Intravenously administered tissue plasminogen activator (tPA) has proved an effective therapy for ischemic stroke if initiated within 3 hours of symptom onset [1]. Fifty percent of treated patients, however, remain disabled or die despite therapy. One likely explanation for this limited effect is late or ineffective recanalization. Recanalization rates range from 25% to 40% with systemic tPA alone [2,3]. Recent evidence suggests that early reperfusion is the key to thrombolytic benefit [4–6]. This article addresses the evolving role of transcranial Doppler (TCD) in acute stroke, with emphasis on its (1) monitoring of recanalization and (2) therapeutic potential to augment recanalization.

Transcranial Doppler advantages and limitations

Ultraearly neuroimaging may provide crucial information for individual patients by determining the status of arterial occlusion and collateral perfusion and the extent and severity of ischemia in the earliest stages of treatment [7]. Noncontrast CT could provide some information regarding the extent and severity of ischemic injury by visualization of early ischemic changes. Hyperdense middle cerebral artery (MCA) sign and the M2-MCA "dot" sign [8] give some clues to location of occlusion and clot burden, but it is CT angiography or, to a slightly lesser degree, MR angiography, that can assess vessel patency most accurately in acute stroke [9,10]. Both these imaging methods, however, provide only "snapshots in time" and are not able to provide continuous information about arterial patency during or after intravenous (IV) tPA treatment.

TCD is ideal for such bedside monitoring. It is inexpensive, portable, and noninvasive and requires minimal patient cooperation. Despite this, TCD has not been accepted widely for use in acute stroke, because of the belief that it is too operator dependent to be applied to decision making. Several studies compare TCD in the acute stroke setting with digital subtraction arteriography, CT angiography, and MR angiography—with variable results [11–14]. Based on a battery of detailed diagnostic TCD criteria using specific flow findings, however, accuracy can be improved. TCD accuracy for detecting proximal MCA occlusion is superior to that at other intracranial locations, such as the vertebral and basilar arteries [15,16].

Two major limitations exist with TCD, impeding its widespread use. First, it is a truly operator-dependent, hand-held technique, requiring detailed 3-D knowledge of the intracranial arterial anatomy. More critically, however, TCD is hampered by a 10% to 15% rate of inadequate temporal windows—most commonly seen in elderly female patients. This is related to thickness and porosity of the temporal bone

---

* Corresponding author. Calgary Stroke Program, Department of Clinical Neurosciences, University of Calgary, Foothills Medical Centre, 1403 29th Street NW, Room 1162, Calgary, AB, Canada T2N 2T9.
    E-mail address: ademchuk@ucalgary.ca (A.M. Demchuk).

attenuating ultrasound energy transmission. Squamous temporal bone thickness greater than or equal to 5 mm produces marked signal attenuation [17].

A newer technology, called power motion-mode Doppler (PMD) TCD, seems to improve window detection/penetration and simplifies the operator dependence of TCD by providing multigate flow information simultaneously in the PMD display [18]. In other words, PMD/TCD also facilitates alignment of the ultrasound beam to permit visualization of blood flow from multiple vessels simultaneously without additional auditory or spectral clues [19].

Focused fast track insonation protocol in acute stroke

Using a fast track insonation protocol [20], emergency room TCD studies can be completed and interpreted within minutes at the bedside by a treating clinician, nurse, or technologist. The choice of fast-track insonation steps is determined by the location of the presumed ischemic arterial territory.

Insonation generally begins with locating the proximal MCA on the nonaffected side to establish the presence of a temporal window with detection of a normal MCA waveform and velocity range. The normal, unaffected, MCA mean flow velocity (MFV) can be used as a comparator for all corresponding MFV recordings from the affected side. Next, the MCA on the affected side is located with insonation, starting at the proximal to mid–M1-MCA depth range, usually 50 to 60 mm. The waveform, systolic flow acceleration and MFV are compared with that of the nonaffected side. If normal ipsilateral MCA flow is revealed, the more distal MCA segments are insonated successively (range 40–50 mm), followed by the internal carotid artery (ICA) bifurcation (range 60–70 mm). A low MCA MFV compared with unaffected MCA MFV usually represents MCA occlusion.

Confirmation of MCA occlusion is made by detection of secondary flow abnormalities, such as reversal of anterior communicating artery flow. A higher MFV for the anterior cerebral artery (ACA) than MCA also can be confirmatory (Fig. 1). A very proximal MCA or terminal ICA occlusion can be associated with absent MCA flow signal, which must be distinguished from absence of temporal window. Detectable PCA signal rules out an inadequate temporal bone window. The absence of MCA flow signal also can be confirmed by insonation across the midline from the contralateral window (depths 80–100 mm) when feasible.

A quick TCD examination of a patient who has hyperacute stroke may require insonation of only the unaffected MCA, affected MCA, and ipsilesional ACA. Ratios can be used to determine the likelihood

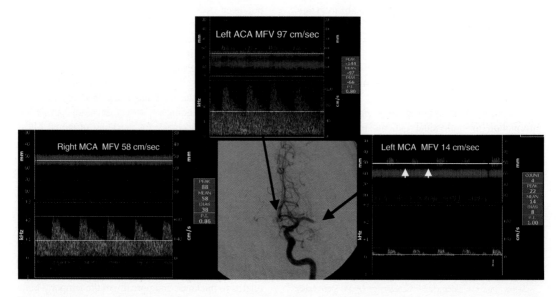

Fig. 1. Left MCA M1 occlusion. Affected MCA high-resistance PMD signature (*small arrows*) showing no flow in diastole. Flow diversion to ACA with ACA-MFV > MCA-MFV. Affected MCA MFV:unaffected MCA-MFV ratio = 0.24 (< 0.5). Black arrows correspond to arterial occlusions on subsequent angiogram.

of proximal intracranial occlusion. A ratio of affected MCA MFV:contralesional MCA MFV less than 0.6 is highly specific and sensitive for a proximal intra-cranial occlusions amenable to intra-arterial (IA) lysis (see Fig. 1) [21]. This MCA ratio is used to decide if catheter angiography and possible IA rescue therapy should be considered during IV recombinant tPA (rtPA) infusion, if proximal occlusion persists.

The orbital bony window can be helpful when intracranial ICA disease must be evaluated. Reversal of ophthalmic artery flow signifies severe proximal ICA obstruction [22]. Alternatively, carotid imag-ing can be performed after TCD, in a combined extra-cranial/intracranial assessment [23]. Insonation of the basilar and vertebral arteries, or other vessels on the contralesional side, usually is not required unless ischemic lesion localization is uncertain or posterior circulation disease is suspected. Most examinations can be accomplished within minutes, without time delays to therapy, as TCD often can be performed during the neurologic examination, blood draws, and vital signs monitoring.

Grading of residual flow by transcranial Doppler

The thrombolysis in myocardial infarction (TIMI) scale, an angiographic residual flow classification developed by cardiologists, provides significant insight into how quickly and effectively coronary thrombolysis can be accomplished [24–26]. Gener-ally, higher amounts of residual flow around the clot predict better success of coronary thrombolysis. The TIMI scale has been used in stroke trials and corre-lates with likelihood of recanalization [27].

The authors developed a similar residual flow grading scale for TCD. The thrombolysis in brain ischemia (TIBI) flow grading system allows real time assessment of residual flow [28]. The TIBI classi-fication rates TCD blood flow waveforms according to six groups: grade 0 = absent, grade 1 = minimal, grade 2 = blunted, grade 3 = dampened, grade 4 = ste-notic, and grade 5 = normal (Fig. 2). The TIBI flow grades correlate with stroke severity and correspond to the degree of arterial recanalization on angiog-raphy as measured by the TIMI scale [29]. TIBI flow grades can be measured in all vessels, with particu-lar attention to the regions at or just distal to the presumed sites of arterial occlusion. Patients who have acute stroke and some residual flow signal are twice as likely as those without to experience early recanalization with IV tPA. For comparison, patients who do not have detectable residual flow signal have

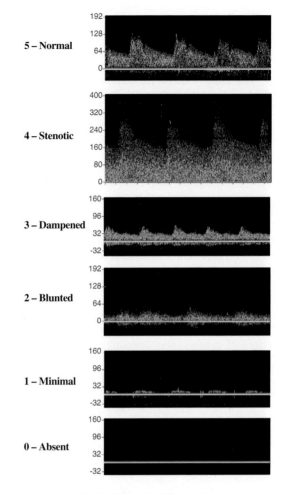

Fig. 2. TIBI residual flow grades.

a less than 20% chance for complete early recanali-zation with IV rtPA alone [30].

Transcranial Doppler monitoring for recanalization

Prolonged TCD monitoring has been performed for years. No adverse biologic effects are documented at the frequencies and power ranges used in diag-nostic ultrasound if applied according to safety guide-lines [31]. Recent work demonstrates a role for TCD monitoring in acute stroke, to follow the evolution of the MCA occlusion in real time [32] and to determine the speed of clot lysis [33]. Obtaining continuous in-formation about the status of an arterial occlusion in acute stroke has the potential to facilitate further decision making regarding thrombolytic therapy [34]. Some sites of arterial occlusion are demonstrated to respond less well to tPA than others; for example, terminal ICA or tandem ICA/MCA arterial occlusions are less likely to undergo complete recanalization [35].

The timing of arterial recanalization after IV rtPA, as determined with TCD, correlates with clinical recovery from stroke, which reflects the accepted 300-minute window to achieve early complete recovery [36]. Rapid arterial recanalization is associated with better short-term improvement, whereas slow (≥ 30 minutes) progression of flow improvement and dampened flow signal are associated with less favorable prognosis [37]. Overall, the degree of recanalization by TCD is an independent predictor of outcome, which, when combined with stroke severity and CT early ischemic changes, predicts outcome best soon after IV tPA administration [38].

Early reocclusion is another curious finding of TCD monitoring during thrombolysis, suggesting failure of systemic tPA therapy. Up to 34% of tPA-treated patients who achieve recanalization go on to develop reocclusion. This total accounts for two thirds of patients who deteriorate clinically after initial improvement [39,40].

Transcranial Doppler monitoring for microemboli

TCD also is able to detect high-intensity transient signals, also known as microembolic signals (MES), which represent emboli traversing through the major intracranial vessels (Fig. 3). These MES correspond to true emboli in animal models [41]. TCD can monitor for emboli by continuous bilateral insonation of the MCAs.

These MES are frequent, following soon after acute stroke onset [42]. MES represent an independent predictor of early ischemic recurrence, when the stroke etiology seems related to large artery atherosclerosis, such as carotid or MCA stenosis [43–47]. Emboli detection also is shown to help optimize management of carotid endarterectomy patients, with reduced emboli counts after postoperative dextran therapy [48]. Similarly, embolic monitoring during carotid stenting demonstrates reduced embolic counts when a proximal endovascular-clamping device is used, compared with a filter device [49].

MES monitoring can be used to guide preventive therapy in patients who have active embolization and who are at high stroke risk from carotid artery occlusive disease. Acetylsalicylic acid [50,51], clopidogrel [52], and tirofiban/heparin [53] all seem effective in reducing MES counts and show trends toward efficacy in reducing clinical ischemic events (transient ischemic attack or stroke). Combinations of these therapies seem most effective at abolishing microembolization. Large-scale clinical trials are needed, with clinical outcomes as the primary endpoint.

Therapeutic transcranial Doppler

Experimental evidence suggests that ultrasound enhances thrombolysis and increases the lytic effect

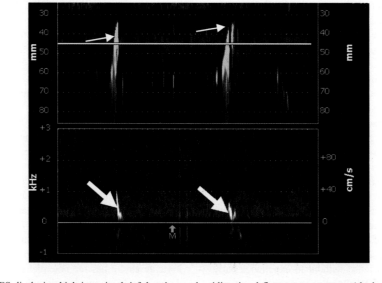

Fig. 3. Two MES displaying high intensity, brief duration, and unidirectional flow on spectrogram (*thick white arrows*), with movement over time on M mode (*thin white arrows*).

of tPA, particularly if used in the low MHz-kHz frequency range [54–64]. Basic research shows that ultrasound exposure can cause various changes, such as reversible disaggregation of noncrosslinked fibrin fibers, microcavity formation in the shallow layer of thrombus, increased enzymatic transport of TPA, improved uptake and penetration of tPA into clots, and flow enhancement with microstreaming and vessel dilation. The effect on lysis does not seem mediated by thermal or cavitation effects.

TCD always transmits some degree of ultrasound energy to the intracranial vessels—even at 2 MHz frequency and power output less than 750 mW—raising the possibility that this diagnostic modality also could enhance tPA activity [54]. Recent in vitro studies shows that 1 hour of 1 MHz TCD augments tPA in the recanalization of 90% of clots, compared with a 30% rate when TCD exposure is limited to 30 minutes [55].

Critics argue that TCD delivers insufficient energy to the clot to achieve this effect, because of tremendous attenuation of ultrasound energy through the bony skull, and that lower-frequency/low-power insonation accelerates tPA-mediated thrombolysis better. Some energy clearly reaches the clot/residual flow interface, as signals are detected successfully that reveal residual flow and recanalization. A study using 2 MHz TCD with a temporal bone window at an average power of 135 mW shows that most skulls allow transmission of at least 10% of beam energy [56]. The maximum portion of energy successfully transmitted through the temporal bone was 35%.

Pilot work in patients who had acute stroke demonstrated an unusually high rate of "on-the-table" clinical responders with early complete recanalization when continuous 2 MHz TCD was combined with IV tPA. This raises the possibility that ultrasonic energy transmission by TCD was facilitating more rapid thrombolysis [57]. This observation soon led to a phase II randomized controlled trial, called CLOTBUST, to assess whether or not such therapeutic effect is relevant clinically [58].

The purpose of CLOTBUST was to determine the safety and the degree of lysis augmentation attributable to diagnostic TCD, to estimate the magnitude of the potential clinical benefit for a subsequent phase III efficacy trial. A total of 126 patients were assigned randomly to receive continuous ultrasonography or placebo. Symptomatic intracerebral hemorrhage occurred in three patients in each group (4.8%). Complete recanalization or dramatic clinical recovery within 2 hours after tPA bolus occurred in 49% of the target group compared with 30% of the control group ($P = 0.03$). At 3 months, 42% of the target

group and 29% of the control group had favorable outcomes ($P = 0.20$). Continuous TCD monitoring seemed to augment tPA-induced arterial recanalization safely, with a nonsignificant trend toward an increased rate of recovery from stroke compared with placebo [58]. A phase III efficacy trial would require an estimated 274 patients per group to replicate these results with sufficient power.

Future developments

Recent developments in nanobubble augmented ultrasound thrombolysis seem promising. Nanobubbles adhere to the clot surface, where ultrasound energy causes the nanobubbles to cavitate and burst. As they fragment, jets of fluid and particles erode the adjacent clot [59]. Because ultrasound destroys the nanobubbles rapidly, repeat applications of nanobubbles are required. Nanobubble augmented ultrasound thrombolysis has proved effective in animal models of stroke [60] and clotted dialysis grafts [61,62], with phase I/II trials in human dialysis grafts, arteries, and veins ongoing.

The first generation of galactose-based air-bubble contrast agent accelerates the effects of thrombolysis. A recent study compares 103 consecutive patients who had stroke and occluded MCAs who received either tPA alone, tPA plus ultrasound, or tPA with ultrasound and galactose-based SHU 508 A delivered at 2, 20, and 40 minutes after tPA. The rate of rapid recanalization, defined as occurring within 1 minute, was 21.4% in the SHU 508 A/ultrasound/tPA group, 10.7% in the ultrasound/tPA group, and 4.3% in the tPA-only group. Complete recanalization at 2 hours was 54.5% in the SHU 508 A/ultrasound/tPA group, 40.8% in the ultrasound/tPA group, and 23.9% in the tPA-alone group. Neurologic improvement was significantly better in the SHU 508 A/ultrasound/tPA group [63]. The first multicenter Food and Drug Administration–registered safety study of therapeutic MRX-815 nanobubble platform combined with IV tPA and ultrasound is underway [65].

Summary

TCD is an evolving neurovascular ultrasound technique that has an established diagnostic and potential therapeutic role in acute stroke management [64]. Angiographically validated criteria for circle-of-Willis occlusion and TIBI classification of residual flow have set the stage for the further development of this technique. TCD has shown its clinical value in thrombolysis monitoring and early emboli detection. The therapeutic effect requires confirmation and may be enhanced further by nanobubble technologies.

References

[1] The National Institutes of Neurological Disorders and Stroke rt-PA Stroke Study Group. Tissue plasminogen activator for acute ischemic stroke. N Engl J Med 1995;333:1581–7.

[2] del Zoppo GJ, Poeck K, Pessin MS, et al. Recombinant tissue plasminogen activator in acute thrombotic and embolic stroke. Ann Neurol 1992;32:78–86.

[3] Uchino K, Molina C, Saqqur M, et al for the CLOTBUST Collaborators. Likelihood of early arterial recanalization with intravenous TPA a Multicenter Transcranial Doppler Study. Stroke 2003; 34:247 [abstract].

[4] Ringelstein EB, Biniek R, Weiller C, et al. Type and extent of hemispheric brain infarctions and clinical outcome in early and delayed middle cerebral artery recanalization. Neurology 1992;42:289–98.

[5] Heiss W-D, Grond M, Thiel A, et al. Tissue at risk of infarction rescued by early reperfusion: a positron emission tomography study in systemic recombinant tissue plasminogen activator thrombolysis of acute stroke. J Cereb Blood Flow Metab 1998;18:1298–307.

[6] Alexandrov AV, Demchuk AM, Felberg RA, et al. High rate of complete recanalization and dramatic clinical recovery during TPA infusion when continuously monitored by 2 MHz transcranial Doppler monitoring. Stroke 2000;31:610–4.

[7] Caplan LR, Mohr JP, Kistler JP, et al. Should thrombolytic therapy be the first-line treatment for acute ischemic stroke? Thrombolysis—not a panacea for ischemic stroke. N Engl J Med 1997;337:1309–10.

[8] Barber PA, Demchuk AM, Hudon ME, et al. Hyperdense sylvian fissure MCA "dot" sign: a CT marker of acute ischemia. Stroke 2001;32:84–8.

[9] Wildermuth S, Knauth M, Brandt T, et al. Role of CT angiography in patient selection for thrombolytic therapy in acute hemispheric stroke. Stroke 1998;29: 935–8.

[10] Kenton AR, Martin PJ, Abbott RJ, et al. Comparison of transcranial color-coded sonography and magnetic resonance angiography in acute stroke. Stroke 1997; 28:1601–6.

[11] Fieschi C, Argentino C, Lenzi GL, et al. Clinical and instrumental evaluation of patients with ischemic stroke within six hours. J Neurol Sci 1989;91:311–22.

[12] Zanette EM, Fieschi C, Bozzao L, et al. Comparison of cerebral angiography and transcranial Doppler sonography in acute stroke. Stroke 1989;20:899–903.

[13] Kaps M, Link A. Transcranial sonographic monitoring during thrombolytic therapy. AJNR Am J Neuroradiol 1998;19:758–60.

[14] Razumovsky AY, Gillard JH, Bryan RN, et al. TCD, MRA, and MRI in acute cerebral ischemia. Acta Neurol Scand 1999;99:65–76.

[15] Demchuk AM, Christou I, Wein TH, et al. Accuracy and criteria for localizing arterial occlusion with transcranial Doppler. J Neuroimaging 2000;10:1–12.

[16] Demchuk AM, Christou I, Wein TH, et al. Specific transcranial Doppler flow findings related to the presence and site of arterial occlusion with transcranial Doppler. Stroke 2000;31:140–6.

[17] Jarquin-Valdivia AA, McCartney J, Palestrant D, et al. The thickness of the temporal squama and its implication for transcranial sonography. J Neuroimaging 2004;14:139–42.

[18] Moehring MA, Spencer MP. Power M-mode Doppler (PMD) for observing cerebral blood flow and tracking emboli. Ultrasound Med Biol 2002;28:49–57.

[19] Alexandrov AV, Demchuk AM, Burgin WS. Insonation method and diagnostic flow signatures for transcranial power motion (M-mode) Doppler. J Neuroimaging 2002;12:236–44.

[20] Alexandrov AV, Demchuk AM, Wein TH, et al. The yield of transcranial Doppler in acute cerebral ischemia. Stroke 1999;30:1605–9.

[21] Saqqur M, Shuaib A, Alexandrov AV, et al. Derivation of transcranial doppler criteria for rescue intra-arterial thrombolysis: multicenter experience from the Interventional Management of Stroke Study. Stroke 2005; 36:865–8.

[22] Saqqur M, Demchuk AM, Hill MD, et al. Bedside emergency TCD diagnosis of severe carotid disease using orbital window examination. J Neuroimaging 2005;15:138–43.

[23] Chernyshev OY, Garami Z, Calleja S, et al. Yield and accuracy of urgent combined carotid/transcranial ultrasound testing in acute cerebral ischemia. Stroke 2005; 36:32–7.

[24] The TIMI Study Group. The Thrombolysis in Myocardial Infarction (TIMI) trial: phase I findings. N Engl J Med 1985;312:932–6.

[25] Anderson JL. Why does thrombolysis fail? Breaking through the reperfusion ceiling. Am J Cardiol 1997; 80:1588–90.

[26] Hackworthy RA, Sorensen SG, Fitzpatrick PG, et al. Dependence of assessment of coronary artery reperfusion during acute myocardial infarction on angiographic criteria and interobserver variability. Am J Cardiol 1988;62:538–42.

[27] Furlan A, Higashida R, Wechsler L, et al. Intra-arterial prourokinase for acute ischemic stroke. The PROACT II study: a randomized controlled trial. Prolyse in acute cerebral thromboembolism. JAMA 1999;282: 2003–11.

[28] Demchuk AM, Burgin WS, Christou I, et al. Thrombolysis in Brain Ischemia (TIBI) transcranial Doppler flow grades predict clinical severity, early recovery, and mortality in patients treated with tissue plasminogen activator. Stroke 2001;32:89–93.

[29] Burgin WS, Malkoff M, Felberg RA, et al. Transcranial Doppler ultrasound criteria for recanalization

after thrombolysis for middle cerebral artery stroke. Stroke 2000;31:1128–32.

[30] Labiche LA, Malkoff M, Alexandrov AV. Residual flow signals predict complete recanalization in stroke patients treated with TPA. J Neuroimaging 2003;13: 28–33.

[31] Barnett SB, Ter Haar GR, Ziskin MC, et al. International recommendations and guidelines for the safe use of diagnostic ultrasound in medicine. Ultrasound Med Biol 2000;26:355–66.

[32] Demchuk AM, Wein TH, Felberg RA, et al. Evolution of rapid middle cerebral artery recanalization during intravenous thrombolysis for acute ischemic stroke. Circulation 1999;100:2282–3.

[33] Alexandrov AV, Burgin WS, Demchuk AM, et al. Speed of intracranial clot lysis with intravenous TPA therapy: sonographic classification and short term improvement. Circulation 2001;103:2897–902.

[34] Christou I, Burgin WS, Alexandrov AV, et al. Arterial status after intravenous TPA therapy for ischemic stroke: a need for further interventions. Int Angiol 2001;20:208–13.

[35] Kim YS, Garami Z, Mikulik R, et al and the CLOTBUST Collaborators. Early recanalization rates and clinical outcomes in patients with tandem internal carotid artery/middle cerebral artery occlusion and isolated middle cerebral artery occlusion. Stroke 2005; 36:869–71.

[36] Christou I, Alexandrov AV, Burgin WS, et al. Timing of recanalization after tissue plasminogen activator therapy determined by transcranial doppler correlates with clinical recovery from ischemic stroke. Stroke 2000;31:1812–6.

[37] Alexandrov AV, Burgin WS, Demchuk AM, et al. Speed of intracranial clot lysis with intravenous tissue plasminogen activator therapy: sonographic classification and short-term improvement. Circulation 2001; 103:2897–902.

[38] Molina C, Alexandrov AV, Uchino K, et al for the CLOTBUST Collaborators. MOST: a grading scale for ultra-early prediction of stroke outcome after thrombolysis. Stroke 2004;35:51–6.

[39] Alexandrov AV, Grotta JC. Arterial reocclusion in stroke patients treated with intravenous tissue plasminogen activator. Neurology 2002;59:862–7.

[40] Rubiera M, Alvarez-Sabin J, Ribo M, et al. Predictors of early arterial reocclusion after tissue plasminogen activator-induced recanalization in acute ischemic stroke. Stroke 2005;36:1452–6.

[41] Russell D, Madden KP, Clark WM, et al. Detection of arterial emboli using Doppler ultrasound in rabbits. Stroke 1991;22:253–8.

[42] Sliwka U, Lingnau L, Stohlmann WD, et al. Prevalence and time course of microembolic signals in patients with acute stroke. Stroke 1997;28:358–63.

[43] Valton L, Larrue V, Pavy le Traon A, et al. Microembolic signals and risk of early recurrence inpatients with stroke or transient ischemic attack. Stroke 1998; 29:2125–8.

[44] Forteza AM, Babikian VL, Hyde C, et al. Effect of time and cerebrovascular symptoms on the prevalence of microembolic signals in patients with cervical carotid stenosis. Stroke 1996;27:687–90.

[45] Babikian VL, Hyde C, Winter MR. Cerebral microembolism and early recurrent cerebral or retinal ischemic events. Stroke 1997;28:1314–8.

[46] Molloy J, Markus HS. Asymptomatic embolization predicts stroke and TIA risk in patients with carotid artery stenosis. Stroke 1999;30:1440–3.

[47] Gao S, Wong KS, Hansberg T, et al. Microembolic signal predicts recurrent cerebral ischaemic events in acute stroke patients with middle cerebral artery stenosis. Stroke 2004;35:2832–6.

[48] Levi CR, Stork JL, Chambers BR, et al. Dextran reduces embolic signals after carotid endarterectomy. Ann Neurol 2001;50:544–7.

[49] Schmidt A, Diederich KW, Scheinert S, et al. Effect of two different neuroprotection systems on microembolization during carotid artery stenting. J Am Coll Cardiol 2004;44:1966–9.

[50] Goertler M, Baeumer M, Kross R, et al. Rapid decline of cerebral microemboli of arterial origin after intravenous acetylsalicylic acid. Stroke 1999;30:66–9.

[51] Goertler M, Blaser T, Krueger S, et al. Cessation of embolic signals after antithrombotic prevention is related to reduced risk of recurrent arterioembolic transient ischaemic attack and stroke. J Neurol Neurosurg Psychiatry 2002;72:338–42.

[52] Markus HS, Droste DW, Kaps M, et al. Dual antiplatelet therapy with clopidogrel and aspirin in symptomatic carotid stenosis evaluated using Doppler embolic signal detection. Circulation 2005;111: 2233–40.

[53] Junghans U, Siebler M. Cerebral microembolism is blocked by tirofibran, a selective nonpeptide platelet glycoprotein IIb/IIIa receptor antagonist. Circulation 2003;107:2717–21.

[54] Moehring MA, Voie AH, Spencer MP, et al. Investigation of transcranial Doppler (TCD) power output for potentiation of tissue plasminogen activator (tPA) therapy in stroke [abstract]. Cerebrovasc Dis 2000; 10(Suppl 1):9.

[55] Spengos K, Behrens S, Daffertshofer M, et al. Acceleration of thrombolysis with ultrasound through the cranium in a flow model. Ultrasound Med Biol 2000;26:889–95.

[56] Grolimund P. Transmission of ultrasound through the temporal bone. In: Aaslid R, editor. Transcranial Doppler sonography. Wien/New York (NY): Springer Verlag; 1986. p. 10–21.

[57] Alexandrov AV, Demchuk AM, Felberg RA, et al. Dramatic improvement during intravenous tPA infusion combined with 2 Mhz transcranial Doppler monitoring is associated with complete recanalization. Stroke 2000;31:610–4.

[58] Alexandrov AV, Molina CA, Grotta JC, et al. Ultrasound-enhanced systemic thrombolysis for acute ischemic stroke. N Engl J Med 2004;351:2170–8.

[59] Porter TR, LeVeen RF, Fox R, et al. Thrombolytic enhancement with perfluorocarbon-exposed sonicated dextrose albumin microbubbles. Am Heart J 1996;132: 964–8.

[60] Culp WC, Erdem E, Roberson PK, et al. Microbubble potentiated ultrasound as a method of stroke therapy in a pig model: preliminary findings. J Vasc Interv Radiol 2003;14:1433–6.

[61] Culp WC, Porter TR, Xie F, et al. Microbubble potentiated ultrasound as a method of declotting thrombosed dialysis grafts: experimental study in dogs. Cardiovasc Intervent Radiol 2001;24:407–12.

[62] Culp WC, Porter TR, McCowan TC, et al. Microbubble-augmented ultrasound declotting of throm-

bosed arteriovenous dialysis grafts in dogs. J Vasc Interv Radiol 2003;14:343–7.

[63] Molina C, Ribo M, Arenillas JF, et al. Microbubbles administration accelerates clot lysis during continuous 2 MHz ultrasound monitoring in stroke patients treated with intravenous tPA [abstract]. Stroke 2005; 36:419.

[64] Sloan MA, Alexandrov AV, Tegeler CH, et al. Assessment: transcranial Doppler ultrasonography: report of the Therapeutics and Technology Assessment Subcommittee of the American Academy of Neurology. Neurology 2004;62:1468–81.

[65] ImaRx Therapeutics. Available at: http://www.imarx. com/ImaRx/product3_1. Accessed October 3, 2005.

ELSEVIER
SAUNDERS

Neuroimag Clin N Am 15 (2005) 481 – 501

NEUROIMAGING
CLINICS OF
NORTH AMERICA

CT Perfusion in Acute Stroke

Sanjay K. Shetty, MD[a,*], Michael H. Lev, MD[a,b]

[a]Department of Radiology, Massachusetts General Hospital, Boston, MA, USA
[b]Harvard Medical School, Boston, MA, USA

Acute stroke is a common cause of morbidity and mortality worldwide. It is the third leading cause of death in the United States (responsible for approximately 1 in 15 deaths in 2001) and affects approximately 700,000 individuals within the United States annually [1]. The ability to treat patients in the acute setting with thrombolytics has created a pressing need for improved detection and evaluation of acute stroke, with a premium placed on rapid acquisition and generation of data that are practically useful in the clinical setting [2–4]. Clinical examination and unenhanced CT, the existing imaging standard for acute stroke, are limited in their ability to identify individuals likely to benefit from successful recanalization [3,5–11]. Advanced imaging techniques extend traditional anatomic applications of imaging and offer additional insight into the pathophysiology of acute stroke by providing information about the arterial level cerebral vasculature, capillary level hemodynamics, and brain parenchyma. CT perfusion (CTP) expands the role of CT in the evaluation of acute stroke by providing insight into areas in which CT has traditionally suffered in comparison to MR imaging—capillary level hemodynamics and the brain parenchyma—and in doing so forms a natural complement to the strengths of CT angiography (CTA) [12–15]. The imaging of acute stroke demands answers to four critical questions [10,16,17] (Box 1).

CTP attempts to address the latter two of these questions so as to guide management in the acute setting (Box 2).

CTP imaging techniques are relatively new compared with MR imaging–based methods; their clinical applications are therefore less thoroughly reported in the literature [18–20]. Despite this, because the general principles underlying the computation of perfusion parameters, such as cerebral blood flow (CBF), cerebral blood volume (CBV), and mean transit time (MTT), are the same for MR imaging and CT, the overall clinical applicability of perfusion imaging using both of these modalities is likely to be similar.

CTA with CTP provides quantitative data and is fast [12], increasingly available [21], safe [22], and affordable [23]. It typically adds no more than 10 minutes to the time required to perform a standard unenhanced head CT scan and does not hinder intravenous thrombolysis. Like diffusion-weighted imaging (DWI) and MR perfusion-weighted imaging (PWI), CTA/CTP has the potential to serve as a surrogate marker of stroke severity, likely exceeding the NIH Stroke Scale (NIHSS) score or Alberta Stroke Program Early CT Score (ASPECTS) as a predictor of outcome [24–32]. Because of these advantages, the addition of CTP to the imaging armamentarium in acute stroke could have implications for the management of stroke patients worldwide [33–36].

CT perfusion technical considerations

Acute stroke protocol

A protocol for the imaging of acute stroke should address the central questions necessary to triage patients appropriately (see Box 2). The acute stroke protocol used at our institution has three components: unenhanced CT, arch-to-vertex CTA, and dynamic

---

* Corresponding author. Division of Neuroradiology, Department of Radiology, Massachusetts General Hospital, 55 Fruit Street, Boston, MA 02114.

E-mail address: sshetty@partners.org (S.K. Shetty).

Box 1. Four key questions in the imaging
of acute stroke

- Is there hemorrhage?
- Is there intravascular thrombus that can
  be targeted for thrombolysis?
- Is there a core of critically ischemic irreversibly infarcted tissue?
- Is there a penumbra of severely ischemic but potentially salvageable tissue?

CT perfusion acquisition

The cine acquisition of CTP forms the final step in the acute stroke imaging evaluation. With dynamic quantitative CTP, an additional contrast bolus is administered (at a rate of 4–7 mL/s) during continuous cine imaging over a single brain region. Using the standard cine technique, imaging occurs for a total of 45 to 60 seconds, which is sufficient to track the first pass of the contrast bolus through the intracranial vasculature without recirculation effects. Our current scanner (General Electric Lightspeed 16; General Electric Medical Systems, Milwaukee, Wisonconsin) offers 2 cm of coverage per bolus (two 10-mm-thick or four 5-mm-thick slices) [49–51]; however, the coverage volume of each acquisition depends greatly on the manufacturer and generation of the CT scanner and continues to increase with enlarging detector arrays and improving technology. The maximum degree of vertical coverage could potentially be doubled with each bolus using a toggle table technique, in which the scanner table moves back and forth, switching between two different cine views, albeit at a reduced temporal resolution of data acquisition [52]. Our current protocol uses two boluses to acquire two slabs of CTP data at different levels, increasing overall coverage [53]. Importantly, at least one image slice in each acquisition must include a major intracranial artery for CTP map reconstruction. Because the previously acquired CTA data are available before CTP acquisition, one can target the tissue of interest with the CTP acquisition, which is particularly important given the relatively restricted coverage obtained even with two CTP acquisitions. An appropriate image plane allows even multiple vascular territories to be imaged with

first-pass cine CTP. A similar CTA/CTP protocol, or its equivalent, could be applied using any commercially available multidetector-row helical CT scanner with only minor variations.

The role of unenhanced CT in stroke triage is principally to exclude hemorrhage before thrombolytic treatment [37]. A greater than one-third middle cerebral artery (MCA) territory hypodensity at presentation is considered by most to be a contraindication to thrombolysis [38]. CT remains suboptimal in its ability to subtype stroke, localize embolic clot, predict outcome, or assess hemorrhagic risk correctly [3,5–11]. Early ischemic signs of stroke are typically absent or subtle, and their interpretation is prone to significant inter- and intraobserver dependency [11, 31,39–42].

In addition to providing important information about the large caliber vessels of the head and neck, the CTA portion of the acute stroke protocol creates source images from the CTA acquisition (CTA-SI) that provide relevant data concerning tissue level perfusion. It has been theoretically modeled that the CTA-SI are predominantly blood volume weighted rather than blood flow weighted [20,43,44]. The potential utility of the CTA-SI series in the assessment of brain perfusion is discussed in detail elsewhere in this article. This perfused blood volume technique requires the assumption of an approximately steady-state level of contrast during the period of image acquisition [44]. It is for this reason—to approach a steady state—that our CTA protocols call for biphasic contrast injection, which can achieve a better approximation of the steady state [45,46]. More complex methods of achieving uniform contrast concentration with smaller doses have been proposed and may eventually become standard, such as exponentially decelerated injection rates [47] and biphasic boluses constructed after analysis of test bolus kinetics [46,48].

Box 2. Four key questions in the imaging
evaluation of acute stroke and the roles of
various CT techniques

- Is there hemorrhage? *Unenhanced CT*
- Is there intravascular thrombus that
  can be targeted for thrombolysis? *CTA*
- Is there a core of critically ischemic
  irreversibly infarcted tissue?
  CTP (CBV/CTA-SI)
- Is there a penumbra of severely ische-
  mic but potentially salvageable tissue?
  CTP (CBF)

appropriate slab placement [13,54,55]. An important consideration in the design of an acute stroke protocol is the total contrast dose; with our protocol, the contrast used for the CTA has been restricted to allow two 40-mL boluses during the CTP acquisitions.

Because CTP imaging has only recently gained acceptance as a clinical tool and because construction of perfusion maps is dependent on the specific mathematic model used to analyze the dynamic contrast-enhanced data sets, considerable variability exists in the protocols used for CTP scanning. Algorithm-dependent differences in contrast injection rates exist; for example, models that assume no venous outflow necessitate extremely high injection rates (which can be difficult to achieve in practice) to achieve peak arterial enhancement before venous opacification occurs [56]. Considerably slower injection rates can be used with deconvolution-based models [57]. Regardless of injection rate, however, higher contrast concentrations are likely to produce maps with improved signal-to-noise ratios [58].

One accepted deconvolution CTP imaging protocol calls for scanning at 80 kV rather than at a more conventional 120 to 140 kV. Theoretically, given a constant milliamperes per second, this kilovoltage setting would not only reduce the administered radiation dose to the patient but would increase the conspicuity of intravenous contrast, attributable, in part, to greater importance of the photoelectric effect for 80-kV photons, which are closer to the k-edge of iodine [51]. Images are acquired in cine mode at a rate of approximately one image per second. Improved temporal resolution is possible with some scanners, with acquisition rates as fast as one image per half second, although the resulting moderate improvement in tissue-density curve noise may not justify the increased radiation dose. More recent work suggests that lengthening the sampling interval can provide satisfactory results if compensatory changes in contrast bolus volume are used; this has the potential to decrease radiation dose and possibly increase coverage [59].

Comparison with MR–perfusion-weighted imaging

Advantages

Quantitation and resolution

Although CTP and MR-PWI both attempt to evaluate the intricacies of capillary level hemodynamics, the differences in technique create several important distinctions that should be considered (Fig. 1). Although dynamic susceptibility contrast (DSC) MR-PWI techniques rely on the indirect T2* effect induced in adjacent tissues by high concentrations of intravenous gadolinium, CTP relies on direct visualization of the contrast material. The linear relation between contrast concentration and attenuation in CT more readily lends itself to quantitation, which is not possible with MR-PWI techniques. MR-PWI may also be more sensitive to contamination by large vascular structures and is also limited in some areas because of susceptibility effects from adjacent structures. In addition, CTP has greater spatial resolution than MR-PWI. These factors contribute to the possibility that visual evaluation of core/penumbra mismatch is more reliable with CTP than with MR perfusion [60,61].

Availability and safety

CT also benefits from the practical availability and relative ease of scanning, particularly when dealing with critically ill patients and the attendant monitors or ventilators. CT may be the only option for a subgroup of patients with an absolute contraindication to MR scanning, such as a pacemaker, and is a safe option when the patient cannot be screened for MR safety.

Disadvantages

Limited coverage

A major disadvantage of current CTP techniques is the relatively limited coverage; although MR-PWI is capable of delivering information about the whole brain, the coverage afforded by CTP depends greatly on the available CT technology.

Ionizing radiation

CTA/CTP also requires ionizing radiation and iodinated contrast. The safety issues involved are no different from those of any patient group receiving contrast-enhanced head CT scanning and are discussed at length in multiple articles [13,62]. The CTP protocol, in particular, has been optimized to provide maximum perfusion signal with minimum dose [51].

Iodinated contrast

Our current protocol uses two 40-mL boluses of iodinated contrast material for the CTP cine acquisitions, in addition to the contrast required for the CTA acquisition. This is a not insignificant dose of iodinated contrast, particularly in the relatively older population most at risk for stroke, and the dose may be of even higher concern if the patient sub-

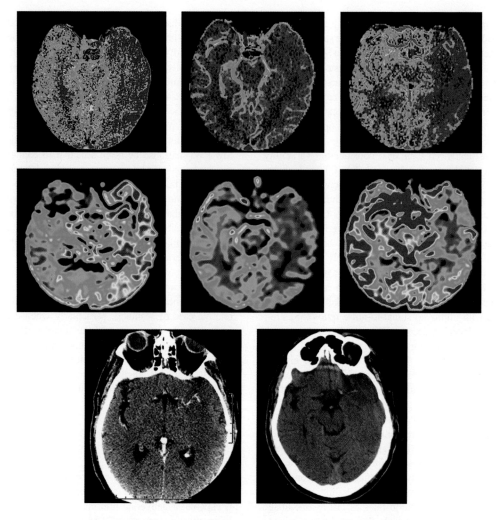

Fig. 1. Correlation of CTP and MR perfusion images. Perfusion images obtained in a patient presenting with lower left extremity weakness. CTP images (*top row, from left:* MTT, CBV, and CBF) and MR perfusion images (*middle row, from left:* MTT, CBV, and CBF) were obtained 1 hour apart (11 and 12 hours after the onset of symptoms, respectively) and demonstrate a large perfusion abnormality in the left MCA distribution. (*Bottom row*) Corresponding CTA-SI (11 hours after ictus) and unenhanced CT (25 hours after ictus) are also shown.

sequently requires additional contrast for endovascular intervention. Nonionic iodinated contrast has been shown to not worsen stroke outcome, however [63–65]. In patients with preexisting renal dysfunction (creatinine greater than 2 mg/dL) or insulin-dependent diabetes, our protocol calls for nonionic iso-osmolar contrast administration, minimizing the chance of nephrotoxicity [66].

Complex postprocessing

Postprocessing of CTA and CTP images is more labor-intensive than that of MR angiography and MR perfusion images, although with training and quality control, three-dimensional reconstructions of CTA data sets as well as quantitative CTP maps can be constructed rapidly and reliably [67–69].

CT perfusion: general principles

Perfusion-weighted CT and MR imaging techniques—as opposed to those of MR angiography and CTA, which detect bulk vessel flow—are sensitive to capillary tissue level blood flow [70]. This evaluation of capillary level hemodynamics extends the traditional anatomic role of imaging to provide insight into the delivery of blood to brain parenchyma. The idea of contrast-enhanced CTP imaging emerged as early as 1976, when a computerized subtraction technique was used to measure relative cerebral blood volume (rCBV) using the EMI scanner. Before the advent of helical CT scanning, time-to-peak analysis of cerebral perfusion was proposed as a means of evaluating stroke patients; however, this dynamic CT study took 10 to 15 minutes longer to perform than a conventional CT examination, and given the absence of an approved treatment for acute stroke at the time, this method never gained clinical acceptance [71].

The generic term *cerebral perfusion* refers to tissue level blood flow in the brain. This flow can be described using a variety of parameters, which primarily include CBF, CBV, and MTT (Table 1). Understanding the dynamic relations between these parameters as cerebral perfusion pressure drops in the setting of acute stroke is crucial to the accurate interpretation of perfusion maps. Definitions of these parameters follow.

CBV is defined as the total volume of blood in a given unit volume of the brain. This definition includes blood in the tissues as well as blood in the large-capacitance vessels, such as arteries, arterioles, capillaries, venules, and veins. CBV has units of milliliters of blood per 100 g of brain tissue.

CBF is defined as the volume of blood moving through a given unit volume of brain per unit time. CBF has units of milliliters of blood per 100 g of brain tissue per minute.

MTT is defined as the average of the transit time of blood through a given brain region. The transit time of blood through the brain parenchyma varies depending on the distance traveled between arterial inflow and venous outflow, Mathematically, MTT is related to CBV and CBF according to the central volume principle, which states that MTT = CBV/CBF [72,73].

Table 1
Normal values for perfusion parameters in brain tissue

Brain tissue	CBF	CBV	MTT
Gray matter	60 mL/100 g/min	4 mL/100 g	4 s
White matter	25 mL/100 g/min	2 mL/100 g	4.8 s

Adapted from Calamante F, Gadian DG, Connelly A. Delay and dispersion effects in dynamic susceptibility contrast MRI: simulations using singular value decomposition. Magn Reson Med 2000;44(3):466–73; with permission.

CT perfusion theory and modeling

Although easy to define in theory, the perfusion parameters of CBV, CBF, and MTT can be difficult to quantify in practice. The dynamic first-pass approach to CTP measurement involves the dynamic intravenous administration of an intravascular contrast agent, which is tracked with serial imaging during its first-pass circulation through the brain tissue capillary bed. Depending on the assumptions regarding the arterial inflow and the venous outflow of the tracer, the perfusion parameters of CBV, CBF, and MTT can then be computed mathematically. Dynamic first-pass contrast-enhanced CTP models assume that the tracer (ie, the contrast) used for perfusion measurement is nondiffusible, neither metabolized nor absorbed by the tissue bed through which it traverses. Leakage of contrast material outside the intravascular space, which can occur in cases of blood-brain barrier (BBB) breakdown associated with tumor, infection, or inflammation, requires a different model to be used and therefore adds an additional layer of complexity to the calculations. Other means of assessing cerebral perfusion, including positron emission tomography (PET) and xenon CT imaging, for example, use diffusible tracer models, which generally involve fewer assumptions regarding steady-state CBF than do the dynamic first-pass contrast-enhanced models used with MR and CT imaging. The two major types of mathematic models involved in performing these calculations are the deconvolution-based and nondeconvolution-based methods.

Nondeconvolution techniques

Nondeconvolution-based perfusion methods rely on the application of the Fick principle to a given region of interest (ROI) within the brain parenchyma. After a time-density curve (TDC) is derived for each pixel, CBF can be calculated based on the concept of conservation of flow. The ease of the mathematic solution to this differential equation, however, is highly dependent on the assumptions made regarding inflow and outflow to the region. One common model assumes no venous outflow, which simplifies the calculation at the cost of necessitating an extremely high injection dose.

CBV can be approximated as the area under the fitted (smoothed) tissue TDC divided by the area under the fitted arterial TDC [43]. Note that when it is assumed that contrast concentration in the arteries and capillaries is at a steady state, this equation forms the basis for the quantitative computation of CBV using the whole-brain perfused blood volume method of Hamberg and colleagues [20] and Hunter and coworkers [44] described previously. After soft tissue components have been removed by coregistration and subtraction of the precontrast scan, CBV then simply becomes a function of the density of tissue contrast normalized by the density of arterial contrast.

Deconvolution techniques

Direct calculation of CBF, applicable for even relatively slow injection rates, can be accomplished using the deconvolution theory [57], which compensates for the inability to deliver a complete and instantaneous bolus of contrast into the artery supplying a given region of the brain. In reality, a contrast bolus (particularly when administered in a peripheral vein) undergoes delay and dispersion before arriving in the cerebral vasculature; deconvolution attempts to correct for this by calculating the residue function. CBF can then be obtained directly as proportional to the maximum height of this scaled residue function curve, whereas CBV is reflected as the area under the scaled residue function curve. Once CBF and CBV are known, MTT can be calculated using the central volume principle.

Mathematically, deconvolution of the arterial (arterial input function [AIF]) and tissue curves can be accomplished using a variety of techniques, including the Fourier transform and the singular value decomposition methods. These methods vary in their sensitivity to such factors as (1) the precise vascular anatomy of the underlying tissue bed being studied and (2) the degree of delay, or dispersal, of the contrast bolus between the measured arterial and tissue TDCs [74]. In current clinical software, the singular value decomposition method, which is more sensitive to contrast dispersal factors than to specific local arterial anatomy, is the more commonly used technique.

The creation of accurate quantitative maps of CBV, CBF, and MTT using the deconvolution method has been validated in a number of studies [49,50, 74–80]. Specifically, validation has been accomplished by comparison with xenon [80,81], PET [82], and MR perfusion [83–85] in human beings as well as with microspheres in animals [49,50,76].

CT perfusion postprocessing

In urgent clinical cases, perfusion changes can often be observed immediately after scanning by direct visual inspection of the axial source images at the CT scanner console. Soft copy review at a workstation using movie or cine mode can reveal relative perfusion changes over time, although advanced postprocessing is required to appreciate subtle changes and to obtain quantification. Axial source images acquired from a cine CTP study are networked to a freestanding workstation for detailed analysis.

The computation of quantitative first-pass cine cerebral perfusion maps typically requires some combination of the following user inputs (Fig. 2):

- *Arterial input ROI:* A small ROI is placed over the central portion of a large intracranial artery, preferably orthogonal to the imaging plane to minimize volume averaging. An attempt should be made to select an arterial ROI with maximal peak contrast intensity. An essential caveat in selecting a CTP slab is that the imaged level must contain a major intracranial artery to generate the AIF. The ROI selection can be completed in a semiautomated manner on some systems.
- *Venous outflow ROI:* A small venous ROI with similar attributes is selected, most commonly at the superior sagittal sinus. With some software packages, selection of an appropriate venous ROI is critical in producing quantitatively accurate perfusion maps, whereas others are less sensitive to this selection [69].
- *Baseline:* The baseline is the flat portion of the arterial TDC, before the upward sloping of the curve caused by contrast enhancement. The baseline typically begins to rise after 4 to 6 seconds.
- *Postenhancement cutoff:* Data should be truncated to remove the tail portion of the TDC, which may slope upward toward a second peak value if recirculation effects are present.

Other user-defined inputs, such as threshold or resolution values, are dependent on the specific software package used for image reconstruction. It is worth noting that major variations in the input values described here may not only result in perfusion maps of differing image quality but, potentially, in perfusion maps with variation in their quantitative values for CBF, CBV, and MTT.

In general, deconvolution is also less sensitive to variations in underlying vascular anatomy than are the nondeconvolution-based methods. This is because, for simplicity, the fundamental assumption of most nondeconvolution cerebral perfusion models is that a single feeding artery and a single draining vein support all blood flow to and from a given tissue bed and that the precise arterial, venous, and tissue

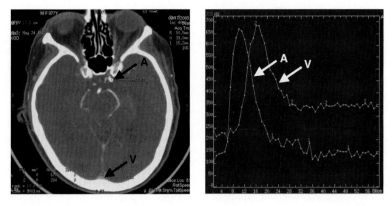

Fig. 2. CTP postprocessing. (*Left*) Appropriate ROI placement on an artery (A, *arrow*; a major vessel running perpendicular to the plane of section to avoid volume averaging) and on a vein (V, *arrow*; superior sagittal sinus, also running perpendicular to the plane of section and placed to avoid the inner table of the skull). (*Right*) TDCs generated from this artery (A, *arrow*) and vein (V, *arrow*) show the arrival, peak, and passage of the contrast bolus over time. These TDCs serve as the AIF and the venous output for the subsequent deconvolution step.

TDCs can be uniquely identified by imaging. This assumption is clearly an oversimplification. Although MR-PWI maps (CBF and MTT) have been shown to have increased accuracy with a bolus delay-corrected (BDC) technique [86], a delay correction is built into most available CTP processing software, so this is less of a concern in CTP.

Potential imaging pitfalls in the computation of CBF using the deconvolution method include patient motion and partial volume averaging, which can cause the AIF to be underestimated. The effects of these pitfalls can be minimized by the use of image coregistration software to correct for patient motion as well as by careful choice of ROIs for the AIF. In addition, comparison with the contralateral (normal) side to establish a percentage change from normal is a useful interpretive technique, because reliability of quantitative data is in the range of 20% to 25% variation.

Clinical applications of CT perfusion

Indications (and potential indications) for advanced functional imaging of stroke in the first 12 hours include the following: (1) exclusion of patients most likely to hemorrhage and inclusion of patients most likely to benefit from thrombolysis; (2) extension of the time window beyond 3 hours for intravenous and 6 hours for anterior circulation intra-arterial thrombolysis; (3) triage to other available therapies, such as hypertension or hyperoxia

administration; (4) disposition decisions regarding neurologic intensive care unit (NICU) admission or emergency department discharge; and (5) rational management of wake-up strokes, for which the precise time of onset is unknown [87]. The Desmoteplase in Acute Ischemic Stroke (DIAS) trial suggests that the intravenous use of desmoteplase can be extended to a therapeutic window of 3 to 9 hours after ictus, with significantly improved reperfusion rates and clinical outcomes achieved in patients with a diffusion/perfusion mismatch on MR imaging [88]. Indeed, based on this evidence and while awaiting information from other large trials, such as the Echoplanar Imaging Thrombolysis Evaluation Trial (EPITHET), some authors have cautiously proposed the use of advanced MR imaging or CT for extending the traditional therapeutic time window [16,89], pointing to evidence of a relevant volume of salvageable tissue present in the 3- to 6-hour time frame in more than 80% of stroke patients [90–92]. Methods that accurately distinguish salvageable from nonsalvageable brain tissue are being increasingly promoted as a means to select patients for thrombolysis beyond the 3-hour window for intravenous therapy.

CT perfusion interpretation: infarct detection

A number of groups have suggested that CTA source images, such as DWI, can sensitively detect tissue destined to infarct despite successful recanalization (Fig. 3) [29,93,94]. Theoretic modeling indicates that CTA-SI, assuming an approximately steady state of contrast in the brain arteries and parenchyma during image acquisition, are predominantly blood volume weighted rather than blood flow weighted, although this has yet to be validated empirically in a large series [20,43,44,85]. An early report indicated that CTA-SI typically define minimal final infarct size and, hence, like DWI and CBV, can be used to identify infarct core in the acute setting [93]. Coregistration and subtraction of the conventional unenhanced CT brain images from the axial postcontrast CTA source images should result in quantitative blood volume maps of the entire brain [13,20,44]. CTA-SI subtraction maps, obtained by coregistration and subtraction of the unenhanced head CT scan from the CTA source images, are particularly appealing for clinical use, because, unlike quantitative first-pass CTP maps, they provide whole-brain coverage (Fig 4). Rapid and convenient coregistra-

tion/subtraction software is now commercially available on multiple platforms, allowing generation of these maps outside the research arena [95,96]. Subtraction maps, despite the improved conspicuity of blood volume lesions, may be limited by increased image noise [97]. A pilot study in 20 consecutive patients with MCA stem occlusion who underwent intra-arterial thrombolysis after imaging demonstrated that CTA-SI and CTA-SI subtraction maps improve infarct conspicuity over that of unenhanced CT in patients with hyperacute stroke. True reduction in blood pool (as reflected by CTA-SI subtraction) rather than increase in tissue edema (as reflected by unenhanced CT) may explain much of the improved infarct delineation in CTA-SI. Concurrent review of unenhanced CT, CTA-SI, and CTA-SI subtraction images may be indicated for optimal CT assessment of hyperacute MCA stroke.

In another study, CTA-SI preceding DWI was performed in 48 consecutive patients with clinically

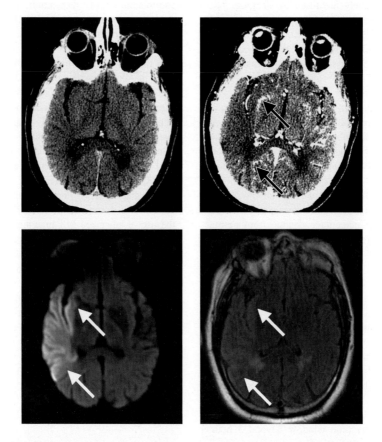

Fig. 3. Increased infarct conspicuity on CTA-SI. An infarct in the right MCA distribution is more conspicuous on the CTA-SI *(top right, arrows)* than on the unenhanced CT *(top left)* performed in the acute setting. Subsequent DWI *(bottom left)* and fluid-attenuated inversion recovery images (FLAIR; *bottom right*) confirm the territory of infarction seen on CTA-SI *(arrows)*.

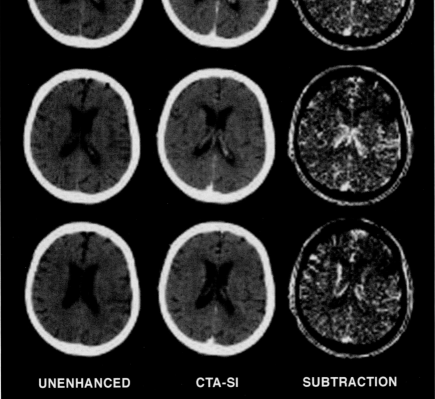

UNENHANCED   CTA-SI   SUBTRACTION

Fig. 4. Value of CTA-SI and CTA-SI subtraction images. Unenhanced, CTA-SI, and CTA-SI subtraction images demonstrate the value of the CTA-SI and CTA-SI subtraction images in improving conspicuity of acute stroke. The infarct is most obvious on the subtraction image, although the contrast-to-noise is increased on the other images as well. (Courtesy of Nat Alpert, PhD, MGH PET Lab.)

suspected stroke presenting within 12 hours of symptom onset (42 patients within 6 hours) [29]. CTA-SI and DWI lesion volumes were independent predictors of final infarct volume, and the overall sensitivity and specificity for parenchymal stroke detection were 76% and 90% for CTA-SI and 100% and 100% for DWI, respectively (Fig. 5). When cases with an initial DWI lesion volume less than 15 mL (small lacunar and distal infarctions) were excluded from analysis, CTA-SI sensitivity and specificity increased to 95% and 100%, respectively. Although DWI is more sensitive than CTA-SI for parenchymal

stroke detection of small lesions, DWI and CTA-SI are highly accurate predictors of final infarct volume. DWI tends to underestimate final infarct size, whereas CTA-SI more closely approximates final infarct size, despite the bias toward DWI being obtained after the CTA-SI in this cohort of patients with unknown recanalization status.

Finally, it is noteworthy that as with DWI, not every acute CTA-SI hypodense ischemic lesion is destined to infarct [98,99]. In the presence of early complete recanalization, dramatic sparing of regions with reduced blood pool on CTA source images can

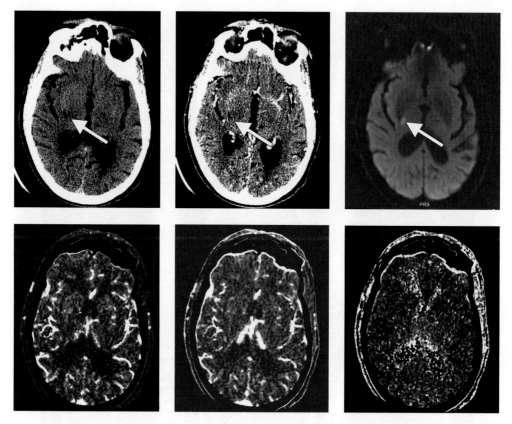

Fig. 5. A false-negative CTA-SI attributable to early imaging of a small infarct, retrospectively seen to be present on the unenhanced CT and CTA-SI *(white arrows)*. A 62-year-old man presented with left-sided weakness. *(Top row)* Unenhanced CT at 3 hours CTA-SI at 3 hours, and DWI at 5 hours show a small infarct in the posterior limb of the right internal capsule *(white arrow)*. *(Bottom row)* CTP images (CBF, CBV, and MTT) obtained 3 hours after onset of symptoms are normal.

sometimes occur. Hunter and colleagues [100] studied the normalized blood volume on CTA-SI from 28 acute stroke patients at the extremely thin boundary between infarcted and spared tissue. They found that the probability of infarction in the core, inner boundary, and outer boundary were .99, .96, and .11 respectively, supporting the concept that CTA-SI thresholds predictive of tissue outcome exist.

The processed CTP maps can also improve the detection of infarct in the acute setting, improving sensitivity (MTT maps) and specificity (relative cerebral blood flow [rCBF] and rCBV maps) for the detection of infarct relative to unenhanced CT [101]. Perfusion maps were also more accurate in determining the extent of infarct, particularly when used to determine the percentage of MCA territory infarct [101]. In one study that measured final infarct volume on follow-up fluid-attenuated inversion recovery (FLAIR) images, the rCBV map correlated

better with final infarct volume than admission DWI [102].

CT perfusion interpretation: ischemic penumbra and infarct core

An important goal of advanced stroke imaging is to provide an assessment of ischemic tissue viability that transcends an arbitrary clock-time [103–105]. The original theory of penumbra stems from experimental studies in which two thresholds were characterized [106]. One threshold identified a CBF value below which there was cessation of cortical function, without increase in extracellular potassium or reduction in pH. A second lower threshold identified a CBF value below which there was disruption of cellular integrity. With the advent of advanced neuroimaging and modern stroke therapy, a more clinically relevant operationally-defined penumbra, which identifies hypoperfused but potentially salvageable tissue, has gained acceptance [103,107–109].

Ischemic penumbra

Cine single-slab CTP imaging, which can provide quantitative maps of CBF, CBV, and MTT, has the potential to describe regions of ischemic penumbra, ischemic but still viable tissue. In the simplest terms, the operationally defined penumbra is the volume of tissue contained within the region of CBF/CBV mismatch on CTP maps, where the region of CBV abnormality represents the core of infarcted tissue and the CBF/CBV mismatch represents the surrounding region of tissue that is hypoperfused but salvageable (Figs. 6–9). The few reports that have investigated

the role of CTP in acute stroke triage have typically assumed predefined threshold values for the core and penumbra based on human and animal studies from the PET, MR imaging, single photon emission computed tomography (SPECT), or xenon literature and have determined the accuracy of these in predicting outcome [53]. By assuming cutoff values greater than or equal to a 34% reduction from baseline CT-CBF for penumbra and less than or equal to 2.5 mL per 100 g CT-CBV for core, Wintermark and coworkers [53] found good correlation between DWI and CT-CBV infarct core ($r = 0.698$) and the MR-MTT and CT-CBF ischemic penumbra ($r = 0.946$) (see Table 1 for normal values of these parameters). Of note, the CT-CBV maps suffer from decreased signal-to-noise relative to the CT-CBF maps, suggesting that the interpretation of CBV maps may benefit from a semiautomated thresholding approach to segmentation to gauge the size of infarct more

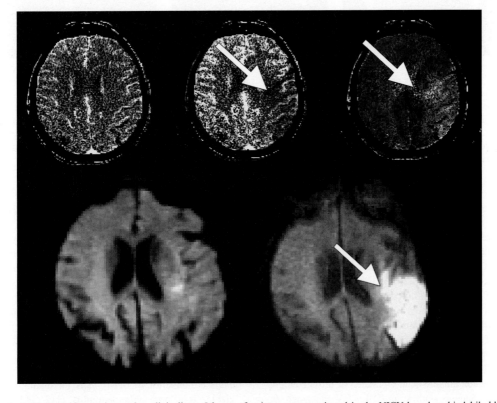

Fig. 6. A 65-year-old man, improving clinically at 5 hours after ictus, was monitored in the NICU based on his labile blood pressure, a fixed left M2 occlusion on CTA, and a significant core/penumbra mismatch on CTP. His 24-hour follow-up DWI showed a small infarction; however, 24 hours after cessation of hypertensive therapy, there was infarct growth into the region of penumbra. CTP (CBV/CBF/MTT) at 4.5 hours (*top row*), DWI at 24 hours (*bottom left*), and follow-up DWI at 48 hours (*bottom right*). The CTP demonstrate a mismatch between the CBV (no abnormality) and the CBF/MTT penumbra (*arrows*). After cessation of hypertensive therapy, the DWI abnormality grows into the region predicted by the CBF/MTT maps (*arrow*).

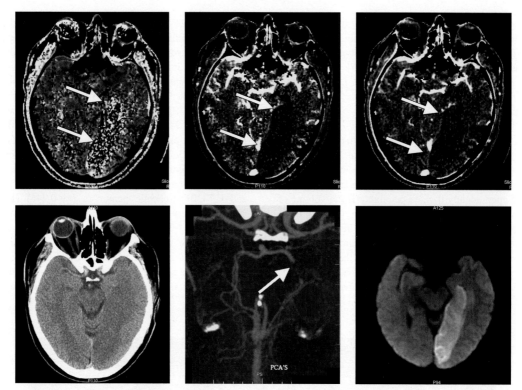

Fig. 7. A 49-year-old man presented with a right homonymous hemianopsia and aphasia. A dense left posterior cerebral artery (PCA) infarct was identified with no evidence of additional territory at risk on CTP performed 5 hours after symptom onset. No change in the infarct territory was seen on subsequently performed MR imaging. (*Top row*) CTP images (MTT, CBF, and CBV) show a matched region of abnormal perfusion (*arrows*) in the left occipital and medial temporal lobes, corresponding to an infarct in the left PCA distribution. (*Bottom row*) Corresponding unenhanced CT (*left*) shows a subtle area of hypodensity in the same region, representing infarct. Reformatted CTA image (*middle*) shows occlusion of the left P2 segment (*arrow*). DWI (*right*) from subsequently performed MR imaging shows no change in the region of the infarction.

accurately [61]. CTP values derived from coregistered images in regions of DWI hyperintensity and apparent diffusion coefficient (ADC) hypointensity revealed decreased absolute CBF values of 8.9 mL per 100 g/min and 7.8 mL per 100 g/min, respectively, and absolute perfused CBV values of 1.0 mL per 100 g and 0.9 mL per 100 g, respectively, values that were significantly different compared with those of a contralateral control region. The interpretation of CTP in the setting of acute stroke is summarized in Box 3.

CT-CBF/CBV mismatch correlates significantly with lesion enlargement. Untreated or unsuccessfully treated patients with large CBF/CBV mismatch exhibit substantial lesion growth on follow-up, whereas those patients without significant mismatch or those with early complete recanalization do not exhibit lesion progression of their admission CTA-SI lesion volume (see Figs. 6–9). CTP-defined mis-

match might therefore serve as a marker of salvageable tissue and thus prove useful in patient triage for thrombolysis [110]. This result clearly has implications for the utility of a CTP-based model for predicting outcome in patients without robust recanalization. Similarly, in an earlier pilot study of CTP imaging, ultimate infarct size was most strongly correlated with CT-CBF lesion size in 14 embolic stroke patients without robust recanalization [111], again demonstrating the importance of the mismatch region as tissue at risk for infarction.

Several studies of MR-PWI suggest that CBF maps are superior to MTT maps for distinguishing viable from nonviable penumbra [112–114]. The reason for this relates to the fact that MTT maps display circulatory derangements that do not necessarily reflect ischemic change, including large vessel occlusions with compensatory collateralization and reperfusion hyperemia after revascularization.

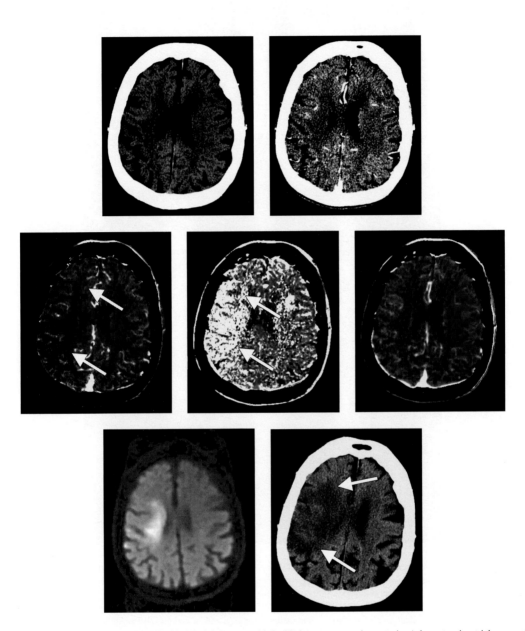

Fig. 8. A 96-year-old woman with left-sided facial droop and left-sided upper extremity paresis. A hypertensive trial was not successful in improving symptoms, and anticoagulation was not initiated because of the high risk of hemorrhagic transformation. Subsequent CT shows expansion of the right MCA territory infarct into the region of the mismatch. (*Top row*) Unenhanced and CTA-SI show a region of hypodense infarct in the right corona radiata, with relative sparing of the cortex. (*Middle row*) Concurrently performed CTP shows a larger region of decreased CBF (*left, white arrows*) and prolonged MTT (*middle, white arrows*) that described the entire right MCA territory, although the same region shows mildly increased CBV (*right*); this represents perfusion mismatch and indicates tissue at risk. (*Bottom row*) MR imaging performed 3 hours (*left*) later confirms the region of the infarct, and follow-up CT performed 2 days later (*right*) shows expansion of the infarct into the region of the mismatch (*white arrows*).

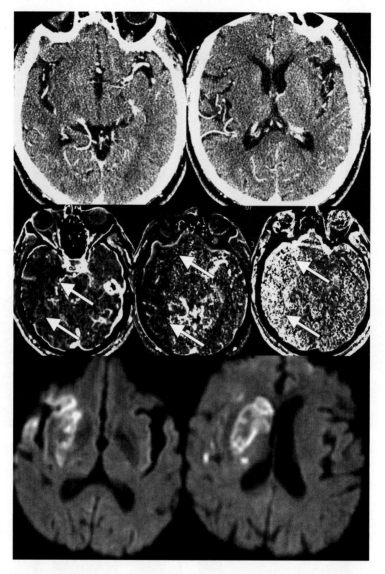

Fig. 9. A 77-year-old man presented with left-sided facial droop. Subtle changes of the right insula and right lentiform nucleus were seen on CTA-SI, and CTP demonstrated an ischemic penumbra involving the entire right MCA territory, consistent with a large territory at risk for subsequent infarction. Successful intra-arterial thrombolysis was performed at 3 hours. Follow-up DWI showed an infarct limited to the initial CTA-SI abnormality. CTA-SI (*top row*), CTP (CBV, *inferiorly*; CBF, *superiorly*; and MTT, *superiorly* showing large area of perfusion abnormality [*arrows*]), and follow-up DWI at 36 hours (*bottom row*).

Refinements of the traditional penumbra model

The operationally defined penumbra oversimplifies reality, however, because not all tissue contained within the operationally defined penumbra is destined to infarct. There is a region of benign oligemia contained within the region of the CBV/CBF mismatch that is not expected to infarct even in the absence

of reperfusion. This refinement of the traditional model has important clinical implications, because treatment regimens that are based on an overestimated volume of tissue at risk are likely too aggressive, exposing the patient to the risks and complications of treatment for tissue that would not likely have proceeded to infarct even without intervention. Few studies have reported specific CBF thresholds for

Box 3. Summary of CT perfusion interpretation pearls

- CBV, CBF match:
  - No treatment regardless of lesion size
- Large CBV, larger CBF:
  - Possible treatment based on time after ictus, size
  - Consider no treatment if CBV > 100 mL
- Small CBV, larger CBF:
  - Typically a good candidate for treatment
  - Consider no treatment if prolonged time after ictus

distinguishing penumbra likely to infarct in the absence of early recanalization (nonviable penumbra) from penumbra likely to survive despite persistent vascular occlusion (viable penumbra) [112,114]. Fewer still have addressed this problem using CTP. Previous work from our group and others has detected a significant difference between the MR-CBF thresholds for penumbra likely to infarct and penumbra likely to remain viable [112,114] and has also revealed a good correlation between MR perfusion and CTP parameter values [35,83–85,115]. In a pilot study of CTP thresholds for infarction, we found that normalized CBF, or rCBF, is the most robust parameter for distinguishing viable from nonviable penumbra. In rough approximation, CT-CBF penumbra with less than 50% reduction from baseline values has a high probability of survival, whereas penumbra with a greater than two thirds reduction from baseline values has a high probability of infarction. No region with a mean rCBV less than 0.68, absolute CBF less than 12.7 mL per 100 g/min, or absolute CBV less than 2.2 mL per 100 g survived. The latter compares well with the CBV threshold of 2.5 mL per 100 g selected by Wintermark and colleagues [53] to define core. Because of differences in CBV and CBF between gray and white matter (see Table 1), it is essential that the contralateral ROI used for normalization have the same gray matter/white matter ratio as the ipsilateral ischemic region under study. Moreover, a number of studies suggest that because of different cellular populations, gray and white matter may respond differently to ischemic injury.

There is little literature addressing perfusion thresholds in patients undergoing intra-arterial recanalization procedures [116,117]. Our results for mean rCBF thresholds are in agreement with those of SPECT and MR imaging studies performed in patients who received other stroke therapies [112, 118–120].

Imaging predictors of clinical outcome

Predicting outcome is perilous. The penumbra is dynamic, and several factors influence its fate, including time after ictus, residual and collateral blood flow, admission glucose, temperature, hematocrit, systolic blood pressure, and treatment (including hyperoxia) [121]. As already mentioned, CTA/CTP has the potential to serve as a surrogate marker of stroke severity, likely exceeding the NIHSS score or ASPECTS as a predictor of outcome [24–32].

Infarct core and clinical outcome

As noted earlier, measuring the penumbra is technically challenging. Flow thresholds for various states of tissue perfusion vary considerably among studies and techniques applied [122]. Infarct core is crucial. Multiple studies examining heterogeneous cohorts of patients receiving varied treatments consistently find that ultimate clinical outcome is strongly correlated with admission core lesion volume, be it measured by DWI, CT-CBV, subthreshold xenon CT-CBF, or unenhanced CT [123–127]. One of these studies is especially noteworthy, because results were stratified by degree of recanalization at 24 hours. This study revealed "...that 2 factors mainly influenced clinical outcome: (1) recanalization ($P = .0001$) and (2) day-0 DWI lesion volume ($P = .03$)" [128]. In a study of CTP in patients with MCA stem occlusions, patients with admission whole-brain CTP lesion volumes greater than 100 mL (equal to approximately one third the volume of the MCA territory) had poor clinical outcomes, regardless of recanalization status. Moreover, in those patients from the same cohort who had early complete MCA recanalization, final infarct volume was closely approximated by the size of the initial whole-brain CTP lesion [93].

Risk of hemorrhage

The degree of early CBF reduction in acute stroke may also help to predict hemorrhagic risk. Preliminary results from our group suggest that severe hypoattenuation, relative to normal tissue, on whole-brain CTP images may also identify ischemic regions more likely to bleed after intra-arterial thrombolysis [129]. In a SPECT study of 30 patients who had complete recanalization within 12 hours of stoke onset, those with less than 35% of normal cerebellar flow at the infarct core were at significantly higher risk for hemorrhage [117]. Indeed, multiple studies have suggested that severely ischemic regions with early reperfusion are at the highest risk for hemorrhagic transformation [125,130]. Of note, there is a suggestion that the presence of punctate microhemorrhage is correlated with the risk of hemorrhagic transformation; these small foci of hemorrhage are seen on gradient echo (susceptibility-weighted) MR imaging sequences and are not visible on unenhanced CT [131]. It remains to be seen, however, whether these microbleeds serve as a contraindication to thrombolytic therapy.

Experimental applications of CT perfusion in stroke

The additional information about capillary level hemodynamics afforded by CTP could be particularly important in future clinical trials of acute stroke therapy, in which CTP could refine the selection of subjects to include only those patients most likely to benefit from treatment; this imaging-guided patient selection may help to demonstrate beneficial effects that would be obscured if patients without salvageable tissue were included. CTA combined with CTP could be used to identify patients with proximal large vessel occlusive thrombus, who are the most appropriate candidates for intra-arterial treatment [12,44, 132]. The ability of perfusion imaging to determine in a quantitative manner ischemic brain regions that are viable but at risk for infarction if blood flow is not quickly restored might provide a more rational basis for establishing the maximum safe time window for administering thrombolytic agents than the current arbitrary cutoffs of 3 hours after ictus for intravenous thrombolysis and 6 hours after ictus for intra-arterial thrombolysis (see Box 3) [24,133]. MR perfusion has already been used to support extending the therapeutic time window in a subset of patients with a DWI/MR-PWI mismatch: the DIAS trial of patients with an NIHSS of 4 to 20 and an MR diffusion/perfusion mismatch (where the perfusion abnormality was defined using MTT) showed significantly improved rates of reperfusion and clinical outcome when intravenous desmoteplase was administered between 3 and 9 hours of ictus onset in an escalating dose range of 62 to 125 μg/kg [92]. CTP could serve a similar role in rationally extending the therapeutic time window for stroke intervention.

Despite a multitude of animal studies that have demonstrated a benefit from neuroprotective agents, the only therapy proven in human beings to improve outcome has been thrombolysis (intravenous and intra-arterial) [2,3,133]. There is growing literature positing that ischemic but potentially salvageable penumbral tissue is an ideal target for neuroprotective agents [30,103,134], suggesting that CTP or other perfusion techniques may be suited to selection of patients in trials of these agents. Kidwell and Warach [135] argue that enrollment in clinical trials should require a definitive diagnosis of stroke confirmed by imaging and laboratory studies.

Summary

As new treatments are developed for stroke, the potential clinical applications of CTP imaging in the diagnosis, triage, and therapeutic monitoring of these diseases are certain to increase.

Technical advances in scanner hardware and software should no doubt continue to increase the speed, coverage, and resolution of CTP imaging. CTP offers the promise of efficient use of imaging resources and, potentially, of decreased morbidity. Most importantly, current CT technology already permits the incorporation of CTP as part of an all-in-one acute stroke examination to answer the four fundamental questions of stroke triage quickly and accurately, further increasing the contribution of imaging to the diagnosis and treatment of acute stroke.

References

[1] American Heart Association. Heart disease and stroke statistics—2004 update. Dallas, TX: American Heart Association; 2003. Available at: http://www.aha.org. Accessed February 2005.

[2] Tissue plasminogen activator for acute ischemic stroke. The National Institute of Neurological Disorders and Stroke rt-PA Stroke Study Group. N Engl J Med 1995;333:1581–7.

[3] Furlan A, Higashida R, Wechsler L, et al. Intra-arterial prourokinase for acute ischemic stroke. JAMA 1999;282:2003–21.

[4] Marler JR, Tilley BC, Lu M, et al. Early stroke treatment associated with better outcome: the NINDS rt-PA stroke study. Neurology 2000;55(11):1649–55.

[5] del Zoppo GJ, Poeck K, Pessin MS, et al. Recombinant tissue plasminogen activator in acute thrombotic and embolic stroke. Ann Neurol 1992;32(1):78–86.

[6] Hacke W, Kaste M, Fieschi C, et al. Intravenous thrombolysis with recombinant tissue plasminogen activator for acute hemispheric stroke. The European Cooperative Acute Stroke Study (ECASS). JAMA 1995;274(13):1017–25.

[7] Madden KP, Karanjia PN, Adams Jr HP, et al. Accuracy of initial stroke subtype diagnosis in the TOAST study. Trial of ORG 10172 in Acute Stroke Treatment. Neurology 1995;45(11):1975–9.

[8] Ezzeddine MA, Lev MH, McDonald CT, et al. CT angiography with whole brain perfused blood volume imaging: added clinical value in the assessment of acute stroke. Stroke 2002;33(4):959–66.

[9] Dubey N, Bakshi R, Wasay M, et al. Early computed tomography hypodensity predicts hemorrhage after intravenous tissue plasminogen activator in acute ischemic stroke. J Neuroimaging 2001;11(2):184–8.

[10] Lev MH, Nichols SJ. Computed tomographic angiography and computed tomographic perfusion imaging of hyperacute stroke. Top Magn Reson Imaging 2000;11(5):273–87.

[11] Wardlaw J, Dorman P, Lewis S, et al. Can stroke physicians and neuroradiologists identify signs of early cerebral infarction on CT? J Neurol Neurosurg Psychiatry 1999;67:651–3.

[12] Lev MH, Farkas J, Rodriguez VR, et al. CT angiography in the rapid triage of patients with hyperacute stroke to intraarterial thrombolysis: accuracy in the detection of large vessel thrombus. J Comput Assist Tomogr 2001;25(4):520–8.

[13] Lev MH, Gonzalez RGCT. Angiography and CT perfusion imaging. In: Toga AW, Mazziotta JC, editors. Brain mapping: the methods. 2nd edition. San Diego, CA: Academic Press; 2002. p. 427–84.

[14] Wildermuth S, Knauth M, Brandt T, et al. Role of CT angiography in patient selection for thrombolytic therapy in acute hemispheric stroke. Stroke 1998; 29(5):935–8.

[15] Knauth M, von Kummer R, Jansen O, et al. Potential of CT angiography in acute ischemic stroke [see comments]. AJNR Am J Neuroradiol 1997;18(6): 1001–10.

[16] Schellinger PD, Fiebach JB, Hacke W. Imaging-based decision making in thrombolytic therapy for ischemic stroke: present status. Stroke 2003;34(2):575–83.

[17] Warach S. Tissue viability thresholds in acute stroke: the 4-factor model. Stroke 2001;32(11):2460–1.

[18] Roberts HC, Roberts TP, Dillon WP. CT perfusion flow assessment: "up and coming" or "off and running"? AJNR Am J Neuroradiol 2001;22(6): 1018–9.

[19] Hamberg LM, Hunter GJ, Halpern EF, et al. Quantitative high resolution measurement of cerebrovascular physiology with slip-ring CT. AJNR Am J Neuroradiol 1996;17(4):639–50.

[20] Hamberg LM, Hunter GJ, Kierstead D, et al. Measurement of cerebral blood volume with subtraction three-dimensional functional CT. AJNR Am J Neuroradiol 1996;17(10):1861–9.

[21] Fox SH, Tanenbaum LN, Ackelsberg S, et al. Future directions in CT technology. Neuroimaging Clin N Am 1998;8(3):497–513.

[22] Smith WS, Roberts HC, Chuang NA, et al. Safety and feasibility of a CT protocol for acute stroke: combined CT, CT angiography, and CT perfusion imaging in 53 consecutive patients. AJNR Am J Neuroradiol 2003;24(4):688–90.

[23] Gleason S, Furie KL, Lev MH, et al. Potential influence of acute CT on inpatient costs in patients with ischemic stroke. Acad Radiol 2001;8(10): 955–64.

[24] Albers GW. Expanding the window for thrombolytic therapy in acute stroke. The potential role of acute MRI for patient selection. Stroke 1999;30(10): 2230–7.

[25] Barber PA, Demchuk AM, Zhang J, et al. Validity and reliability of a quantitative computed tomography score in predicting outcome of hyperacute stroke before thrombolytic therapy. ASPECTS Study Group. Alberta Stroke Programme Early CT Score. Lancet 2000;355(9216):1670–4.

[26] Broderick JP, Lu M, Kothari R, et al. Finding the most powerful measures of the effectiveness of tissue plasminogen activator in the NINDS tPA stroke trial. Stroke 2000;31(10):2335–41.

[27] Schellinger PD, Jansen O, Fiebach JB, et al. Monitoring intravenous recombinant tissue plasminogen activator thrombolysis for acute ischemic stroke with diffusion and perfusion MRI. Stroke 2000;31(6):1318–28.

[28] Tong D, Yenari M, Albers G, et al. Correlation of perfusion- and diffusion weighted MRI with NIHSS score in acute (<6.5 hour) ischemic stroke. Neurology 1998;50(4):864–70.

[29] Berzin T, Lev M, Goodman D, et al. CT perfusion imaging versus MR diffusion weighted imaging: prediction of final infarct size in hyperacute stroke [abstract]. Stroke 2001;32:317.

[30] Warach S. New imaging strategies for patient selection for thrombolytic and neuroprotective therapies. Neurology 2001;57(Suppl 2):S48–52.

[31] von Kummer R, Holle R, Grzyska U, et al. Interobserver agreement in assessing early CT signs of middle cerebral artery infarction. AJNR Am J Neuroradiol 1996;17:1743–8.

[32] Grotta JC, Chiu D, Lu M, et al. Agreement and variability in the interpretation of early CT changes in stroke patients qualifying for intravenous rtPA therapy [see comments]. Stroke 1999;30(8):1528–33.

[33] Koroshetz WJ, Gonzales RG. Imaging stroke in progress: magnetic resonance advances but computed tomography is poised for counterattack. Ann Neurol 1999;46(4):556–8.

[34] Koroshetz WJ, Lev MH. Contrast computed tomography scan in acute stroke: "you can't always get what you want but you get what you need." Ann Neurol 2002;51(4):415–6.

[35] Lev MH. CT versus MR for acute stroke imaging: is

the "obvious" choice necessarily the correct one? AJNR Am J Neuroradiol 2003;24(10):1930–1.

[36] Lev MH, Koroshetz WJ, Schwamm LH, et al. CT or MRI for imaging patients with acute stroke: visualization of "tissue at risk"? Stroke 2002;33(12): 2736–7.

[37] von Kummer R, Allen KL, Holle R, et al. Acute stroke: usefulness of early CT findings before thrombolytic therapy [see comments]. Radiology 1997; 205(2):327–33.

[38] von Kummer R. Early major ischemic changes on computed tomography should preclude use of tissue plasminogen activator. Stroke 2003;34(3):820–1.

[39] Fiorelli M, von Kummer R. Early ischemic changes on computed tomography in patients with acute stroke. JAMA 2002;287(18):2361–2 [author reply: 2362].

[40] Mullins ME, Lev MH, Schellingerhout D, et al. Influence of availability of clinical history on detection of early stroke using unenhanced CT and diffusion-weighted MR imaging. AJR Am J Roentgenol 2002;179(1):223–8.

[41] Lev M, Farkas J, Gemmete J, et al. Acute stroke: improved nonenhanced CT detection—benefits of softcopy interpretation by using variable window width and center level settings. Radiology 1999;213:150–1.

[42] Fiorelli M, Toni D, Bastianello S, et al. Computed tomography findings in the first few hours of ischemic stroke: implications for the clinician. J Neurol Sci 2000;173(1):10–7.

[43] Axel L. Cerebral blood flow determination by rapidsequence computed tomography. Radiology 1980; 137:679–86.

[44] Hunter GJ, Hamberg LM, Ponzo JA, et al. Assessment of cerebral perfusion and arterial anatomy in hyperacute stroke with three-dimensional functional CT: early clinical results. AJNR Am J Neuroradiol 1998;19:29–37.

[45] Bae KT, Tran HQ, Heiken JP. Multiphasic injection method for uniform prolonged vascular enhancement at CT angiography: pharmacokinetic analysis and experimental porcine model. Radiology 2000;216(3): 872–80.

[46] Fleischmann D, Rubin GD, Bankier AA, et al. Improved uniformity of aortic enhancement with customized contrast medium injection protocols at CT angiography. Radiology 2000;214(2):363–71.

[47] Bae KT, Tran HQ, Heiken JP. Uniform vascular contrast enhancement and reduced contrast medium volume achieved by using exponentially decelerated contrast material injection method. Radiology 2004; 231(3):732–6.

[48] Fleischmann D, Hittmair K. Mathematical analysis of arterial enhancement and optimization of bolus geometry for CT angiography using the discrete Fourier transform. J Comput Assist Tomogr 1999; 23(3):474–84.

[49] Cenic A, Nabavi DG, Craen RA, et al. Dynamic CT measurement of cerebral blood flow: a validation study. AJNR Am J Neuroradiol 1999;20(1):63–73.

[50] Nabavi DG, Cenic A, Craen RA, et al. CT assessment of cerebral perfusion: experimental validation and initial clinical experience. Radiology 1999;213(1): 141–9.

[51] Wintermark M, Maeder P, Verdun FR, et al. Using 80 kVp versus 120 kVp in perfusion CT measurement of regional cerebral blood flow. AJNR Am J Neuroradiol 2000;21(10):1881–4.

[52] Roberts HC, Roberts TP, Smith WS, et al. Multisection dynamic CT perfusion for acute cerebral ischemia: the "toggling-table" technique. AJNR Am J Neuroradiol 2001;22(6):1077–80.

[53] Wintermark M, Reichhart M, Thiran JP, et al. Prognostic accuracy of cerebral blood flow measurement by perfusion computed tomography, at the time of emergency room admission, in acute stroke patients. Ann Neurol 2002;51(4):417–32.

[54] Aksoy FG, Lev MH. Dynamic contrast-enhanced brain perfusion imaging: technique and clinical applications. Semin Ultrasound CT MR 2000;21(6): 462–77.

[55] Eastwood JD, Lev MH, Provenzale JM. Perfusion CT with iodinated contrast material. AJR Am J Roentgenol 2003;180(1):3–12.

[56] Klotz E, Konig M. Perfusion measurements of the brain: using the dynamic CT for the quantitative assessment of cerebral ischemia in acute stroke. Eur J Radiol 1999;30(3):170–84.

[57] Wintermark M, Maeder P, Thiran JP, et al. Quantitative assessment of regional cerebral blood flows by perfusion CT studies at low injection rates: a critical review of the underlying theoretical models. Eur Radiol 2001;11(7):1220–30.

[58] Lev MH, Kulke SF, Weisskoff RM, et al. Dose dependence of signal to noise ratio in functional MRI of cerebral blood volume mapping with sprodiamide. J Magn Reson Imaging 1997;7:523–7.

[59] Wintermark M, Smith WS, Ko NU, et al. Dynamic perfusion CT: optimizing the temporal resolution and contrast volume for calculation of perfusion CT parameters in stroke patients. AJNR Am J Neuroradiol 2004;25(5):720–9.

[60] Coutts SB, Simon JE, Tomanek AI, et al. Reliability of assessing percentage of diffusion-perfusion mismatch. Stroke 2003;34(7):1681–3.

[61] Roccatagliata L, Lev MH, Mehta N, et al. Estimating the size of ischemic regions on CT perfusion maps in acute stroke: is freehand visual segmentation sufficient? In: Proceedings of the 89th Scientific Assembly and Annual Meeting of the Radiological Society of North America. Chicago, Illinois, 2003. p. 1292.

[62] Mullins ME, Lev MH, Bove P, et al. Comparison of image quality between conventional and low-dose nonenhanced head CT. AJNR Am J Neuroradiol 2004;25(4):533–8.

[63] Kendell B, Pullicono P. Intravascular contrast injection in ischemic lesions, II. Effect on prognosis. Neuroradiology 1980;19:241–3.

[64] Doerfler A, Engelhorn T, von Kommer R, et al. Are iodinated contrast agents detrimental in acute cerebral ischemia? An experimental study in rats. Radiology 1998;206:211–7.

[65] Palomaki H, Muuronen A, Raininko R, et al. Administration of nonionic iodinated contrast medium does not influence the outcome of patients with ischemic brain infarction. Cerebrovasc Dis 2003; 15(1–2):45–50.

[66] Aspelin P, Aubry P, Fransson SG, et al. Nephrotoxic effects in high-risk patients undergoing angiography. N Engl J Med 2003;348(6):491–9.

[67] Fiorella D, Heiserman J, Prenger E, et al. Assessment of the reproducibility of postprocessing dynamic CT perfusion data. AJNR Am J Neuroradiol 2004; 25(1):97–107.

[68] Kealey SM, Loving VA, Delong DM, et al. User-defined vascular input function curves: influence on mean perfusion parameter values and signal-to-noise ratio. Radiology 2004;231(2):587–93.

[69] Sanelli PC, Lev MH, Eastwood JD, et al. The effect of varying user-selected input parameters on quantitative values in CT perfusion maps. Acad Radiol 2004;11(10):1085–92.

[70] Villringer A, Rosen BR, Belliveau JW, et al. Dynamic imaging with lanthanide chelates in normal brain: contrast due to magnetic susceptibility effects. Magn Reson Med 1988;6:164–74.

[71] Shih TT, Huang KM. Acute stroke: detection of changes in cerebral perfusion with dynamic CT scanning. Radiology 1988;169(2):469–74.

[72] Meier P, Zieler K. On the theory of the indicator-dilution method for measurement of blood flow and volume. J Appl Physiol 1954;6:731–44.

[73] Roberts G, Larson K. The interpretation of mean transit time measurements for multi-phase tissue systems. J Theor Biol 1973;39:447–75.

[74] Wirestam R, Andersson L, Ostergaard L, et al. Assessment of regional cerebral blood flow by dynamic susceptibility contrast MRI using different deconvolution techniques. Magn Reson Med 2000; 43(5):691–700.

[75] Cenic A, Nabavi DG, Craen RA, et al. CT method to measure hemodynamics in brain tumors: validation and application of cerebral blood flow maps. AJNR Am J Neuroradiol 2000;21(3):462–70.

[76] Nabavi DG, Cenic A, Dool J, et al. Quantitative assessment of cerebral hemodynamics using CT: stability, accuracy, and precision studies in dogs. J Comput Assist Tomogr 1999;23(4):506–15.

[77] Nabavi DG, Cenic A, Henderson S, et al. Perfusion mapping using computed tomography allows accurate prediction of cerebral infarction in experimental brain ischemia. Stroke 2001;32(1):175–83.

[78] Ostergaard L, Weisskoff RM, Chesler DA, et al. High resolution of cerebral blood flow using intravascular tracer bolus passages. Part I: Mathematical approach ad statistical analysis. Magn Reson Med 1996;36(5): 715–25.

[79] Ostergaard L, Chesler DA, Weisskoff RM, et al. Modeling cerebral blood flow and flow heterogeneity from magnetic resonance residue data. J Cereb Blood Flow Metab 1999;19(6):690–9.

[80] Wintermark M, Thiran JP, Maeder P, et al. Simultaneous measurement of regional cerebral blood flow by perfusion CT and stable xenon CT: a validation study. AJNR Am J Neuroradiol 2001;22(5):905–14.

[81] Furukawa M, Kashiwagi S, Matsunaga N, et al. Evaluation of cerebral perfusion parameters measured by perfusion CT in chronic cerebral ischemia: comparison with xenon CT. J Comput Assist Tomogr 2002;26(2):272–8.

[82] Gillard JH, Antoun NM, Burnet NG, et al. Reproducibility of quantitative CT perfusion imaging. Br J Radiol 2001;74(882):552–5.

[83] Eastwood JD, Lev MH, Wintermark M, et al. Correlation of early dynamic CT perfusion imaging with whole-brain MR diffusion and perfusion imaging in acute hemispheric stroke. AJNR Am J Neuroradiol 2003;24(9):1869–75.

[84] Wintermark M, Reichhart M, Cuisenaire O, et al. Comparison of admission perfusion computed tomography and qualitative diffusion- and perfusion-weighted magnetic resonance imaging in acute stroke patients. Stroke 2002;33(8):2025–31.

[85] Schramm P, Schellinger PD, Klotz E, et al. Comparison of perfusion computed tomography and computed tomography angiography source images with perfusion-weighted imaging and diffusion-weighted imaging in patients with acute stroke of less than 6 hours' duration. Stroke 2004;35(7):1652–8.

[86] Rose SE, Janke AL, Griffin M, et al. Improved prediction of final infarct volume using bolus delay-corrected perfusion-weighted MRI. Implications for the ischemic penumbra. Stroke 2004;35(11):2466–71.

[87] Serena J, Davalos A, Segura T, et al. Stroke on awakening: looking for a more rational management. Cerebrovasc Dis 2003;16(2):128–33.

[88] Hacke W, Albers G, Al-Rawi Y, et al. The Desmoteplase in Acute Ischemic Stroke Trial (DIAS): a phase II MRI-based 9-hour window acute stroke thrombolysis trial with intravenous desmoteplase. Stroke 2005;36(1):66–73.

[89] Rother J. Imaging-guided extension of the time window: ready for application in experienced stroke centers? Stroke 2003;34(2):575–83.

[90] Rother J, Schellinger PD, Gass A, et al. Effect of intravenous thrombolysis on MRI parameters and functional outcome in acute stroke < 6 hours. Stroke 2002; 33(10):2438–45.

[91] Parsons MW, Barber PA, Chalk J, et al. Diffusion- and perfusion-weighted MRI response to thrombolysis in stroke. Ann Neurol 2002;51(1):28–37.

[92] Hacke W, Albers G, Al-Rawi Y, et al. The Desmoteplase in Acute Ischemic Stroke Trial (DIAS): a phase II MRI-based 9-hour window acute stroke thrombolysis trial with intravenous desmoteplase. Stroke 2005;36(1):66–73.

[93] Lev MH, Segal AZ, Farkas J, et al. Utility of perfusion-weighted CT imaging in acute middle cerebral artery stroke treated with intra-arterial thrombolysis: prediction of final infarct volume and clinical outcome. Stroke 2001;32(9):2021–8.

[94] Schramm P, Schellinger PD, Fiebach JB, et al. Comparison of CT and CT angiography source images with diffusion-weighted imaging in patients with acute stroke within 6 hours after onset. Stroke 2002;33(10):2426–32.

[95] Alpert NM, Berdichevsky D, Levin Z, et al. Performance evaluation of an automated system for registration and postprocessing of CT scans. J Comput Assist Tomogr 2001;25(5):747–52.

[96] Schellingerhout D, Lev MH, Bagga RJ, et al. Coregistration of head CT comparison studies: assessment of clinical utility. Acad Radiol 2003;10(3):242–8.

[97] Bove P, Lev M, Chaves T, et al. CT perfusion imaging improves infarct conspicuity in hyperacute stroke [abstract]. Stroke 2001;32:325.

[98] Kidwell CS, Saver JL, Mattiello J, et al. Thrombolytic reversal of acute human cerebral ischemic injury shown by diffusion/perfusion magnetic resonance imaging. Ann Neurol 2000;47(4):462–9.

[99] Kidwell CS, Saver JL, Starkman S, et al. Late secondary ischemic injury in patients receiving intraarterial thrombolysis. Ann Neurol 2002;52(6):698–703.

[100] Hunter GJ, Silvennoinen HM, Hamberg LM, et al. Whole-brain CT perfusion measurement of perfused cerebral blood volume in acute ischemic stroke: probability curve for regional infarction. Radiology 2003;227(3):725–30.

[101] Wintermark M, Fischbein NJ, Smith WS, et al. Accuracy of dynamic perfusion CT with deconvolution in detecting acute hemispheric stroke. AJNR Am J Neuroradiol 2005;26(1):104–12.

[102] Bisdas S, Donnerstag F, Ahl B, et al. Comparison of perfusion computed tomography with diffusion-weighted magnetic resonance imaging in hyperacute ischemic stroke. J Comput Assist Tomogr 2004; 28(6):747–55.

[103] Warach S. Measurement of the ischemic penumbra with MRI: it's about time. Stroke 2003;34(10):2533–4.

[104] Wu O, Koroshetz WJ, Ostergaard L, et al. Predicting tissue outcome in acute human cerebral ischemia using combined diffusion- and perfusion-weighted MR imaging. Stroke 2001;32(4):933–42.

[105] Barber PA, Darby DG, Desmond PM, et al. Prediction of stroke outcome with echoplanar perfusion- and diffusion-weighted MRI. Neurology 1998;51(2): 418–26.

[106] Astrup J, Siesjo BK, Symon L. Thresholds in cerebral ischemia—the ischemic penumbra. Stroke 1981; 12(6):723–5.

[107] Sorensen AG, Buonanno FS, Gonzalez RG, et al. Hyperacute stroke: evaluation with combined multi-section diffusion-weighted and hemodynamically weighted echo-planar MR imaging. Radiology 1996; 199(2):391–401.

[108] Sunshine JL, Tarr RW, Lanzieri CF, et al. Hyperacute stroke: ultrafast MR imaging to triage patients prior to therapy. Radiology 1999;212:325–32.

[109] Schlaug G, Benfield A, Baird AE, et al. The ischemic penumbra: operationally defined by diffusion and perfusion MRI. Neurology 1999;53(7): 1528–37.

[110] Mehta N, Lev MH, Mullins ME, et al. Prediction of final infarct size in acute stroke using cerebral blood flow/cerebral blood volume mismatch: added value of quantitative first pass CT perfusion imaging in successfully treated versus unsuccessfully treated/untreated patients. In: Proceedings of the 41st Annual Meeting of the American Society of Neuroradiology. Washington, DC, 2003. Oak Brook (IL): American Society of Neuroradiology; 2003.

[111] Aksoy FG, Lev MH, Eskey CJ, et al. CT perfusion imaging of acute stroke: how well do CBV, CBF, and MTT maps predict final infarct size? In: Proceedings of the 86th Scientific Assembly and Annual Meeting of the Radiological Society of North America. Chicago, Illinois, 2000.

[112] Rohl L, Ostergaard L, Simonsen CZ, et al. Viability thresholds of ischemic penumbra of hyperacute stroke defined by perfusion-weighted MRI and apparent diffusion coefficient. Stroke 2001;32(5): 1140–6.

[113] Grandin CB, Duprez TP, Smith AM, et al. Usefulness of magnetic resonance-derived quantitative measurements of cerebral blood flow and volume in prediction of infarct growth in hyperacute stroke. Stroke 2001;32(5):1147–53.

[114] Schaefer PW, Ozsunar Y, He J, et al. Assessing tissue viability with MR diffusion and perfusion imaging. AJNR Am J Neuroradiol 2003;24(3):436–43.

[115] Lev MH, Hunter GJ, Hamberg LM, et al. CT versus MR imaging in acute stroke: comparison of perfusion abnormalities at the infarct core. In: Proceedings of the 40th Annual Meeting of the American Society of Neuroradiology. Vancouver, British Columbia, Canada, 2002.

[116] Sasaki O, Takeuchi S, Koizumi T, et al. Complete recanalization via fibrinolytic therapy can reduce the number of ischemic territories that progress to infarction. AJNR Am J Neuroradiol 1996;17(9): 1661–8.

[117] Ueda T, Sakaki S, Yuh W, et al. Outcome in acute stroke with successful intra-arterial thrombolysis procedure and predictive value of initial single-photon emission-computed tomography. J Cereb Blood Flow Metab 1999;19:99–108.

[118] Liu Y, Karonen JO, Vanninen RL, et al. Cerebral hemodynamics in human acute ischemic stroke: a study with diffusion- and perfusion-weighted magnetic resonance imaging and SPECT. J Cereb Blood Flow Metab 2000;20(6):910–20.

[119] Hatazawa J, Shimosegawa E, Toyoshima H, et al. Cerebral blood volume in acute brain infarction: a combined study with dynamic susceptibility con-

trast MRI and 99mTc-HMPAO-SPECT. Stroke 1999; 30(4):800–6.

[120] Shimosegawa E, Hatazawa J, Inugami A, et al. Cerebral infarction within six hours of onset: prediction of completed infarction with technetium-99m-HMPAO SPECT. J Nucl Med 1994;35(7): 1097–103.

[121] Koennecke HC. Editorial comment—challenging the concept of a dynamic penumbra in acute ischemic stroke. Stroke 2003;34(10):2434–5.

[122] Heiss WD. Ischemic penumbra: evidence from functional imaging in man. J Cereb Blood Flow Metab 2000;20(9):1276–93.

[123] Jovin TG, Yonas H, Gebel JM, et al. The cortical ischemic core and not the consistently present penumbra is a determinant of clinical outcome in acute middle cerebral artery occlusion. Stroke 2003; 34(10):2426–33.

[124] Lev MH, Roccatagliata L, Murphy EK, et al. A CTA based, multivariable "benefit of recanalization" model for acute stroke triage: core infarct size on CTA source images independently predicts outcome. In: Proceedings of the 42nd Annual Meeting of the American Society of Neuroradiology. Seattle, Washington, 2004.

[125] Suarez J, Sunshine J, Tarr R, et al. Predictors of clinical improvement, angiographic recanalization, and intracranial hemorrhage after intra-arterial thrombolysis for acute ischemic stroke. Stroke 1999;30: 2094–100.

[126] Molina CA, Alexandrov AV, Demchuk AM, et al. Improving the predictive accuracy of recanalization on stroke outcome in patients treated with tissue plasminogen activator. Stroke 2004;35(1):151–6.

[127] Baird AE, Dambrosia J, Janket S, et al. A three-item scale for the early prediction of stroke recovery. Lancet 2001;357(9274):2095–9.

[128] Nighoghossian N, Hermier M, Adeleine P, et al. Baseline magnetic resonance imaging parameters and stroke outcome in patients treated by intravenous tissue plasminogen activator. Stroke 2003;34(2): 458–63.

[129] Swap C, Lev M, McDonald C, et al. Degree of oligemia by perfusion-weighted CT and risk of hemorrhage after IA thrombolysis. In: Stroke—Proceedings of the 27th International Conference on Stroke and Cerebral Circulation. San Antonio, Texas, 2002.

[130] Ogasawara K, Ogawa A, Ezura M, et al. Brain single-photon emission CT studies using 99mTc-HMPAO and 99mTc-ECD early after recanalization by local intraarterial thrombolysis in patients with acute embolic middle cerebral artery occlusion. AJNR Am J Neuroradiol 2001;22(1):48–53.

[131] Kidwell CS, Chalela JA, Saver JL, et al. Hemorrhage early MRI evaluation (HEME) study [abstract]. Stroke 2003;34:239.

[132] del Zoppo G. Acute stroke—on the threshold of a therapy. N Engl J Med 1995;333(13):1632–3.

[133] Muir KW, Grosset DG. Neuroprotection for acute stroke: making clinical trials work. Stroke 1999; 30(1):180–2.

[134] Grotta J. Neuroprotection is unlikely to be effective in humans using current trial designs. Stroke 2002; 33(1):306–7.

[135] Kidwell CS, Warach S. Acute ischemic cerebrovascular syndrome: diagnostic criteria. Stroke 2003;34(12): 2995–8.

ELSEVIER
SAUNDERS

Neuroimag Clin N Am 15 (2005) 503 – 530

**NEUROIMAGING
CLINICS OF
NORTH AMERICA**

Diffusion-Weighted Imaging in Acute Stroke

Pamela W. Schaefer, MD[a,b,*], Wiliam A. Copen, MD[b],
Michael H. Lev, MD[a,b], R. Gilberto Gonzalez, MD, PhD[a,b]

[a]*Massachusetts General Hospital, Boston, MA, USA*
[b]*Harvard Medical School, Boston, MA, USA*

This review begins by explaining the pulse sequences and postprocessing techniques that are used to create diffusion-weighted images (DWI). Subsequently, the pathophysiology of ischemic stroke is discussed, with emphasis on processes that result in changes in water diffusion. Finally, the use of DWI in the care of patients who have actute stroke is discussed, including optimal integration of DWI with other imaging data to facilitate clinical decision making.

Self-diffusion and the apparent diffusion coefficient

DWI, like almost all other clinical MR imaging techniques, creates images based on signals arising from hydrogen nuclei. In the context of magnetic resonance (MR) physics, hydrogen nuclei often are called spins, because the axis of orientation of their magnetic spins is a critically defining property. Because most spins in living tissue exist as part of water molecules, signal intensity in MR imaging is determined largely by differences in the local magnetic environments surrounding water.

In brain tissue, or in any other environment with a temperature above absolute zero, water molecules exhibit random motion (Fig. 1) whose rate is determined by D, the diffusion coefficient (or diffusivity coefficient) as expressed in Fick's law. DWI seeks to

quantify D, although it cannot do so directly. Instead, DWI pulse sequences measure the change in position of water molecules that occurs during a short time interval, Δ, which lasts only a fraction of a second. During the period Δ, the random motion of each water molecule causes it to become displaced from its initial position by a distance L. The value of L varies randomly among different water molecules, and DWI cannot measure L for any individual molecule. DWI can, however, measure $\bar{L}$, the mean displacement for all water molecules in a particular imaging voxel. $\bar{L}$ is greater when the D is greater, according to the following relationship (Eq. 1), described by Einstein:

$$\bar{L} = \sqrt{2D\Delta} \tag{1}$$

DWI pulse sequences, because they are sensitive to differences in $\bar{L}$, are capable of estimating the D of water in each voxel of tissue. Because this estimate is only an indirect one, it is called the apparent diffusion coefficient (ADC).

The Stejskal-Tanner pulse sequence

Most DWI pulse sequences are based on the work of Stejskal and Tanner [1]. The Stejskal-Tanner pulse sequence represents a small modification to the typical spin-echo pulse sequence that is used most often for clinical imaging. For DWI, long time to repetition (TR) and time to echo (TE) values usually are used, so that DWI has T2 and diffusion weighting. Also, because DWI is sensitive to patient motion, ultrafast spin-echo, echoplanar techniques are used.

* Corresponding author. Division of Neuroradiology, Department of Radiology, Massachusetts General Hospital, 55 Fruit Street, Gray B285, Boston, MA 02114.

E-mail address: pschaefer@partners.org (P.W. Schaefer).

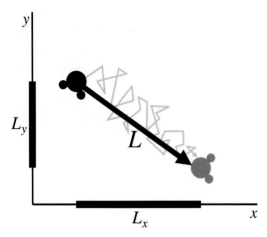

Fig. 1. Self-diffusion. During a period D lasting a fraction of a second, random motion causes each water molecule to become displaced by a path length L. DWI is capable of measuring $\bar{L}$, the average path length traversed by all water molecules within an imaging voxel. The magnitude of $\bar{L}$ is related to the magnitude of the D (see Eq. 1). Note that each individual DWI acquisition is capable of measuring only that component of each path that is parallel to the direction in which the diffusion gradients are oriented. For example, if the diffusion gradients are oriented along the X axis, only L_x, the projection of L on the X axis, can be measured. Therefore, accurate estimation of D requires image acquisition in at least three orthogonal directions.

The novel aspect of the Stejskal-Tanner pulse sequence that results in images with diffusion weighting is the addition of two pulsed magnetic field gradients to the spin-echo sequence (Fig. 2) [1]. The two gradients have identical direction, steepness, and temporal duration and are separated in time by a period Δ. The 180°-radiofrequency pulse that defines the spin-echo pulse sequence occurs exactly in the middle of D.

The Stejskal-Tanner pulse sequence, like a conventional spin-echo pulse sequence, begins with a 90°-radiofrequency pulse that forces all spins to precess in the transverse plane at the same rate and in phase with one another. Subsequently, when the first of the two magnetic field gradients unique to DWI is turned on, its effect is to alter the rate of precession of each spin temporarily, to a degree that depends on its position along the axis of the field gradient. Then, when the gradient is turned off, all spins again precess at the same rate, but they have acquired differences in phase that reflect their position. In effect, their position has been "labeled" by their phase. For this reason, the first of the extra magnetic field gradients used for DWI sometimes is called the labeling gradient.

During the period Δ, the spins are free to diffuse freely within the voxel, carrying with them the differences in phase that reflect their original positions at the time of the labeling gradient. The 180°-radiofrequency pulse preserves these phase differences, but reverses their signs, so that initially "leading" spins become "lagging" ones.

The second unique aspect of the Stejskal-Tanner pulse sequence is the unlabeling gradient, which is a pulsed magnetic field gradient of the same direction, steepness, and temporal duration as the labeling gradient. The unlabeling gradient once again changes the rate of precession of each spin temporarily, to a degree reflecting its position along the axis of the gradient. Accordingly, when the gradient is turned off, each spin resumes precession at its original rate but has experienced a second, location-dependent change in phase.

For a spin that has not moved since the time of the labeling gradient, the changes in phase induced by the labeling and unlabeling gradients negate one another, and the spin precesses as if the labeling and unlabeling gradients never were present. Spins that have moved along the axis of the gradients during the period Δ, however, accumulate differences in phase, relative to one another, that cause a drop in the overall signal intensity arising from the voxel. The loss of signal intensity is described by Eq. 2.

$$S_{DWI} = S_0 e^{-bD} \qquad\qquad (2)$$

for which S_{DWI} is the signal intensity on DWI, S_0 is the signal intensity that would have been measured by an identical T2-weighted spin-echo pulse sequence without diffusion gradients, e is the natural logarithm base which equals approximately 2.71828, D is the ADC, and b, the gradient factor, colloquially called the b value, which describes the degree of diffusion-weighting in the image. The gradient factor is a function of the strength and duration of the diffusion gradients and of the time Δ that elapses between them. The user usually specifies the b value that is desired for the pulse sequence rather than individually designating the strength, duration, and temporal separation of the diffusion gradients.

To summarize, a typical clinical diffusion-weighted pulse sequence is a spin-echo sequence that has been modified to produce T2-weighted images in which signal intensity in each voxel is attenuated by a degree that depends on the ADC in the voxel. Larger values of ADC result in greater degrees of signal attenuation. The degree of T2 weighting in the image is determined by the TR and TE chosen for the pulse sequence, and the degree of diffusion weighting is

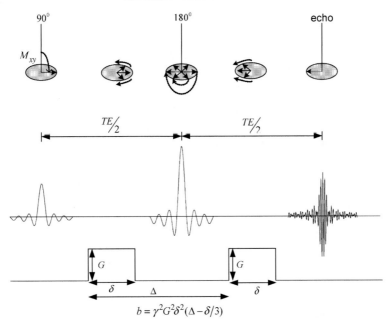

$$b = \gamma^2 G^2 \delta^2 (\Delta - \delta/3)$$

Fig. 2. Stejskal-Tanner diffusion spin-echo sequence. Spins accumulate phase shift during the first gradient pulse. The 180° pulse inverts the phase of all spins. The second gradient lobe induces another phase shift that effectively is opposite to the first gradient pulse as a result of the effect of the spin echo. The phase shifts are identical in magnitude and cancel each other out. For moving or diffusing spins, the translation of the spins to different locations in a time t results in an incomplete refocusing and, hence, the attenuation of the resulting echo. D, diffusion coefficient; γ, gyromagnetic ratio; and G, magnitude of, δ, width of, and Δ, time between the two balanced diffusion gradient pulses.

determined by an exponential function of the gradient factor, or b value, which is specified by the user as part of the pulse sequence.

Multiple image acquisitions and measurement of apparent diffusion coefficient

A single DWI acquired in the manner described previously is not, by itself, able to measure ADC and quantify water diffusion. There are two reasons for this. The first is that in a single DWI, the contributions to signal intensity of T2 and diffusion cannot be separated. In Eq. 2, if a particular voxel exhibits higher-than-normal signal intensity in a DWI (ie, S_{DWI} is large), it is unclear if ADC is low (ie, D is small) or if this voxel simply exhibits relatively long T2 and is, therefore, hyperintense on T2-weighted images (ie, S_0 is large). The latter situation often is called "T2 shine-through" and can lead to the misinterpretation of a hyperintense lesion in DWI as representing a focus of low ADC.

The simplest way to differentiate a lesion with low ADC from one that is merely T2 hyperintense is to obtain DWI with at least two different values of b.

When this is done, Eq. 2 can be solved for D, and ADC can be calculated. Then, maps of ADC can be synthesized in which each pixel's brightness is assigned to represent the ADC calculated for the corresponding voxel of brain tissue. A lesion that appears dark on the ADC map is one in which ADC truly is lower than normal.

Although any two or more values of b can be chosen, for reasons related to noise propagation, the most accurate estimates of D are obtained when only two values of b are used: a maximum value on the order of 1000 s/mm^2 and zero. It can be seen from Eq. 2 that the second image, in which $b = 0$, is just a T2-weighted image, acquired using the same imaging parameters and voxel locations as the high–b-value DWI.

The second reason why a single high-b DWI is incapable of measuring ADC is because of the anisotropy of water diffusion. In a single DWI acquisition, the pulse sequence uses labeling and unlabeling gradients that are oriented in only one direction. Therefore, signal attenuation in DWI does not actually depend on $\bar{L}$, but rather on that component of $\bar{L}$ that lies along the direction of the labeling and unlabeling gradients. This is acceptable if imaging water molecules in a beaker, in which molecules are equally likely to diffuse in any direction and diffusion is, therefore, isotropic. In brain tissue, however, water diffusion is anisotropic; water molecules diffuse at different rates in different directions. White matter diffusion is especially anisotropic. Because cell membranes and myelin form a significant barrier to diffusion, water molecules are more likely to diffuse in a direction parallel to axonal orientation than in a perpendicular direction. Therefore, a single DWI acquired with labeling and unlabeling gradients oriented parallel to axonal orientation measures ADC values that are relatively high, whereas an image acquired with gradients oriented perpendicular to axonal orientation measures ADC values that are relatively low. In clinical practice, acquisition of a single high−b-value image results in patchy areas of white matter hyperintensity that simulate low ADC and can be mistaken for acute infarctions.

The solution to this problem is to acquire at least three separate high−b-value images, with labeling and unlabeling gradients applied in orthogonal directions. The resulting images are combined mathematically into a single image, in which signal intensity for each voxel is assigned the geometric mean of signal intensity in the three component images. In the composite image, tissue appears hyperintense because of either decreased ADC or T2 abnormalities but not because of artifacts related to the orientation of the diffusion gradients and white matter tracts.

Diffusion MR imaging for acute stroke

For acute stroke studies, DWI, exponential images, ADC maps, and T2-weighted images should be reviewed (Fig. 3). In lesions, such as acute ischemic strokes, the T2 and diffusion effects cause increased signal on DWI and regions of decreased diffusion are identified best on DWI. The exponential image and ADC maps are used to exclude "T2 shine-through" as the cause of the increased signal on DWI (Fig. 4). Truly decreased diffusion is hypointense on ADC and hyperintense on exponential images (Fig. 5). The exponential and ADC images also are useful for detecting areas of increased diffusion that may be masked by T2 effects on DWI. On DWI, regions with elevated diffusion may be slightly hypointense, isointense, or slightly hyperintense, depending on the strength of the diffusion and T2 components. Regions with elevated diffusion are hyperintense on ADC maps and hypointense on exponential images.

Ischemic stroke and water diffusion

Although DWI has proved useful in studying a variety of different diseases, the technique first gained widespread use because of its unparalleled sensitivity in the detection of acute stroke and its specificity in distinguishing acute infarctions from other lesions. These capabilities can be understood by reviewing the patholophysiologic changes that occur in ischemic brain tissue and by considering their effects on the ADC.

Fig. 6A depicts cellular organization in normal gray matter schematically. Approximately 80% of gray matter volume is composed of cells, with the remaining 20% composed of the interstitial space and blood vessels. The intracellular space and the inter-

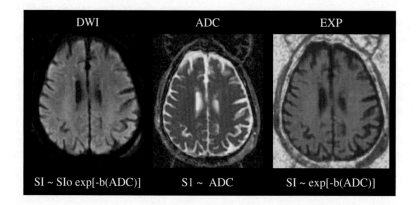

Fig. 3. Typical diffusion MR maps. The appearances on DWI, exponential (EXP) image, and ADC map and the corresponding mathematic expressions for their signal intensities are shown. Image parameters are $b = 1,000$ s/mm^2; effective gradient, 25 mT/m; repetition time, 7500 msec; minimum echo time; matrix, 128 × 128; field of view, 200 × 200 mm; section thickness, 5 mm with 1-mm gap. SI, signal intensity, SIo, signal intensity on T2-weighted image.

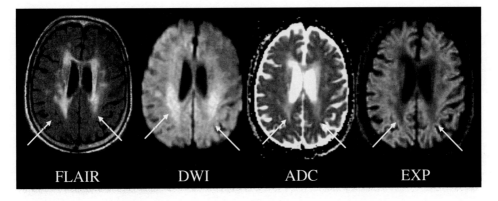

FLAIR DWI ADC EXP

Fig. 4. "T2 shine-through." Seventy-eight-year-old man who had dizziness. DWI hyperintense lesions in the right posterior frontal subcortical white matter and bilateral posterior corona radiata are hyperintense on FLAIR images and ADC maps and hypointense on exponential images. These findings are consistent with elevated diffusion secondary to microangiopathic change rather than acute infarction suggested by DWI alone.

stitial space differ with respect to their concentrations of various ionic species, and energy-dependent membrane ion pumps maintain these differences. The operation of membrane ion pumps is dependent on cellular synthesis of adenosine triphosphate (ATP) and other high-energy phosphate compounds, which in turn require delivery of oxygen and metabolites.

The collective effect of energy-dependent ion pumps is to extract ions from the intracellular space and deposit them in the extracellular interstitial space. In ischemic conditions, when ATP concentrations and membrane ion pumps, such as the sodium-ATPase pump, begin to fail, there is a net migration of ions from the extracellular space to the intracellular space. Water follows by osmosis, resulting in cellular

swelling (see Fig. 6B). This swelling is called cytotoxic edema, which begins within minutes after stroke onset. It results in no change in the mass, volume, or overall water content of affected tissue, because it reflects not an addition of water but a shift of water from the extracellular to the intracellular space. In an acute gray matter infarction, cytotoxic edema increases the fraction of water molecules that are in the intracellular space, from approximately 80% to approximately 95%.

Cytotoxic edema results in a characteristic decrease in ADC and, therefore, an increase in signal intensity on DWI that can be detected minutes after stroke onset. Several theories are proposed to explain this change in ADC. The predominant theory is that

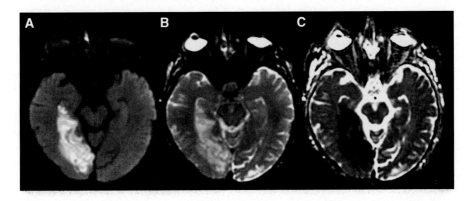

Fig. 5. Example images produced by a diffusion-weighted pulse sequence. (A) DWI, obtained by geometrically averaging the individual high−b-value images, demonstrates a large hyperintense lesion in the right temporal and occipital lobes. Because this image is T2 weighted and diffusion weighted, it cannot be determined if this lesion is hyperintense because of T2 prolongation or because of low ADC values or both. (B) T2-weighted image, obtained by arithmetically averaging several images acquired with the diffusion gradients turned off, demonstrates that the lesion does have prolonged T2. (C) In an ADC map, obtained by solving Eq. 2 for ADC on a pixel-by-pixel basis using the values depicted in images (A) and (B), the lesion is darker than surrounding brain tissue and, therefore, has lower ADC.

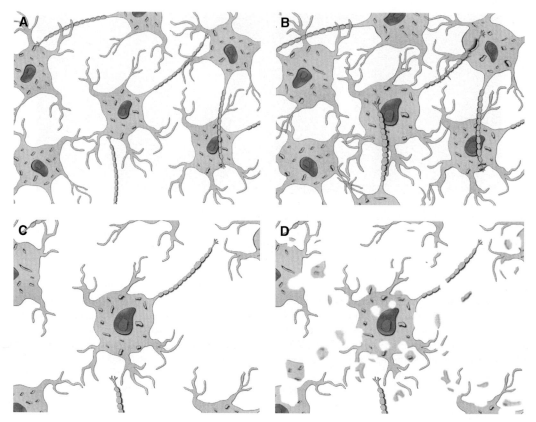

Fig. 6. Stages of ischemic damage to brain tissue. (*A*) Normal gray matter. (*B*) Cytotoxic edema. Within minutes after onset of ischemia, failure of energy-dependent membrane ion pumps causes an accumulation of ions in the intracellular space. Water follows by osmosis, resulting in cellular swelling. This process is associated with a decrease in ADC and accounts for DWI's superior sensitivity in the detection of acute infarcts. (*C*) Vasogenic edema. Release of inflammatory mediators results in efflux of new water from the vasculature, which is associated with an increase in ADC. Vasogenic edema becomes evident on MR imaging within approximately 6 hours after stroke onset and peaks approximately 3 to 5 days thereafter. (*D*) Cellular breakdown. During the ensuing weeks, months, and years, breakdown of cellular membranes and gradual phagocytosis of necrotic debris further remove restrictions on water diffusion, resulting in further increases in ADC.

water movement is more restricted in the intracellular compared with the extracellular space [2–4]. In the intracellular space, cellular organelles, cytoskeletal macromolecules, and other subcellular structures serve as barriers to the random motion of water molecules. In addition, intracellular metabolite ADCs are reduced significantly in ischemic rat brain. Proposed explanations are increased intracellular viscosity as a result of microtubule dissociation and fragmentation of other cellular components as a result of collapse of the energy-dependent cytoskeleton; increased tortuosity of the intracellular space; and decreased cytoplasmic mobility [5–7].

Furthermore, changes in the extracellular space may contribute to the decreased diffusion associated with acute stroke. With cellular swelling, there is reduced extracellular space volume and a decrease in

the diffusion of low-molecular-weight tracer molecules in animal models [8,9]. This is believed to result from a greater tortuosity of the paths that extracellular molecules must traverse to avoid contact with the relatively impermeable cell membranes. Other factors, such as temperature decrease and cell membrane permeability, play a minor role in explaining ADC decreases in ischemic brain tissue [10–12].

Time course of diffusion lesion evolution

Decreased diffusion in ischemic brain tissue is observed as early as 30 minutes after arterial occlusion and progresses through a stereotypic sequence of ADC reduction, followed by subsequent increase, pseudonormalization and, finally, permanent eleva-

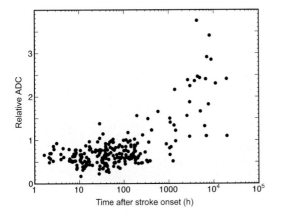

Fig. 7. Time course of ADC in stroke. In the core of an infarction, relative ADC (ADC expressed as a fraction of its normal value) begins to decrease from its normal value of 1 soon after stroke onset. It reaches its minimum within the first day and then begins to increase again, passing through normal values, and ultimately remaining permanently elevated. Note that the X axis is a logarithmic scale. (*From* Copen WA, et al. Ischemic stroke: effects of etiology and patient age on the time course of the core apparent diffusion coefficient. Radiology 2001;221:27–34; with permission.)

tion. (Figs. 7 and 8) [13–18]. Initially, the ADC continues to decrease with maximal signal reduction at 1 to 4 days. There is marked hyperintensity on DWI (a combination of T2 and diffusion weighting), less hyperintensity on exponential images, and hypointensity on ADC images. Subsequently, release of inflammatory mediators from ischemic brain tissue leads to vasogenic edema with extravasation of water molecules from blood vessels to expand the interstitial space (see Fig. 6C), where water molecule diffusion is highly unrestricted. Consequently, after approximately 4 days, the ADC begins to rise and returns to baseline at 1 to 2 weeks. This process is called pseudonormalization to reflect the fact that the tissue is irreversibly necrotic despite normal ADC values. At this point, a stroke usually is mildly hyperintense on DWI because of the T2 component and isointense on the ADC and exponential images. Thereafter, the ADC is elevated secondary to increasing extracellular water, cell membrane breakdown and disintegration, gradual phagocytosis of necrotic debris that takes place over months to years, and gliosis. There is slight hypointensity, isointensity, or hyperintensity on DWI (depending on

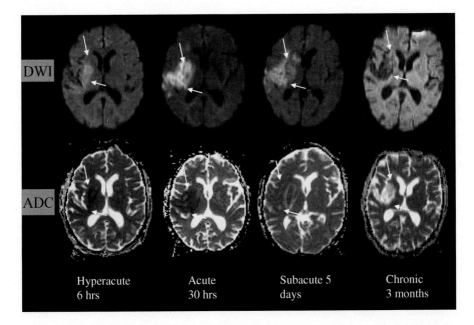

Fig. 8. DWI and ADC time course of stroke evolution. Seventy-two-year-old woman who had acute left hemiparesis. At 6 hours, the right MCA infarction is hyperintense on DWI and hypointense on ADC images secondary to early cytotoxic edema. At 30 hours, DWI hyperintensity and ADC hypointensity are more pronounced secondary to increased cytotoxic edema. At 5 days, the ADC hypointensity is mild, indicating that the ADC has nearly pseudonormalized. This is secondary to cell lysis and the development of vasogenic edema. The lesion remains markedly hyperintense on DWI because the T2 and diffusion components are combined. At 3 months, the infarction is DWI hypointense and ADC hyperintense, indicating elevation of diffusion due to gliosis and tissue cavitation.

the strength of the T2 and diffusion components), increased signal intensity on ADC maps, and decreased signal on exponential images.

The time course is influenced by several factors. Early reperfusion can lead to pseudonormalization at 1 to 2 days in patients who receive intravenous recombinant tissue plasminogen activator (rtPA) within 3 hours after stroke onset [19]. Furthermore, there are different temporal rates of tissue evolution toward infarction within a single ischemic lesion. In one study, although the average ADC of an ischemic lesion was depressed within 10 hours, different zones within an ischemic lesion demonstrated low, pseudonormal, or elevated ADCs [20]. Stroke type also is an important factor. Minimum ADC is reached more slowly and transition from decreasing to increasing ADC is later in lacunes versus other stroke types (nonlacunes) [18]. In nonlacunes, the subsequent rate of ADC increase is more rapid in younger versus older patients. In spite of these variations, in the absence of thrombolysis, tissue with reduced ADC nearly always progresses to infarction.

Reliability

Because detection of hypoattenuation on CT and hyperintensity on T2-weighted and FLAIR MR images requires marked increases in tissue water, conventional CT and MR imaging cannot detect hyperacute infarctions (less than 6 hours) reliably. CT is 38% to 45% sensitive and conventional MR imaging sequences are 18% to 46% sensitive for the detection of hyperacute infarctions [21,22]. For infarctions imaged within 24 hours, one study reports a sensitivity of 58% for CT and 82% for MR imaging [23]. Conversely, DWI are highly sensitive and specific in the detection of hyperacute and acute infarctions [21,24–26]. They are sensitive to the detection of decreased diffusion of water molecules that occurs early in ischemia, and they have a much higher contrast-to-noise ratio compared with CT, FLAIR, and T2-weighted sequences. Reported sensitivities range from 88% to 100% and reported specificities range from 86% to 100%.

Most false-negative DWI occur with punctate brainstem, thalamic, or basal ganglia infarctions (Fig. 9) [21,24,25,27]. Some lesions are seen on follow-up MR imaging and some lesions are not seen at follow-up but are presumed on the basis of an abnormal neurologic examination. False-negative DWI also occur in patients who have regions with increased mean transit time (MTT) or decreased relative cerebral blood flow (CBF) that demonstrate

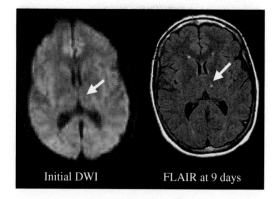

Initial DWI   FLAIR at 9 days

Fig. 9. False-negative DWI. Thalamic lacune without an acute DWI abnormality. Forty-five-year-old woman who had sensory syndrome. Initial DWI demonstrates no definite acute infarction. Follow-up FLAIR image at 9 days demonstrates a punctate hyperintense left thalamic lacunar infarction (*arrow*).

hyperintensity on follow-up DWI; that is, initially, they have brain regions with ischemic but viable tissue that eventually progresses to infarction.

False-positive DWI occurs in patients who have subacute or chronic infarctions with "T2 shine-through," specifically, a lesion is hyperintense on DWI resulting from increased T2 signal rather than decreased diffusion. Interpreting DWI with ADC maps or exponential images easily avoids this pitfall. In general, acute lesions demonstrate hypointense signal on ADC maps and hyperintense signal on exponential images, whereas subacute to chronic lesions demonstrate hyperintense signal on ADC maps and hypointense signal on exponential images. False-positive DWI also can be seen with other entities that demonstrate decreased diffusion. These include cerebral abscess (restricted diffusion resulting from increased viscosity), tumor (restricted diffusion resulting from dense cell packing), venous infarctions, demyelinative lesions (decreased diffusion resulting from myelin vacuolization), hemorrhage, herpes encephalitis (decreased diffusion resulting from cell necrosis), and diffuse axonal injury (decreased diffusion resulting from cytotoxic edema or axotomy). Because these lesions typically are reviewed in combination with T1, FLAIR, T2, and gadolinium-enhanced T1-weighted images, they usually can be differentiated easily from acute infarctions.

Diffusion-weighted imaging reversibility

DWI reversible tissue refers to tissue that is abnormal on initial DWI but normal on follow-up images. In the absence of thrombolysis or other intra-arterial (IA) recanalization procedures, DWI reversibility is rare. Grant and colleagues could identify only 21 out of thousands of DWI hyperintense lesions in patients who had acute focal neurologic deficits that resolved or appeared smaller on follow-up images and most had causes other than ischemic stroke [28]. The causes were acute stroke or TIA (three patients), transient global amnesia (TGA) (seven patients), status epilepticus (four patients), hemiplegic migraine (three patients), and venous sinus thrombosis (four patients). ADC ratios (ipsilateral over contralateral normal-appearing brain tissue) were similar to those observed with acute stroke (0.64–0.79 for gray matter and 0.20–0.87 for white matter).

In the setting of intravenous or IA thrombolysis, DWI reversibility is observed in up to 33% of DWI abnormal tissue (Fig. 10) [29]. A normal appearance on follow-up images may not reflect complete tissue recovery, however. Kidwell and coworkers demonstrate a decrease in size from the initial DWI abnormality to the follow-up DWI abnormality immediately after IA thrombolysis in 8 of 18 patients, but DWI lesion volume subsequently increased in five patients. Several studies demonstrate that ADCs are significantly higher in DWI reversible tissue compared with DWI abnormal tissue that progresses to infarction. Mean ADCs range from 663 to 732 $\times$ 10^{-6} mm^2 per second in DWI-reversible regions compared with 608 to 650 $\times$ 10^{-6} mm^2 per second in DWI-abnormal regions that infarct [29,30]. Animal models also show high correlation between threshold ADCs of 550 $\times$ 10^{-6} mm^2 per second and tissue volume with histologic infarction [31].

Other studies suggest that an ADC threshold for tissue infarction does not exist. In one study of patients who had early reperfusion, less than half of the tissue volume with an initial ADC of less than 60% of normal appeared abnormal on T2-weighted images at day 7 [32]. This is well below the threshold ADCs of approximately 80% of normal tissue (discussed previously). It is likely that duration and severity of ischemia, rather than absolute ADC value, determine whether or not tissue recovers. For example, the degree of ADC decrease correlates strongly with degree of CBF decrease, and the CBF threshold for tissue infarction increases with increasing occlusion time (discussed later) [33,34].

Diffusion tensor imaging

Acquisition of three high–b-value images with gradients applied in orthogonal directions plus a fourth image with a low b-value (ideally zero) suffice for measurement of ADC. It can be advantageous (although more time consuming), however, to acquire high–b-value images with gradients applied in a larger number of directions. If at least six diffusion gradient directions are used, then not only ADC but also the entire diffusion tensor can be calculated. This technique is called diffusion tensor imaging (DTI).

The diffusion tensor is an abstract 3-D object that describes the likelihood of a water molecule to diffuse from a central point in every possible direction (Fig. 11). In a beaker of water, the diffusion tensor is spherical, reflecting the equal likelihood of a water molecule to diffuse in any direction. In white

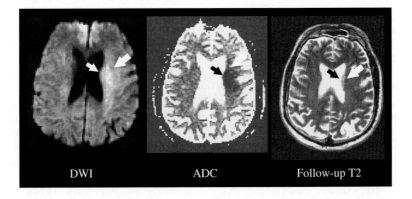

Fig. 10. Acute ischemic stroke with DWI reversibility. Sixty-nine-year-old man who had acute dysarthria and hemiparesis. MRA demonstrates MCA occlusion. He was treated with IA rtPA with complete recanalization. DWI and ADC maps demonstrate acute ischemia involving the left caudate body and corona radiata. Follow-up T2-weighted images demonstrate hyperintensity, consistent with infarction in the caudate body (*small arrow*). Most of the corona radiata (*large arrow*), however, appears normal on follow-up T2-weighted images.

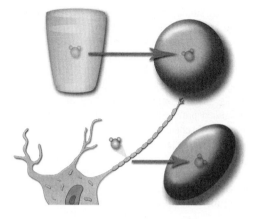

Fig. 11. The diffusion tensor. (*Upper arrow*) For water molecules in a cup of water, diffusion is isotropic, and the tensor is spherical. The graphic representation of the tensor above implies that, during a finite time period, a water molecule is equally likely to move from its original position at the center of the sphere to any point on the surface of the sphere. (*Lower arrow*) For water molecules in white matter, diffusion is anisotropic, and the tensor is cigar-shaped. Water molecules are more likely to diffuse parallel to the axis of traversing axons than perpendicular to that axis.

matter, the tensor is elongated and cigar-shaped, reflecting the greater likelihood of diffusion along the direction of white matter tracts. The tensor is represented mathematically by a 3 × 3 matrix that is axis symmetric and, therefore, has six unique elements (hence, the need for six diffusion gradient directions).

DTI allows the calculation of three parameters that all may be useful in the evaluation of acute ischemic stroke.

1. The trace of the diffusion tensor [Tr(ADC)] or the average diffusivity, $<D>$ ($<D> = [\lambda_1 + \lambda_2 + \lambda_3]/3$, where λ_1, λ_2, and λ_3 are the eigenvalues or three principal directions of the diffusion tensor) that measures the overall diffusion in a region, independent of direction [35].
2. Diffusion anisotropy indices, such as fractional anisotropy (FA) or the lattice index, that measure the amount of difference in diffusion in different directions [36,37].
3. Fiber orientation mapping that provides information on white matter tract structure, integrity, and connectivity [38–40].

Because of its increased signal-to-noise ratio, measurement of average diffusivity, $<D>$, has provided new information on differences between gray and white matter diffusion that were not appreciable

with measurement of diffusion along three orthogonal directions [41,42]. For example, $<D>$ images can identify regions of reduced white matter diffusion that appear normal on DWI. Furthermore, studies demonstrate that $<D>$ decreases are greater in white matter versus gray matter in the acute and subacute periods, whereas $<D>$ increases are higher in white matter versus gray matter in the chronic period. Although gray matter typically is believed to be more vulnerable to ischemia than white matter, recent animal experiments demonstrate that severe histopathologic changes can occur in white matter as early as 30 minutes after acute stroke onset. Furthermore, reduced bulk water motion from cytoskeletal collapse and disruption of fast axonal transport, which do not exist in gray matter, may occur in white matter.

Diffusion anisotropy occurs because water diffusion is different in different directions because of tissue structure [43,44]. Gray matter has relatively low diffusion anisotropy. White matter, however, as a result of highly organized tract bundles, has relatively high diffusion anisotropy, with diffusion much greater parallel, rather than perpendicular, to the fiber tracts [35,43,45,46]. Oligodendrocyte concentration and fast axonal transport also may contribute to white matter diffusion anisotropy. In addition, it is believed that the intracellular compartment is more anisotropic than the extracellular compartment because of the presence of microtubules, organelles, and intact membranes [47,48].

With acute stroke, FA correlates with time of stroke onset [49,50]. In general, FA is elevated in the hyperacute and early acute periods, becomes reduced at approximately 12 to 24 hours, and progressively decreases over time. Because strokes evolve at different rates, however, there is heterogeneity in the change in FA over time within different regions of a single ischemic lesion and between different ischemic lesions [49,50]. Furthermore, the decreases in FA associated with ischemia are significantly greater in white matter compared with gray matter, likely as a result of structural differences [42,50]. In the white matter extracellular space, there are dense arrays of parallel white matter tracts. With acute ischemia, the diffusion decrease is much greater in lambda 1, the eigenvalue that coincides with the long axis of white matter fiber tracts, compared with the other eigenvalues. In the gray matter extracellular space there is a meshwork. With acute ischemia, the diffusion decrease is more similar between eigenvalues.

Yang and colleagues describe three temporally related different phases in the relationship between FA and ADC (Fig. 12). Increased FA and reduced ADC characterize the initial phase; reduced FA and

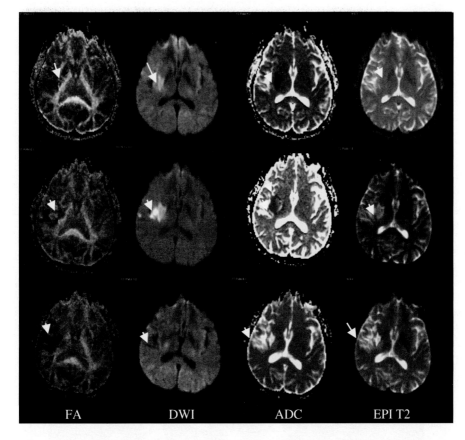

Fig. 12. Temporal evolution of FA changes in acute ischemic stroke. An elderly man who had left hemiparesis was examined at 4 hours, 5 days, and 5 months after onset. At four hours (*row 1*), the right putamen stroke (*arrow*) is hyperintense on FA images, hyperintense on DWI, hypointense on ADC images, and not seen on echo planar T2-weighted images. These findings represent the first stage of FA changes in stroke described by Yang and colleagues. After 5 days (*row 2*), the lesion is hypointense on FA images, hyperintense on DWI, hyperintense on ADC images, and hyperintense on echo planar T2-weighted images. These findings represent the second stage of FA changes in stroke described by Yang and colleagues. At 5 months (*row 3*), the lesion is hypointense on FA images, hypointense on DWI, hyperintense on ADC images and hyperintense on T2-weighted images. These findings represent the third stage of FA changes in stroke described by Yang and colleagues.

reduced ADC characterize a second, intermediate phase; and reduced FA with elevated ADC characterize a more chronic third phase [50]. In addition, FA inversely correlates with T2 signal change [51]. These changes can be explained as follows. As cytotoxic edema develops, there is a shift of water from the extracellular to the intracellular space, but cell membranes remain intact and there is not a significant overall increase in tissue water. This explains elevated FA, reduced ADC, and normal T2. As the ischemic insult continues, cells lyse, the glial reaction occurs, and there is degradation of the blood-brain barrier, an overall increase in tissue water, predominantly in the extracellular space, occurs. This explains reduced FA, elevated ADC, and elevated T2. Reduced FA, reduced ADC, and elevated T2 may

occur when there is an overall increase in tissue water, but the intracellular fraction still is high enough to cause reduced ADC, and the extracellular portion is high enough to cause reduced FA. Other factors, such as loss of axonal transport, loss of cellular integrity, and decreases in interstitial fluid flow, may contribute to decreases in FA over time.

Fiber orientation mapping can provide new information on how strokes affect adjacent white matter tracts. Fiber orientation mapping can detect wallerian degeneration prior to conventional MR imaging and may be useful in predicting motor function in the long term (Fig. 13). One study demonstrates that FA is decreased significantly in the corticospinal tracts in patients who have acute stroke and who have moderate to severe hemiparesis but not in patients who have no

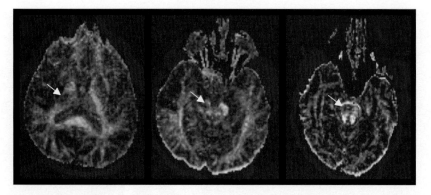

Fig. 13. Wallerian degeneration in the right corticospinal tract 3 months after an infarction in the right MCA territory. FA images demonstrate hypointensity secondary to reduced FA in the right corticospinal tract.

or mild hemiparesis at long-term follow-up [52]. Another study of patients who had subacute stroke demonstrates a significant reduction in the eigenvalues parallel to the corticospinal tract at 2 to 3 weeks in eight patients who had stroke and had poor recovery but not in eight patients who had good recovery [53]. In the chronic period, DTI can distinguish between a primary stroke and a region of wallerian degeneration. A primary chronic stroke has reduced FA and elevated mean diffusivity, whereas the corticospinal tract has reduced FA but preserved or only slightly elevated mean diffusivity [54].

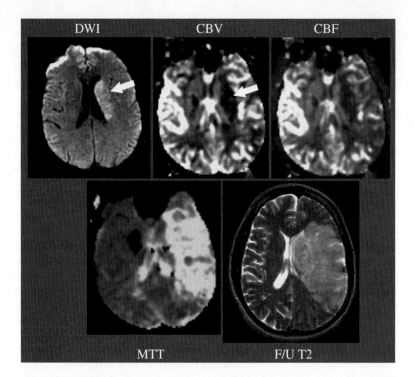

Fig. 14. Diffusion-perfusion mismatch where the infarction grows into nearly all of the tissue at risk of infarction. Fifty-year-old woman who had aphasia and right-sided weakness resulting from a left MCA stem embolus, imaged at 6 hours. DWI demonstrates hyperintensity, consistent with acute infarction, in the left corona radiata and caudate nucleus (*arrow*). The CBV map demonstrates a hypointense lesion similar in size to the DWI abnormality (*arrow*). CBF and MTT images demonstrate much larger abnormal regions (CBF hypointense and MTT hyperintense) involving the left frontal and parietal lobes. The CBF and MTT abnormal but DWI normal tissue reflect the operational ischemic penumbra. In spite of heparin and hypertensive therapy, follow-up T2-weighted image demonstrate growth of the infarction into most of the ischemic penumbra.

Diffusion in combination with perfusion MR imaging in the evaluation of acute stroke

Diffusion and perfusion MR imaging in predicting tissue viability

In the clinical setting, DWI is interpreted in combination with perfusion-weighted images. The most important clinical impact may result from defining the ischemic penumbra, a region that is ischemic but still viable and that may infarct if not treated. Therefore, most investigation is focused on strokes resulting from a proximal occlusion with a perfusion lesion larger than the diffusion lesion (Figs. 14 and 15). Operationally, the diffusion abnormality is believed to represent the ischemic core and the region characterized by normal diffusion, but abnormal perfusion is believed to represent the ischemic penumbra [16,55–60]. Definition of the penumbra is complicated because of the multiple hemodynamic parameters that may be calculated from the perfusion

MR imaging data, such as cerebral blood volume (CBV), CBF, MTT, and other tissue transit time measures (time to peak [TTP], relative peak height, and so forth).

Several articles focus on diffusion and perfusion volumetric data. After arterial occlusion, brain regions with decreased diffusion and decreased perfusion are believed to represent nonviable tissue or the infarction core. The majority of strokes increase in volume on DWI with the peak volumetric measurements achieved at 2 to 3 days post ictus. The initial DWI lesion volume correlates highly with final infarction volume with reported correlation coefficients (r^2) ranging from 0.69 to 0.98 [17,30, 61–63]. The initial CBV lesion volume usually is similar to DWI lesion volume and also correlates highly with final infarction volume, with r^2 ranging from 0.79 to 0.81 [30,62,64]. In one large series, predicted lesion growth from the initial DWI to the follow-up lesion size was 24% and from the initial CBV to the follow-up lesion size was 22% (Fig. 16).

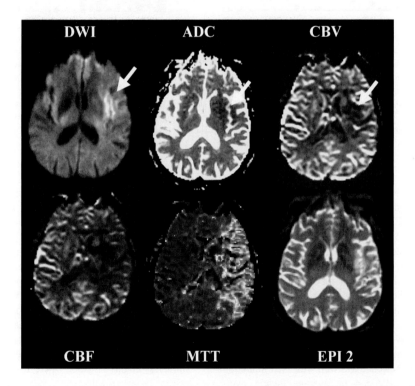

Fig. 15. Diffusion-perfusion mismatch where entire penumbra recovers. Seventy-six-year-old man who had mild right hemiparesis, right facial droop with left MCA stem embolus, imaged at 2 hours. There is hyperintensity on DWI and hypointensity on the CBV maps in the left insula, left putamen, and left inferior frontal lobe (*arrow*). This region is believed to represent the core of ischemic tissue and was abnormal on follow-up T2-weighted images. The CBF and MTT images show larger abnormalities involving most of the visualized left MCA territory. The DWI and CBV are normal but CBF and MTT abnormal tissue is believed to represent the ischemic penumbra. The patient was started on heparin and hypertensive therapy. None of the ischemic penumbra progressed to infarction.

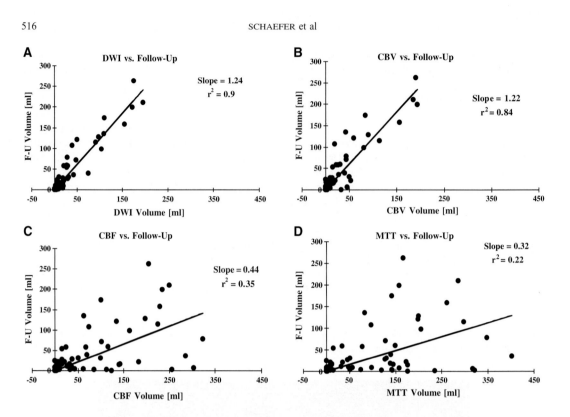

Fig. 16. Initial lesion size versus final lesion size in 81 patients. Scatter plots demonstrate (*A*) initial DWI lesion volume versus final lesion volume, $r^2 = 0.9$ and slope = 1.24 ± 0.08; (*B*) initial CBV lesion volume versus final lesion volume, $r^2 = 0.84$ and slope = 1.22 ± 0.11; (*C*) initial CBF lesion volume versus final lesion volume, $r^2 = 0.35$ and slope = 0.44 ± 0.09; (*D*) initial MTT versus final lesion volume (vertical axis). $r^2 = 0.22$ and slope = 0.32 ± 0.08. The DWI has the highest correlation to a linear fit. Of the perfusion images, the CBV has the highest correlation to a linear fit. (*From* Schaefer PW, et al. Predicting cerebral ischemic infarct volume with diffusion and perfusion MR imaging. AJNR Am J Neuroradiol 2002;23:1785–94; with permission.)

When there is a rare DWI-CBV mismatch, DWI lesion volume still correlates highly with final infarction volume, but the predicted lesion growth increases to approximately 60% [30]. The CBV, in this setting, also correlates highly with final infarction volume with no predicted lesion growth. In other words, when there is a DWI-CBV mismatch, DWI abnormality typically grows into the size of the CBV abnormality.

Many more strokes are characterized by a DWI-CBF or a DWI-MTT mismatch compared with a DWI-CBV mismatch. In general, initial CBF and MTT volumes correlate less well with final infarction volume than CBV and on average greatly overestimate final infarction volume. r^2 range from 0.3 to 0.67 for CBF and from 0.3 to 0.69 for MTT [30,62,64–66]. Predicted final infarction volume was 44% of the initial CBF abnormality and 32% of the initial MTT abnormality in one study [30]. Another study demonstrates that size of the DWI-

CBF and DWI-MTT mismatches correlate with final infarction volume. r^2 for DWI-CBF and DWI-MTT mismatch volume versus final infarction volume were 0.657 and 0.561, respectively [64].

In small vessel infarctions (perforator infarctions and distal embolic infarctions) and in whole-territory, large-vessel infarctions, the initial perfusion (CBV, CBF, and MTT) and diffusion lesion volumes usually are similar and there is little to no lesion growth (Fig. 17). A diffusion lesion larger than the perfusion lesion or a diffusion lesion without a perfusion abnormality usually occurs with early reperfusion. Similarly, in this situation, there usually is no significant lesion growth.

More recently, research has focused on defining diffusion and perfusion MR parameter lesion ratios or absolute values in infarction core, penumbra that progresses to infarction, and penumbra that remains viable. Most papers demonstrate that CBF is the most useful parameter for distinguishing hypo-

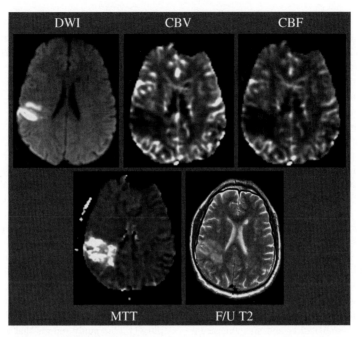

Fig. 17. Diffusion-perfusion match in branch vessel occlusion. Seventy-one-year-old man who had left arm and face weakness. DWI demonstrates an acute infarction in the right inferior parietal region. Defects similar in size are seen on the CBV, CBF, and MTT maps. There is no diffusion-perfusion mismatch. Follow-up T2-weighted image demonstrates no significant lesion growth.

perfused tissue that progresses to infarction from hypoperfused tissue that remains viable in patients not treated with thrombolysis or other IA recanalization parameters (Fig. 18). Reported rCBF ratios for core range from 0.12 to 0.44, for penumbra that progresses to infarction from 0.35 to 0.56, and for penumbra that remains viable from 0.58 to 0.78 [67–71]. Assuming a normal CBF of 50 milliliters per 100 grams per minute [72], these ratios translate to 6 to 22 milliliters per 100 grams per minute for core, 17.5 to 28 per 100 grams per minute for penumbra that progresses to infarction, and 29 to 39 milliliters per 100 grams per minute for penumbra that remains viable.

Variability in CBF ratios likely results from several different factors. The data obtained represents a single time point in a dynamic process. One major factor is variability in timing of tissue reperfusion. Jones and colleagues demonstrate that severity and duration of CBF reduction up to 4 hours define a threshold for tissue infarction in monkeys [34]. For example, the CBF threshold for tissue infarction with reperfusion at 2 to 3 hours was 10 to 12 milliliters per 100 gram per minute, whereas the threshold for tissue infarction with permanent occlusion was 17 to 18 milliliters per 100 gram per minute. Furthermore, Ueda and colleagues, in a study of patients treated

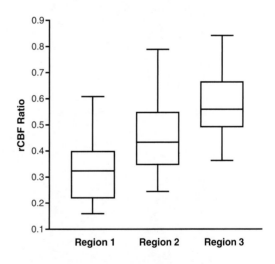

Fig. 18. rCBF ratios. Box and whiskers graph of lesion/contralateral ratio mean values for each patient. Region 1: infarction core with DWI, MTT, and follow-up abnormalities. Region 2: penumbra which infarctions representing tissue that is DWI normal but MTT abnormal and demonstrates infarction at follow-up. Region 3: viable, hypoperfused tissue that recovers representing tissue that is DWI normal but MTT abnormal and appears normal at follow-up. (*From* Schaefer PW, et al. Assessing tissue viability with MR diffusion and perfusion imaging. AJNR Am J Neuroradiol 2003;24:436–43; with permission.)

with thrombolysis, demonstrate that duration of ischemia affects the CBF threshold for tissue viability for up to 5 hours [73]. Another factor is that normal average CBF in human parenchyma varies greatly, from 21.1 to 65.3 milliliters per 100 gram per minute, depending on age and location in gray matter versus white matter [72,74–77]. Other factors include variability in methodologies, variability in initial and follow-up imaging times, and variability in post-ischemic tissue responses.

Low CBV ratios are highly predictive of infarction. Elevated CBV is not predictive of tissue viability and CBV ratios for the two different penumbral regions may not be significantly different (Fig. 19). Lesion ratios range from 0.25 to 0.89 for lesion core, 0.69 to 1.44 for penumbra that progresses to infarction, and 0.94 to 1.29 for penumbra that remains viable [67–71,78]. The finding of elevated CBV in the ischemic penumbra is in accordance with positron emission tomographic studies demonstrating that initially decreased cerebral perfusion pressure produces vasodilatation and an increase in the CBV in order to maintain constant CBF and oxygen extraction fraction [79]. With further decreases in cerebral perfusion pressure, the compensatory vasodilatation reaches a maximum and CBF begins to fall. CBV initially continues to rise and then falls as capillary beds collapse. Thus, elevated CBV appears to represent an unstable situation and is not sustainable over time.

Some studies demonstrate no statistically significant differences in MTT between infarction core and the two (viable and nonviable) penumbral regions, whereas others demonstrate differences between all three regions or between the viable and nonviable penumbral regions [67–71,78]. Reported MTT ratios for core range from 1. 70 to 2.53, for penumbra that progresses to infarction range from 1.74 to 2.19, and for penumbra that remains viable range from 1.65 to 1.66. Previous studies demonstrated that only DWI normal tissue with a TTP of greater than or equal to 6 seconds is at risk of significant lesion enlargement and that tissue with TTP of greater than 6 to 8 seconds correlates highly with final infarction volume [80,81]. One study reports that a greater proportion of severely hypoperfused (>6 seconds MTT) tissue

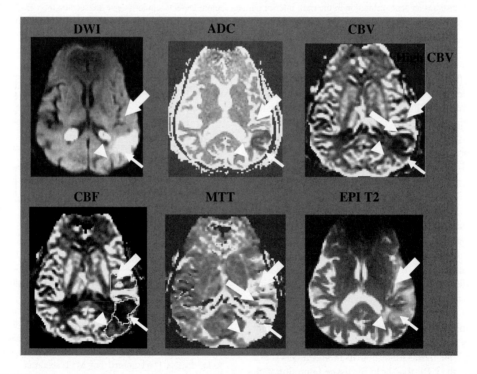

Fig. 19. Diffusion-perfusion mismatch, where a region with elevated CBV but low CBF that progresses to infarction. Eighty-three-year-old woman who had right hemiparesis and aphasia. Three regions are outlined on the CBF maps. The thin white arrow marks infarction core characterized by decreased diffusion, low CBV, low CBF, elevated MTT, and follow-up infarction. The thick white arrow marks penumbra that infarcts which in this case is a DWI normal region with elevated CBV, low CBF, elevated MTT, and follow-up infarction. The white arrowhead marks penumbra that remains viable, which is a DWI and CBV normal region with low CBF, elevated MTT, and normal follow-up.

recovered in patients who have stroke treated with IV tissue-type plasminogen activator (tPA) versus patients who have stroke treated with conventional therapies [82]. One study that evaluated the ability of CBF, MTT, TTP, and relative peak height to predict infarction growth finds that a combination of TTP and relative peak height provided the best prediction of infarction growth (peak height less than 54% and TTP greater than 5.2 seconds had a sensitivity of 71% and a specificity of 98%) [83].

In general, ADC values are significantly different between the core and the two (viable and nonviable) penumbral regions. Some reports demonstrate significant differences between the ADC values for the penumbral regions, whereas others report no statistically significant difference between these regions. In one large study, absolute mean ADC values for infarction core, penumbra that progresses to infarction, and penumbra that remains viable were 661, 782, and 823×10^{-6} mm^2/s, respectively [84]. Other investigators report ADC ratios for infarction core, penumbra that progresses to infarction, and hypoperfused tissue that remains viable of 0.62 to 0.63, 0.89 to 0.90, and 0.93 to 0.96, respectively [67,69].

The aforementioned approaches focused on regions or volumes of tissue. Because there is heterogeneity in diffusion and perfusion parameters within ischemic tissue, Wu and coworkers performed a voxel by voxel analysis of abnormalities on six maps (T2, ADC, DWI, CBV, CBF, and MTT) compared with follow-up T2-weighted images and developed thresholding and generalized linear model algorithms to predict tissue outcome [85]. They found that at their optimal operating points, thresholding algorithms combining DWI and PWI provided 66% sensitivity and 83% specificity and that generalized linear model algorithms combining DWI and PWI provided 66% sensitivity and 84% specificity.

Diffusion and perfusion MR imaging in predicting hemorrhagic transformation of acute stroke

Hemorrhagic transformation (HT) of cerebral infarction refers to secondary bleeding into ischemic tissue with a natural incidence of 15% to 26% during the first 2 weeks and up to 43% over the first month after cerebral infarction [86–89]. Factors that increase the risk of HT include stroke etiology (HT is more frequent with embolic strokes), reperfusion, good collateral circulation, hypertension, anticoagulant therapy, and thrombolytic therapy. Furthermore, in patients treated with IA thrombolytic therapy, higher National Institutes of Health stroke scale

(NIHSS) scores, longer time to recanalization, lower platelet counts, and higher glucose levels predispose patients to HT [90].

It is commonly believed that HT results from reperfusion into severely ischemic tissue because more severe ischemia leads to greater disruption of the cerebral microvasculature and greater degradation of the blood-brain barrier. Subsequently, reperfusion into the damaged capillaries after clot lysis leads to blood extravasation and petechial hemorrhage or a hematoma. Many studies describe HT in spite of persistent arterial occlusion [86,91]. HT in this setting may result from preservation of collateral flow. Furthermore, rtPA thrombolytic therapy may aggravate ischemia-induced microvascular damage by activation of the plasminogen-plasmin system with activation of metalloproteinases that may cause degradation of the basal lamina [92–94].

Because ADC values are believed to mark the severity of ischemia, several studies have assessed the value of the ADC to predict HT (Fig. 20). One study demonstrates that the volume of the initial DWI lesion and the absolute number of voxels with an ADC value less than or equal to 550×10^{-6} mm^2/s correlates with HT of infarctions treated with intravenous tPA [95]. Another study demonstrates that the mean ADC of ischemic regions with subsequent HT is significantly lower than the mean ADC of all analyzed ischemic regions ($510 \pm 140 \times 10^{-6}$ mm^2/s versus $623 \pm 113 \times 10^{-6}$ mm^2/s) [96]. There also was a significant difference when comparing the hemorrhagic ischemic regions with the bland ischemic regions within the same ischemic lesion. A third study demonstrates 100% sensitivity and 71% specificity for predicting HT when infarctions were separated into those with a mean ADC core of less than 300×10^{-6} mm^2/s) versus those with a mean ADC core of greater than 300×10^{-6} mm^2/s) [97].

CBF may be the best perfusion parameter for identifying ischemic tissue that will undergo HT. With single photon emission CT (SPECT) imaging, Ueda and colleagues demonstrate an increased likelihood of HT in ischemic brain tissue with a cerebral blood flow (CBF) less than 35% of the normal cerebellar blood flow [98]. It also is demonstrated that CBF ratios are significantly lower in middle cerebral artery (MCA) infarctions that undergo HT versus those that do not. In one study, all ischemic tissue with a mean CBF ratio of less than 0.18 developed hemorrhage [99]. Other imaging parameters predictive of HT include: (1) hypodensity in greater than one third of the MCA territory on CT [100]; (2) early parenchymal enhancement on gadolinium-enhanced, T1-weighted images [101], and (3) prior

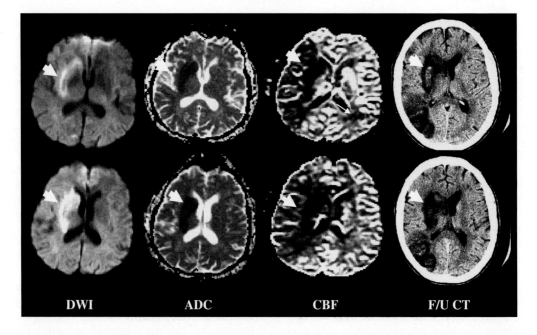

DWI   ADC   CBF   F/U CT

Fig. 20. Acute ischemic stroke with HT. Seventy-six-year-old man who had left hemiparesis, treated with IA rtPA. There is an acute stroke (DWI hyperintense, ADC hypointense) involving the right insula, basal ganglia, and deep white matter. There is marked reduction in ADC and CBF in the basal ganglia and deep white matter (*white arrows*) where there is HT on follow-up CT. Follow-up CT also demonstrates extension of the infarction into the right parietal portion of the ischemic penumbra.

microbleeds detected on T2* gradient-echo imaging [102].

Correlation of diffusion and perfusion MR imaging with clinical outcome

Several studies show how DWI can be used to predict clinical outcome. Some studies demonstrate statistically significant correlations between the acute anterior circulation DWI and ADC lesion volume and acute and chronic neurologic assessment tests, including the NIHSS, the Canadian neurologic scale, the Glasgow outcome score, the Barthel index, and the modified Rankin scale [16,63,103–108]. Correlations between DWI and ADC volume and clinical outcome range from $r = 0.65$ to 0.78. In general, correlations are stronger for cortical strokes than for penetrator artery strokes [16,104]. Lesion location may explain this difference. For example, a small ischemic lesion in the brainstem could produce a worse neurologic deficit than a cortical lesion of the same size. In fact, one study of posterior circulation strokes showed no correlation between initial DWI lesion volume and NIHSS [109]. A significant correlation also is reported between the acute ADC ratio (ADC of lesion/ADC of normal contralateral brain) and chronic neurologic assessment scales [16,103]. Furthermore, one study demonstrates that patients who have a mismatch between the initial NIHSS score (greater than 8) and the initial DWI lesion volume (less than 25 mL) had a higher probability of infarction growth and early neurologic deterioration [110]. Another demonstrates that for ICA and MCA strokes, a DWI volume greater than 89 cm^3 was highly predictive receiver operating characteristic (ROC) curve with 85.7% sensitivity and 95.7% specificity) of early neurologic deterioration [111].

Initial CBV, CBF, MTT, and TTP lesion volumes also correlate with NIHSS, the Canadian neurological scale, the Barthel index, the Scandinavian stroke scale, and the modified Rankin scale. Correlation coefficients range from 0.71 to 0.97 [63,66,107,112,113]. Correlations are widely variable and it is unclear which initial perfusion map best predicts clinical outcome. In one study that compares initial CBV, CBF, and MTT volumes with modified Rankin scale, initial CBF volume had the highest correlation [113]. In another study that compares initial DWI, CBV, and MTT volumes with modified NIHSS, Rankin scale, and Barthel index, initial CBV had the highest correlation [114]. In general, patients who have perfusion lesion volumes larger than diffusion MR lesion volumes (diffusion-perfusion mismatches) have worse outcomes with larger final infarction volumes compared with patients who do not have a diffusion-perfusion mismatch. Furthermore, the size of the diffusion-perfusion mismatch correlates with clinical outcome scales. In one study, patients who had a DWI-MTT mismatch larger than 100 mL had a significantly larger lesion growth and a poorer outcome than patients who had a smaller mismatch [107]. Thrombolytic therapy resulting from early re-canalization with reperfusion can limit lesion growth and alter these correlations. In one study of patients treated with intravenous rtPA, initial MTT volume correlates with the initial NIHSS but does not correlate with the NIHSS measured at 2 to 3 months [82]. In another study, the best independent predictor of excellent outcome in patients treated with IV tPA is an MTT lesion volume decrease of more than 30% 2 hours after IV tPA therapy [115].

Stroke mimics

These syndromes generally fall into four categories: (1) nonischemic lesions with no acute abnormality on routine or DWI; (2) ischemic lesions with reversible clinical deficits that may have imaging abnormalities; (3) vasogenic edema syndromes that may mimic acute infarction clinically and on conventional imaging; and (4) other entities with decreased diffusion.

Nonischemic lesions with no acute abnormality on routine or diffusion-weighted images

Nonischemic syndromes that present with signs and symptoms of acute stroke but have no acute abnormality identified on DWI or routine MR imaging include peripheral vertigo, migraines, seizures, dementia, functional disorders, and metabolic disorders. The clinical deficits associated with these syndromes usually are reversible. If initial imaging is normal and a clinical deficit persists, repeat DWI should be obtained [27]. False-negative DWI and PWI images occur in patients who have small brainstem or deep gray nuclei lacunar infarctions.

Syndromes with reversible clinical deficits that may have decreased diffusion

Transient ischemic attack

An acute neurologic deficit of presumed vascular etiology that resolves within 24 hours is defined as a transient ischemic attack. Of patients who have transient ischemic attacks, 21% to 48% have DWI hyperintense lesions, consistent with small infarctions (Fig. 21) [116–119]. These lesions usually are less than 15 mm in size and are in the clinically appropriate vascular territory. In one study, 20% percent of the lesions were not seen at follow-up; the lesions could have been too small to see on follow-up conventional MR imaging because of atrophy or they could have been reversible [117]. The small DWI lesions most likely are not the cause of patients' symptoms but may represent markers of a more widespread reversible ischemia. Reported statistically significant independent predictors of lesions with decreased diffusion on DWI are previous nonstereotypic TIA, cortical syndrome, an identified stroke mechanism, TIA duration greater than 30 minutes, aphasia, motor deficits, and disturbance of higher brain function [116,117,119,120]. One study demonstrates an increased stroke risk in patients who have

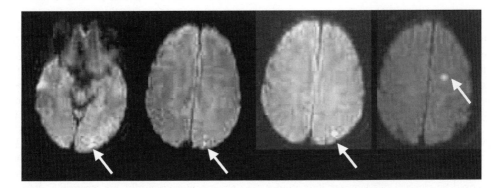

Fig. 21. Transient ischemic attack. Fity-seven-year-old man who had transient right hemiparesis. DWI demonstrate punctate infarctions (*arrows*) in the left occipital, parietal, and frontal lobes.

transient ischemic attacks and abnormalities on DWI [118]. In another study, the information obtained from DWI changed the suspected localization of the ischemic lesion and the suspected etiologic mechanism in more than one third of patients [117].

Transient global amnesia

TGA is a clinical syndrome characterized by sudden onset of profound memory impairment, resulting in retrograde and anterograde amnesia without other neurologic deficits. The symptoms typically resolve in 3 to 4 hours. Many patients who have TGA have no acute abnormality on conventional or DWI [121]. Other studies, however, report punctate lesions with decreased diffusion in the medial hippocampus, the parahippocampal gyrus, and the splenium of the corpus callosum [122–125]. Follow-up T2-weighted sequences in some patients show persistence of these lesions that the investigators conclude were small infarctions. One study, however, reports more diffuse and subtle DWI hyperintense lesions in the hippocampus that resolved on follow-up imaging [126]. The investigators conclude that this phenomenon might be secondary to spreading depression rather than reversible ischemia. A more recent study demonstrates that the detection of DWI changes in TGA is delayed [127]; the investigators observed DWI abnormalities in only 2 of 31 patients who had TGA in the hyperacute phase, but at 48 hours, 26 of 31 patients had DWI abnormalities in the hippocampus. Currently, it is unclear whether or not the TGA patients who have DWI abnormalities have a different prognosis, different etiologic mechanism, or whether or not they should be managed differently compared with patients who have TGA but do not have DWI abnormalities.

Vasogenic edema syndromes

Patients who have these syndromes frequently present with acute neurologic deficits, which raises the question of acute ischemic stroke. Furthermore, conventional imaging cannot reliably differentiate cytotoxic from vasogenic edema because both types of edema produce T2 hyperintensity in gray or white matter. Diffusion MR imaging, however, has become essential in differentiating these syndromes from acute stroke. Whereas cytotoxic edema is characterized by decreased diffusion, vasogenic edema is characterized by elevated diffusion resulting from a relative increase in water in the extracellular compartment [128–130]. Vasogenic edema is hypointense to

slightly hyperintense on DWI, because these images have T2 and diffusion contributions. Vasogenic edema is hyperintense on ADC maps and hypointense on exponential images, whereas cytotoxic edema is hypointense in ADC maps and hyperintense on exponential images.

Posterior reversible encephalopathy syndrome

Posterior reversible encephalopathy syndrome (PRES) is a syndrome that occurs secondary to loss of cerebral autoregulation and capillary leakage in association with a variety of clinical entities [131–143]. These include acute hypertension; treatment with immunosuppressive agents, such as cyclosporin and tacrolimus; treatment with chemotherapeutic agents, such as intrathecal methotrexate, cisplatin, and interferon-α; and hematologic disorders, such as hemolytic uremic syndrome, thrombotic thrombocytopenia purpura, acute intermittent porphyria, and cryoglobulinemia. Typical presenting features are headaches, decreased alertness, altered mental status, seizures, and visual loss, including cortical blindness. The pathophysiology is not entirely clear [130,144]. The predominant hypothesis is that markedly increased pressure or toxins damage endothelial tight junctions. This leads to extravasation of fluid and the development of vasogenic edema. Another, less likely, possibility, based on angiographic findings of narrowing in medium- and large-size vessels, is that vasospasm is the major pathophysiologic mechanism.

T2- and FLAIR-weighted sequences typically demonstrate bilateral symmetric hyperintensity and swelling in cortex and subcortical white matter in the occipital, parietal, and posterior temporal lobes and the posterior fossa. The posterior circulation predominance is believed to result from the fact that there is less sympathetic innervation (which supplies vasoconstrictive protection to the brain in the setting of acute hypertension) in the posterior compared with the anterior circulation. Anterior circulation lesions are not uncommon, however, and frequently are in a border-zone distribution. Acutely, DWI usually show elevated and less frequently normal diffusion (Fig. 22). This is helpful because posterior distribution lesions can mimic basilar tip occlusion with arterial infarctions and border-zone anterior circulation lesions can mimic watershed infarctions clinically and on T2-weighted sequences. Unlike PRES, arterial and watershed infarctions are characterized by decreased diffusion. The clinical deficits and MR abnormalities typically are reversible. Rare small areas of decreased diffusion that progress to infarction are observed, however, and in some cases, tis-

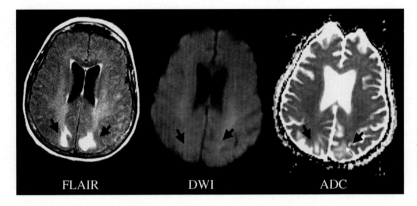

Fig. 22. PRES. Sixty-four-year-old woman who had mental status changes. FLAIR images demonstrate hyperintense lesions in the bilateral parietal occipital regions that suggest acute infarctions (*arrows*). The lesions are isointense on DWI and hyperintense on ADC images. These diffusion MR characteristics are consistent with vasogenic edema.

sue characterized initially by elevated or normal diffusion progresses to infarction [145].

Hyperperfusion syndrome after carotid endarterectomy

In rare cases after carotid endarterectomy, patients may develop a hyperperfusion syndrome [146]. Patients typically present with seizures but may have focal neurologic deficits. T2-weighted images demonstrate hyperintensity in frontal and parietal cortex and subcortical white matter that may mimic arterial infarction. Unlike acute infarctions, however, the lesions have elevated diffusion. Also, there may be increased rather than diminished flow-related enhancement in the ipsilateral MCA. It is believed that similar to PRES, increased pressure damages endothelial tight junctions, leading to a capillary leak syndrome and development of vasogenic edema.

Other syndromes

Rarely, other disease entities, such as HIV or other viral encephalopathies, tumor, and acute demyelination, can present with acute neurologic deficits and patterns of edema on conventional images suggestive of stroke. Similar to PRES and hyperperfusion syndrome after carotid endarterectomy, DWI show increased diffusion.

Other entities with decreased diffusion

Several other entities have decreased diffusion [147]. These include acute demyelinative lesions with decreased diffusion resulting from myelin vacuoliza-

tion; some products of hemorrhage (oxyhemoglobin and extracellular methemoglobin); herpes encephalitis with decreased diffusion resulting from cytotoxic edema from cell necrosis; diffuse axonal injury with decreased diffusion resulting from cytotoxic edema or axotomy with retraction ball formation; abscess with decreased diffusion resulting from the high viscosity of pus; tumors, such as lymphoma and small round cell tumors, with decreased diffusion resulting from dense cell packing; and Creutzfeldt-Jakob disease, with decreased diffusion from myelin vacuolization. When these lesions are reviewed in combination with routine T1, FLAIR, T2, and gadolinium-enhanced T1-weighted images, they usually are differentiated readily from acute infarctions. Occasionally, diffusion and conventional imaging cannot distinguish between a single demyelinative lesion or nonenhancing tumor versus an acute stroke. In these situations, spectroscopy may be helpful.

Venous infarction

Cerebral venous sinus thombosis (CVT) is a rare condition that affects fewer than 1 in 10,000 people. The most common presenting signs and symptoms are headache, seizures, vomiting, and papilledema. Visual changes, altered consciousness cranial nerve palsies, nystagmus, and focal neurologic deficits also are common. Predisposing factors are protein C and S deficiencies; malignancies; pregnancy; medications, such as oral contraceptives, steroids, and hormone replacement therapy; collagen vascular diseases; infection; trauma; surgery; and immobilization [148].

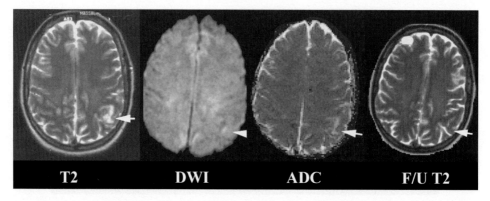

Fig. 23. Thirty-one-year-old woman who had seizures and superior sagittal sinus thrombosis. There is a T2 hyperintense lesion in the left parietal lobe (*arrow*). The lesion is characterized by elevated diffusion (isointense on DWI and hyperintense on ADC), consistent with vasogenic edema and has resolved on follow-up T2-weighted images.

The pathophysiology of CVT is as follows [149–160]. Venous obstruction results in increased venous pressure, increased intracranial pressure, decreased perfusion pressure, and decreased CBF. Increased venous pressure may result in vasogenic edema from breakdown of the blood-brain barrier and extravasation of fluid into the extracellular space. Blood also may extravasate into the extracellular space. Severely decreased blood flow also may result in cytotoxic edema associated with infarction. Increases in CSF production and resorption also are reported.

Parenchymal findings on imaging correlate with degree of venous pressure elevation [161]. With mild to moderate pressure elevations, there is parenchymal swelling with sulcal effacement but without signal abnormality. As pressure elevations become more severe, there is increasing edema and development of intraparenchymal hemorrhage in up to 40%

of patients who have CVT [162,163]. Bilateral parasagittal T2 hyperintense lesions characterize superior sagittal sinus thrombosis. Transverse sinus thrombosis results in T2 hyperintense signal abnormality in the temporal lobe, and deep venous thrombosis is characterized by T2 hyperintense signal abnormalities in the bilateral thalami and basal ganglia.

DWI has proved helpful in the differentiation of venous from arterial infarction and in the prediction of tissue outcome (Figs. 23 and 24). T2 hyperintense lesions may have decreased diffusion, elevated diffusion, or a mixed pattern [164–166]. Lesions with elevated diffusion are believed to represent vasogenic edema and usually resolve. Lesions with decreased diffusion are believed to represent cytotoxic edema. Unlike arterial stroke, some of these lesions resolve and some persist. Resolution of lesions with decreased diffusion may be related to better drainage of blood through collateral pathways in some patients.

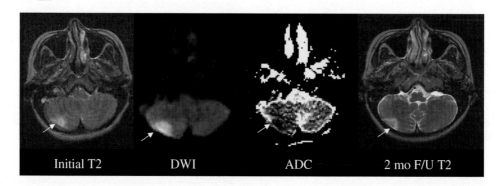

Fig. 24. Superior sagittal, right transverse, and right sigmoid sinus thrombosis. Thirty-one-year-old man who had severe headache and vomiting. MR venogram (not shown) demonstrates thrombosis of the superior sagittal, right transverse, and right sigmoid sinuses. The T2 hyperintense right cerebellar lesion has decreased diffusion (DWI hyperintense and ADC hypointense), consistent with cytotoxic edema (*short white arrow*). The lesion is present at follow-up.

In one study, lesions with decreased diffusion that resolved were seen only in patients who had seizure activity [164].

Summary

Diffusion MR imaging has improved evaluation of acute ischemic stroke vastly. It is highly sensitive and specific in the detection of infarction at early time points when CT and conventional MR sequences are unreliable. The initial DWI lesion is believed to represent infarction core and usually progresses to infarction unless there is early reperfusion. The initial DWI lesion volume and ADC ratios correlate highly with final infarction volume and with acute and chronic neurologic assessment tests. ADC values may be useful in differentiating tissue destined to infarct from that potentially salvageable with reperfusion therapy. ADC values also may be useful for determining tissue at risk of HT after reperfusion therapy. DTI can quantify differences in the responses of gray versus white matter to ischemia. FA may be important in determining stroke onset time, and tractography provides early detection of wallerian degeneration that may be important in determining prognosis. Finally, DWI can determine which patients who have TIA are at risk for subsequent large vessel infarction and can differentiate stroke from stroke mimics. With improvements in MR software and hardware, diffusion MR undoubtedly will continue to improve the management of patients who have acute stroke.

References

[1] Stejskal E, Tanner J. Spin diffusion measurements: spin echos in the presence of time-dependent field gradient. J Chem Phys 1965;42:288–92.

[2] Sevick RJ, Kanda F, Mintorovitch J, et al. Cytotoxic brain edema: assessment with diffusion-weighted MR imaging. Radiology 1992;185:687–90.

[3] Mintorovitch J, Yang GY, Shimuzu H, et al. Diffusion-weighted magnetic resonance imaging of acute focal cerebral ischemia: comparison of signal intensity with changes in brain water and Na+, K(+)-ATPase activity. J Cereb Blood Flow Metab 1994;14: 332–6.

[4] Benveniste H, Hedlund LW, Johnson GA. Mechanism of detection of acute cerebral ischemia in rats by diffusion-weighted magnetic resonance microscopy. Stroke 1992;23:746–54.

[5] Wick M, Nagatomo Y, Prielmeier F, et al. Alteration of intracellular metabolite diffusion in rat brain in vivo during ischemia and reperfusion. Stroke 1995;26: 1930–3 [discussion: 1934].

[6] van der Toorn A, Dijkhuizen RM, Tulleken CA, et al. Diffusion of metabolites in normal and ischemic rat brain measured by localized 1H MRS. Magn Reson Med 1996;36:914–22.

[7] Duong TQ, Ackerman JJ, Ying HS, et al. Evaluation of extra- and intracellular apparent diffusion in normal and globally ischemic rat brain via 19F NMR. Magn Reson Med 1998;40:1–13.

[8] Niendorf T, Dijkuizen RM, Norris DG, et al. Biexponential diffusion attenuation in various states of brain tissue: implications for diffusion-weighted imaging. Magn Reson Med 1996;36:847–57.

[9] Sykova E, Svoboda J, Polak J, et al. Extracellular volume fraction and diffusion characteristics during progressive ischemia and terminal anoxia in the spinal cord of the rat. J Cereb Blood Flow Metab 1994;14:301–11.

[10] Morikawa E, Gingsberg MD, Dietrich WD, et al. The significance of brain temperature in focal cerebral ischemia: histopathological consequences of middle cerebral artery occlusion in the rat. J Cereb Blood Flow Metab 1992;12:380–9.

[11] Le Bihan D, Delannoy J, Levin RL. Temperature mapping with MR imaging of molecular diffusion: application to hyperthermia. Radiology 1989;171: 853–7.

[12] Szafer A, Zhong J, Gore JC. Theoretical model for water diffusion in tissues. Magn Reson Med 1995;33: 697–712.

[13] Warach S, Gaa J, Siewert B, et al. Acute human stroke studied by whole brain echo planar diffusion-weighted magnetic resonance imaging. Ann Neurol 1995;37:231–41.

[14] Schlaug G, Siewert B, Benfield A, et al. Time course of the apparent diffusion coefficient (ADC) abnormality in human stroke. Neurology 1997;49:113–9.

[15] Lutsep HL, Albers GW, DeCrespigny A, et al. Clinical utility of diffusion-weighted magnetic resonance imaging in the assessment of ischemic stroke. Ann Neurol 1997;41:574–80.

[16] Schwamm LH, Koroshetz WJ, Sorensen AG, et al. Time course of lesion development in patients with acute stroke: serial diffusion- and hemodynamic-weighted magnetic resonance imaging. Stroke 1998; 29:2268–76.

[17] Beaulieu C, DeCrispigny A, Tong DC, et al. Longitudinal magnetic resonance imaging study of perfusion and diffusion in stroke: evolution of lesion volume and correlation with clinical outcome. Ann Neurol 1999;46:568–78.

[18] Copen WA, Schwamm LH, Gonzalez RG, et al. Ischemic stroke: effects of etiology and patient age on the time course of the core apparent diffusion coefficient. Radiology 2001;221:27–34.

[19] Marks MP, Tong DC, Beaulieu C, et al. Evaluation of early reperfusion and i.v. tPA therapy using diffusion-

and perfusion-weighted MRI. Neurology 1999;52: 1792–8.

[20] Nagesh V, Welch KM, Windham JP, et al. Time course of ADCw changes in ischemic stroke: beyond the human eye! Stroke 1998;29:1778–82.

[21] Gonzalez RG, Schaefer PW, Buonanno FS, et al. Diffusion-weighted MR imaging: diagnostic accuracy in patients imaged within 6 hours of stroke symptom onset. Radiology 1999;210:155–62.

[22] Mohr J, Biller J, Hial S, et al. Magnetic resonance versus computed tomographic imaging in acute stroke. Stroke 1995;26:807–12.

[23] Bryan R, Levy L, Whitlow W, et al. Diagnosis of acute cerebral infarction: comparison of CT and MR imaging. AJNR Am J Neuroradiol 1991;12:611–20.

[24] Lovblad KO, Laubach HJ, Baird AE, et al. Clinical experience with diffusion-weighted MR in patients with acute stroke. AJNR Am J Neuroradiol 1998;19: 1061–6.

[25] Mullins ME, Schaefer PW, Sorensen AG, et al. CT and conventional and diffusion-weighted MR imaging in acute stroke: study in 691 patients at presentation to the emergency department. Radiology 2002;224:353–60.

[26] Marks MP, DeCrispigny A, Lentz D, et al. Acute and chronic stroke: navigated spin-echo diffusion-weighted MR imaging. Radiology 1996;199:403–8.

[27] Ay H, Buonanno FS, Rordorf G, et al. Normal diffusion-weighted MRI during stroke-like deficits. Neurology 1999;52:1784–92.

[28] Grant PE, He J, Halpern EF, et al. Frequency and clinical context of decreased apparent diffusion coefficient reversal in the human brain. Radiology 2001; 221:43–50.

[29] Kidwell CS, Saver JL, Starkman S, et al. Late secondary ischemic injury in patients receiving intra-arterial thrombolysis. Ann Neurol 2002;52:698–703.

[30] Schaefer PW, et al. Predicting cerebral ischemic infarct volume with diffusion and perfusion MR imaging. AJNR Am J Neuroradiol 2002;23:1785–94.

[31] Dardzinski BJ, Sotak CH, Fisher M, et al. Apparent diffusion coefficient mapping of experimental focal cerebral ischemia using diffusion-weighted echo-planar imaging. Magn Reson Med 1993;30:318–25.

[32] Fiehler J, Foth M, Kucinski T, et al. Severe ADC decreases do not predict irreversible tissue damage in humans. Stroke 2002;33:79–86.

[33] Fiehler J, Knob R, Reichenbacher JR, et al. Apparent diffusion coefficient decreases and magnetic resonance imaging perfusion parameters are associated in ischemic tissue of acute stroke patients. J Cereb Blood Flow Metab 2001;21:577–84.

[34] Jones TH, Morawetz RB, Crowell RM, et al. Thresholds of focal cerebral ischemia in awake monkeys. J Neurosurg 1981;54:773–82.

[35] Le Bihan D, Mangin JF, Poupon C, et al. Diffusion tensor imaging: concepts and applications. J Magn Reson Imaging 2001;13:534–46.

[36] Basser PJ, Pierpaoli C. Microstructural and physio-logical features of tissues elucidated by quantitative-diffusion-tensor MRI. J Magn Reson B 1996;111: 209–19.

[37] Shimony JS, McKinstry RC, Akbudak E, et al. Quantitative diffusion-tensor anisotropy brain MR imaging: normative human data and anatomic analysis. Radiology 1999;212:770–84.

[38] Bammer R, Acar B, Moseley ME. In vivo MR tractography using diffusion imaging. Eur J Radiol 2003;45:223–34.

[39] Conturo TE, Lori NF, Cull TS, et al. Tracking neuronal fiber pathways in the living human brain. Proc Natl Acad Sci USA 1999;96:10422–7.

[40] Makris N, Worth AJ, Sorensen AG, et al. Morphometry of in vivo human white matter association pathways with diffusion-weighted magnetic resonance imaging. Ann Neurol 1997;42:951–62.

[41] Mukherjee P, Bahn MM, McKinstry RC, et al. Differences between gray matter and white matter water diffusion in stroke: diffusion-tensor MR imaging in 12 patients. Radiology 2000;215:211–20.

[42] Sorensen AG, Wu O, Copen WA, et al. Human acute cerebral ischemia: detection of changes in water diffusion anisotropy by using MR imaging. Radiology 1999;212:785–92.

[43] Pierpaoli C, Jezzard P, Basser PJ, et al. Diffusion tensor MR imaging of the human brain. Radiology 1996;201:637–48.

[44] Reese TG, Weisskoff RM, Smith RN, et al. Imaging myocardial fiber architecture in vivo with magnetic resonance. Magn Reson Med 1995;34:786–91.

[45] Moseley ME, Cohen Y, Kucharczyk J, et al. Diffusion-weighted MR imaging of anisotropic water diffusion in cat central nervous system. Radiology 1990;176:439–45.

[46] Moseley ME, Kucharczyk J, Asgari HS, et al. Anisotropy in diffusion-weighted MRI. Magn Reson Med 1991;19:321–6.

[47] Le Bihan D, van Zijl P. From the diffusion coefficient to the diffusion tensor. NMR Biomed 2002; 15:431–4.

[48] Beaulieu C. The basis of anisotropic water diffusion in the nervous system—a technical review. NMR Biomed 2002;15:435–55.

[49] Zelaya F, Flood N, Chalk JB, et al. An evaluation of the time dependence of the anisotropy of the water diffusion tensor in acute human ischemia. Magn Reson Imaging 1999;17:331–48.

[50] Yang Q, Tress BM, Barber PA, et al. Serial study of apparent diffusion coefficient and anisotropy in patients with acute stroke. Stroke 1999;30:2382–90.

[51] Ozsunar Y, Grant PE, Huisman T, et al. Evolution of water diffusion and anisotropy in hyperacute stroke: significant correlation between fractional anisotropy and T2. AJNR Am J Neuroradiol 2004;25: 699–705.

[52] Higano S, Zhong J, Shrier DA, et al. Diffusion anisotropy of the internal capsule and the corona radiata in association with stroke and tumors as measured by

diffusion-weighted MR imaging. AJNR Am J Neuroradiol 2001;22:456–63.

[53] Watanabe T, Honda Y, Fujii Y, et al. Three-dimensional anisotropy contrast magnetic resonance axonography to predict the prognosis for motor function in patients suffering from stroke. J Neurosurg 2001;94:955–60.

[54] Werring DJ, Toosy AT, Clark CA, et al. Diffusion tensor imaging can detect and quantify corticospinal tract degeneration after stroke. J Neurol Neurosurg Psychiatry 2000;69:269–72.

[55] Kucharczyk J, Mintorovitch J, Asgari HS, et al. Diffusion/perfusion MR imaging of acute cerebral ischemia. Magn Reson Med 1991;19:311–5.

[56] Mintorovitch J, Moseley ME, Cohen Y, et al. Comparison of diffusion- and T2-weighted MRI for the early detection of cerebral ischemia and reperfusion in rats. Magn Reson Med 1991;18:39–50.

[57] Moseley ME, Cohen Y, Mintorovitch J, et al. Early detection of regional cerebral ischemia in cats: comparison of diffusion- and T2-weighted MRI and spectroscopy. Magn Reson Med 1990;14:330–46.

[58] Rosen BR, Belliveau JW, Vevea JM, et al. Perfusion imaging with NMR contrast agents. Magn Reson Med 1990;14:249–65.

[59] Rosen BR, Belliveau JW, Buchbinder BR, et al. Contrast agents and cerebral hemodynamics. Magn Reson Med 1991;19:285–92.

[60] Baird AE, Benfield A, Schlaug G, et al. Enlargement of human cerebral ischemic lesion volumes measured by diffusion-weighted magnetic resonance imaging. Ann Neurol 1997;41:581–9.

[61] Rordorf G, Koroshetz WJ, Copen WA, et al. Regional ischemia and ischemic injury in patients with acute middle cerebral artery stroke as defined by early diffusion-weighted and perfusion-weighted MRI. Stroke 1998;29:939–43.

[62] Sorensen AG, Copen WA, Ostergaard L, et al. Hyperacute stroke: simultaneous measurement of relative cerebral blood volume, relative cerebral blood flow, and mean tissue transit time. Radiology 1999;210:519–27.

[63] Tong DC, Yenari MA, Albers GW, et al. Correlation of perfusion- and diffusion-weighted MRI with NIHSS score in acute (<6.5 hour) ischemic stroke. Neurology 1998;50:864–70.

[64] Karonen JO, Liu Y, Vanninen RL, et al. Combined perfusion- and diffusion-weighted MR imaging in acute ischemic stroke during the 1st week: a longitudinal study. Radiology 2000;217:886–94.

[65] Karonen JO, Vanninen RL, Liu Y, et al. Combined diffusion and perfusion MRI with correlation to single-photon emission CT in acute ischemic stroke. Ischemic penumbra predicts infarct growth. Stroke 1999;30:1583–90.

[66] Barber PA, Darby DG, Desmond PM, et al. Prediction of stroke outcome with echoplanar perfusion- and diffusion-weighted MRI. Neurology 1998;51:418–26.

[67] Schaefer PW, Ozsunar Y, He J, et al. Assessing tissue viability with MR diffusion and perfusion imaging. AJNR Am J Neuroradiol 2003;24:436–43.

[68] Schlaug G, Benfield A, Baird AE, et al. The ischemic penumbra: operationally defined by diffusion and perfusion MRI. Neurology 1999;53:1528–37.

[69] Rohl L, Ostergaard L, Simonsen CZ, et al. Viability thresholds of ischemic penumbra of hyperacute stroke defined by perfusion-weighted MRI and apparent diffusion coefficient. Stroke 2001;32:1140–6.

[70] Liu Y, Karonen JO, Vanninen RL, et al. Cerebral hemodynamics in human acute ischemic stroke: a study with diffusion- and perfusion-weighted magnetic resonance imaging and SPECT. J Cereb Blood Flow Metab 2000;20:910–20.

[71] Grandin CB, Duprez JP, Smith AM, et al. Usefulness of magnetic resonance-derived quantitative measurements of cerebral blood flow and volume in prediction of infarct growth in hyperacute stroke. Stroke 2001;32:1147–53.

[72] Lassen NA. Normal average value of cerebral blood flow in younger adults is 50 ml/100 g/min. J Cereb Blood Flow Metab 1985;5:347–9.

[73] Ueda T, Sakaki S, Yuh WT, et al. Outcome in acute stroke with successful intra-arterial thrombolysis and predictive value of initial single-photon emission-computed tomography. J Cereb Blood Flow Metab 1999;19:99–108.

[74] Rempp KA, Brix G, Wenz F, et al. Quantification of regional cerebral blood flow and volume with dynamic susceptibility contrast-enhanced MR imaging. Radiology 1994;193:637–41.

[75] Frackowiak RS, Lenzi GL, Jones T, et al. Quantitative measurement of regional cerebral blood flow and oxygen metabolism in man using 15O and positron emission tomography: theory, procedure, and normal values. J Comput Assist Tomogr 1980;4:727–36.

[76] Furlan M, Marchal G, Viader F, et al. Spontaneous neurological recovery after stroke and the fate of the ischemic penumbra. Ann Neurol 1996;40:216–26.

[77] Marchal G, Beaudouin V, Rioux P, et al. Prolonged persistence of substantial volumes of potentially viable brain tissue after stroke: a correlative PET-CT study with voxel-based data analysis. Stroke 1996;27:599–606.

[78] Hatazawa J, Shimosegawa E, Toyoshima H, et al. Cerebral blood volume in acute brain infarction: A combined study with dynamic susceptibility contrast MRI and 99mTc-HMPAO-SPECT. Stroke 1999;30:800–6.

[79] Powers WJ. Cerebral hemodynamics in ischemic cerebrovascular disease. Ann Neurol 1991;29:231–40.

[80] Wittsack HJ, Ritzl A, Fink GR, et al. MR imaging in acute stroke: diffusion-weighted and perfusion imaging parameters for predicting infarct size. Radiology 2002;222:397–403.

[81] Neumann-Haefelin T, Wittsack HJ, Wenserski F, et al. Diffusion and perfusion-weighted MRI. The DWI/PWI mismatch region in acute stroke. Stroke 1999;8:1591–7.

[82] Parsons MW, Barber PA, Chalk J, et al. Diffusion- and perfusion-weighted MRI response to thrombolysis in stroke. Ann Neurol 2002;51:28–37.

[83] Grandin CB, Duprez TP, Smith AM, et al. Which MR-derived perfusion parameters are the best predictors of infarct growth in hyperacute stroke? Comparative study between relative and quantitative measurements. Radiology 2002;223:361–70.

[84] Oppenheim C, Grandin C, Samson Y, et al. Is there an apparent diffusion coefficient threshold in predicting tissue viability in hyperacute stroke? Stroke 2001; 32:2486–91.

[85] Wu O, et al. Predicting tissue outcome in acute human cerebral ischemia using combined diffusion- and perfusion-weighted MR imaging. Stroke 2001;32: 933–42.

[86] Horowitz SH, Zito JL, Donnarumma R, et al. Computed tomographic-angiographic findings within the first five hours of cerebral infarction. Stroke 1991; 22:1245–53.

[87] Hornig CR, Dorndorf W, Agnoli AL. Hemorrhagic cerebral infarction—a prospective study. Stroke 1986; 17:179–85.

[88] Hakim AM, Ryder-Cooke A, Melanson D. Sequential computerized tomographic appearance of strokes. Stroke 1983;14:893–7.

[89] Calandre L, Ortega JF, Bermejo F. Anticoagulation and hemorrhagic infarction in cerebral embolism secondary to rheumatic heart disease. Arch Neurol 1984; 41:1152–4.

[90] Kidwell CS, Saver JL, Carneado J, et al. Predictors of hemorrhagic transformation in patients receiving intra-arterial thrombolysis. Stroke 2002;33: 717–24.

[91] Ogata J, Yutani C, Imakita M, et al. Hemorrhagic infarct of the brain without a reopening of the occluded arteries in cardioembolic stroke. Stroke 1989; 20:876–83.

[92] Lijnen HR, Silence J, Lemmens G, et al. Regulation of gelatinase activity in mice with targeted inactivation of components of the plasminogen/plasmin system. Thromb Haemost 1998;79:1171–6.

[93] Liotta LA, Goldfarb RH, Brundage R, et al. Effect of plasminogen activator (urokinase), plasmin, and thrombin on glycoprotein and collagenous components of basement membrane. Cancer Res 1981; 41(11 Pt 1):4629–36.

[94] Carmeliet P, Moons L, Lijnen R, et al. Urokinase-generated plasmin activates matrix metalloproteinases during aneurysm formation. Nat Genet 1997;17: 439–44.

[95] Selim M, Fink JN, Kumar S, et al. Predictors of hemorrhagic transformation after intravenous recombinant tissue plasminogen activator: prognostic value of the initial apparent diffusion coefficient and diffusion-weighted lesion volume. Stroke 2002;33:2047–52.

[96] Tong DC, Adami A, Moseley ME, et al. Prediction of hemorrhagic transformation following acute stroke: role of diffusion- and perfusion-weighted magnetic resonance imaging. Arch Neurol 2001;58: 587–93.

[97] Oppenheim C, Samson Y, Dormont D, et al. DWI prediction of symptomatic hemorrhagic transformation in acute MCA infarct. J Neuroradiol 2002; 29:6–13.

[98] Ueda T, Hatakeyama T, Kumon Y, et al. Evaluation of risk of hemorrhagic transformation in local intra-arterial thrombolysis in acute ischemic stroke by initial SPECT. Stroke 1994;25:298–303.

[99] Schaefer PW, Roccatagliata L, Schwamm L, et al. Assessing hemorrhagic transformation with diffusion and perfusion MR imaging. In: Book of abstracts of the 41st annual meeting of the American Society of Neuroradiology, Washington, DC April 28– May 2, 2003.

[100] von Kummer R, Allen KL, Holle R, et al. Acute stroke: usefulness of early CT findings before thrombolytic therapy. Radiology 1997;205:327–33.

[101] Vo KD, Santiago F, Lin W, et al. MR imaging enhancement patterns as predictors of hemorrhagic transformation in acute ischemic stroke. AJNR Am J Neuroradiol 2003;24:674–9.

[102] Kidwell CS, Saver JL, Villablanca JP, et al. Magnetic resonance imaging detection of microbleeds before thrombolysis: an emerging application. Stroke 2002; 33:95–8.

[103] van Everdingen KJ, van der Grond J, Kappelle LJ, et al. Diffusion-weighted magnetic resonance imaging in acute stroke. Stroke 1998;29:1783–90.

[104] Lovblad KO, Baird AE, Schlaug G, et al. Ischemic lesion volumes in acute stroke by diffusion-weighted magnetic resonance imaging correlate with clinical outcome. Ann Neurol 1997;42:164–70.

[105] Engelter S, Provenzale JM, Petrella JR, et al. Infarct volume on apparent diffusion coefficient maps correlates with length of stay and outcome after middle cerebral artery stroke. Cerebrovasc Dis 2003;15: 188–91.

[106] Nighoghossian N, Hermier M, Adeleine P, et al. Baseline magnetic resonance imaging parameters and stroke outcome in patients treated by intravenous tissue plasminogen activator. Stroke 2003;34:458–63.

[107] Rohl L, Geday J, Ostergaard L, et al. Correlation between diffusion- and perfusion-weighted MRI and neurological deficit measured by the Scandinavian Stroke Scale and Barthel Index in hyperacute subcortical stroke (< or = 6 hours). Cerebrovasc Dis 2001;12:203–13.

[108] Thijs V, Lausberg M, Beaulieu C, et al. Is early ischemic lesion volume on diffusion-weighted imaging an independent predictor of stroke outcome? A multivariable analysis. Stroke 2000;31:2597–602.

[109] Engelter S, Wetzel S, Radue E, et al. The clinical significance of diffusion-weighted MR imaging in infratentorial strokes. Neurology 2004;62:474–80.

[110] Davalos A, et al. The clinical-DWI mismatch: a new diagnostic approach to the brain tissue at risk of infarction. Neurology 2004;62:2187–92.

[111] Arenillas J, Rovira A, Molina C, et al. Prediction of early neurologic deterioration using diffusion- and perfusion- weighted imaging in hyperacute middle cerebral artery stroke. Stroke 2002;33:2197–203.

[112] Baird AE, Lovblad KO, Dashe JF, et al. Clinical correlations of diffusion and perfusion lesion volumes in acute ischemic stroke. Cerebrovasc Dis 2000;10: 441–8.

[113] Parsons MW, Yang Q, Barber PA, et al. Perfusion magnetic resonance imaging maps in hyperacute stroke: relative cerebral blood flow most accurately identifies tissue destined to infarct. Stroke 2001;32: 1581–7.

[114] Kluytmans M, van Everdingen KJ, Kappelle LJ, et al. Prognostic value of perfusion- and diffusion-weighted MR imaging in first 3 days of stroke. Eur Radiol 2000;10:1434–41.

[115] Chalela JA, Kang DW, Luby M, et al. Early magnetic resonance imaging findings in patients receiving tissue plasminogen activator predict outcome: insights into the pathophysiology of acute stroke in the thrombolysis era. Ann Neurol 2004;55:105–12.

[116] Ay H, Oliveira-Filho J, Buonanno FS, et al. 'Footprints' of transient ischemic attacks: a diffusion-weighted MRI study. Cerebrovasc Dis 2002;14: 177–86.

[117] Kidwell CS, Alger JR, Di Salle F, et al. Diffusion MRI in patients with transient ischemic attacks. Stroke 1999;30:1174–80.

[118] Purroy F, Montaner J, Rovira A, et al. Higher risk of further vascular events among transient ischemic attack patients with diffusion-weighted imaging acute lesions. Stroke 2004;35(10):2313–9.

[119] Crisostomo R, Garcia M, Tong D. Detection of diffusion-weighted MRI abnormalities in patients with transient ischemic attack: correlation wsith clinical characteristics. Stroke 2003;34:932–7.

[120] Inatomi Y, Kimura K, Yonehara T, et al. DWI abnormalities and clinical characteristics in TIA patients. Neurology 2004;62:376–80.

[121] Huber R, Aschoff AJ, Ludolph AC, et al. Transient Global Amnesia. Evidence against vascular ischemic etiology from diffusion weighted imaging. J Neurol 2002;249:1520–4.

[122] Saito K, Kimura K, Minematsu K, et al. Transient global amnesia associated with an acute infarction in the retrosplenium of the corpus callosum. J Neurol Sci 2003;210:95–7.

[123] Matsui M, Imamura T, Sakamoto S, et al. Transient global amnesia: increased signal intensity in the right hippocampus on diffusion-weighted magnetic resonance imaging. Neuroradiology 2002;44: 235–8.

[124] Ay H, Furie KL, Yamada K, et al. Diffusion-weighted MRI characterizes the ischemic lesion in transient global amnesia. Neurology 1998;51:901–3.

[125] Greer DM, Schaefer PW, Schwamm LH. Unilateral temporal lobe stroke causing ischemic transient global amnesia: role for diffusion-weighted imaging in the initial evaluation. J Neuroimaging 2001;11: 317–9.

[126] Woolfenden AR, O'Brien MW, Schwartzberg RE, et al. Diffusion-weighted MRI in transient global amnesia precipitated by cerebral angiography. Stroke 1997;28:2311–4.

[127] Sedlaczek O, Hirsch J, Grips E, et al. Detection of delayed focal MR changes in the lateral hippocampus in transient global amnesia. Neurology 2004;62: 2165–70.

[128] Ebisu T, Naruse S, Horikawa Y, et al. Discrimination between different types of white matter edema with diffusion-weighted MR imaging. J Magn Reson Imaging 1993;3(6):863–8.

[129] Schaefer PW, Buonanno FS, Gonzalez RG, et al. Diffusion-weighted imaging discriminates between cytotoxic and vasogenic edema in a patient with eclampsia. Stroke 1997;28:1082–5.

[130] Schwartz RB, Mulkern RV, Gudbjartsson H, et al. Diffusion-weighted MR imaging in hypertensive encephalopathy: clues to pathogenesis. AJNR Am J Neuroradiol 1998;19:859–62.

[131] Hinchey J, Nagasaki A, Nakamura K, et al. A reversible posterior leukoencephalopathy syndrome. N Engl J Med 1996;334:494–500.

[132] Nakazato T, et al. Reversible posterior leukoencephalopathy syndrome associated with tacrolimus therapy. Intern Med 2003;42:624–5.

[133] Henderson RD, Rajah H, Nicol AJ, et al. Posterior leukoencephalopathy following intrathecal chemotherapy with MRA-documented vasospasm. Neurology 2003;60:326–8.

[134] Sylvester SL, Diaz LA, Port JD, et al. Reversible posterior leukoencephalopathy in an HIV-infected patient with thrombotic thrombocytopenic purpura. Scand J Infect Dis 2002;34:706–9.

[135] Utz N, Kinkel B, Hedde JP, et al. MR imaging of acute intermittent porphyria mimicking reversible posterior leukoencephalopathy syndrome. Neuroradiology 2001;43:1059–62.

[136] Edwards MJ, Walker R, Vinnicombe S, et al. Reversible posterior leukoencephalopathy syndrome following CHOP chemotherapy for diffuse large B-cell lymphoma. Ann Oncol 2001;12:1327–9.

[137] Soylu A, Kavukcu S, Turkmen M, et al. Posterior leukoencephalopathy syndrome in poststreptococcal acute glomerulonephritis. Pediatr Nephrol 2001;16: 601–3.

[138] Ikeda M, Ito S, Hataya H, et al. Reversible posterior leukoencephalopathy in a patient with minimal-change nephrotic syndrome. Am J Kidney Dis 2001;37(4):E30.

[139] Kamar N, Kany M, Bories P, et al. Reversible posterior leukoencephalopathy syndrome in hepatitis C virus-positive long-term hemodialysis patients. Am J Kidney Dis 2001;37:E29.

[140] Honkaniemi J, Kahara V, Dastidar P, et al. Reversible posterior leukoencephalopathy after combination chemotherapy. Neuroradiology 2000;42:895–9.

[141] Taylor MB, Jackson A, Weller JM. Dynamic susceptibility contrast enhanced MRI in reversible posterior leukoencephalopathy syndrome associated with haemolytic uraemic syndrome. Br J Radiol 2000;73: 438–42.

[142] Lewis MB. Cyclosporin neurotoxicity after chemotherapy. Cyclosporin causes reversible posterior leukoencephalopathy syndrome. BMJ 1999;319:54–5.

[143] Ito Y, Arahata Y, Goto Y, et al. Cisplatin neurotoxicity presenting as reversible posterior leukoencephalopathy syndrome. AJNR Am J Neuroradiol 1998;19: 415–7.

[144] Covarrubias DJ, Luetmer PH, Campeau NG. Posterior reversible encephalopathy syndrome: prognostic utility of quantitative diffusion-weighted MR images. AJNR Am J Neuroradiol 2002;23:1038–48.

[145] Ay H, Buonanno FS, Schaefer PW, et al. Posterior leukoencephalopathy without severe hypertension: utility of diffusion-weighted MRI. Neurology 1998; 51:1369–76.

[146] Breen JC, Caplan LR, DeWitt LD, et al. Brain edema after carotid surgery. Neurology 1996;46:175–81.

[147] Schaefer PW, Grant PE, Gonzalez RG. Diffusion-weighted MR imaging of the brain. Radiology 2000; 217:331–45.

[148] Smith WS, Hauser SL, Easton DJ. Cerebrovascular disease. In: Braunwald E, Fauci AS, Kasper DL, et al, editors. Harrison's principles of internal medicine. McGraw-Hill: New York; 2001. p. 2369–91.

[149] Ameri A, Bousser MG. Cerebral venous thrombosis. Neurol Clin 1992;10:87–111.

[150] Daif A, Awada A, al-Rajeh S, et al. Cerebral venous thrombosis in adults. A study of 40 cases from Saudi Arabia. Stroke 1995;26:1193–5.

[151] Hickey WF, Garnick MB, Henderson IC, et al. Primary cerebral venous thrombosis in patients with cancer—a rarely diagnosed paraneoplastic syndrome. Report of three cases and review of the literature. Am J Med 1982;73:740–50.

[152] Crawford SC, Digre KB, Palmer CA, et al. Thrombosis of the deep venous drainage of the brain in adults. Analysis of seven cases with review of the literature. Arch Neurol 1995;52:1101–8.

[153] Villringer A, Einhaupl KM. Dural sinus and cerebral venous thrombosis. New Horiz 1997;5:332–41.

[154] Lefebvre P, Lierneux B, Lenaerts L, et al. Cerebral venous thrombosis and procoagulant factors—a case study. Angiology 1998;49:563–71.

[155] Ito K, Tsugane R, Ikeda A, et al. Cerebral hemodynamics and histological changes following acute cerebral venous occlusion in cats. Tokai J Exp Clin Med 1997;22:83–93.

[156] Nagai S, Horie Y, Akai T, et al. Superior sagittal sinus thrombosis associated with primary antiphospholipid syndrome–case report. Neurol Med Chir (Tokyo) 1998;38:34–9.

[157] Vielhaber H, Ehrenforth S, Koch HG, et al. Cerebral venous sinus thrombosis in infancy and childhood: role of genetic and acquired risk factors of thrombophilia. Eur J Pediatr 1998;157:555–60.

[158] van den Berg JS, Boerman RH, vd Stolpe A, et al. Cerebral venous thrombosis: recurrence with fatal course. J Neurol 1999;246:144–6.

[159] Forbes KP, Pipe JG, Heiserman JE. Evidence for cytotoxic edema in the pathogenesis of cerebral venous infarction. AJNR Am J Neuroradiol 2001;22:450–5.

[160] Allroggen H, Abbott RJ. Cerebral venous sinus thrombosis. Postgrad Med J 2000;76:12–5.

[161] Tsai FY, Wang AM, Matovich VB, et al. MR staging of acute dural sinus thrombosis: correlation with venous pressure measurements and implications for treatment and prognosis. AJNR Am J Neuroradiol 1995;16:1021–9.

[162] Yuh WT, Simonson TM, Wang AM, et al. Venous sinus occlusive disease: MR findings. AJNR Am J Neuroradiol 1994;15:309–16.

[163] Dormont D, Anxionnat R, Evrad S, et al. MRI in cerebral venous thrombosis. J Neuroradiol 1994;21: 81–99.

[164] Mullins ME, Grant PE, Wang B, et al. Parencyhmal abnormalities associated with cerebral venous thrombosis: assessment with diffusion weighted imaging. AJNR Am J Neuroradiol 2004;25:1666–75.

[165] Ducreux D, Oppenheim C, Vandamme X, et al. Diffusion-weighted imaging patterns of brain damage associated with cerebral venous thrombosis. AJNR Am J Neuroradiol 2001;22:261–8.

[166] Chu K, Kang DW, Yoon BW, et al. Diffusion-weighted magnetic resonance in cerebral venous thrombosis. Arch Neurol 2001;58:1569–76.

ELSEVIER
SAUNDERS

Neuroimag Clin N Am 15 (2005) 531 – 542

NEUROIMAGING
CLINICS OF
NORTH AMERICA

Xenon CT Cerebral Blood Flow in Acute Stroke

Rishi Gupta, MD[a], Tudor G. Jovin, MD[a,b],*, Howard Yonas, MD[c]

[a]Department of Neurology, Stroke Institute, University of Pittsburgh Medical Center, Pittsburgh, PA, USA
[b]Veterans Affairs Pittsburgh Health Care System, Pittsburgh, PA, USA
[c]Department of Neurosurgery, University of New Mexico Health Sciences Center, Albuquerque, NM, USA

Treatment modalities in acute stroke are aimed at reversing the process through which threatened brain tissue supplied by the occluded vessel is destined to undergo infarction. This can be accomplished through two major mechanisms: vessel recanalization and neuroprotection. In recent years, advances have been made in the area of intravenous and intra-arterial recanalization strategies that have translated into improved clinical outcomes. It is hoped that, in part through improved patient selection, recanalization therapy will lead to even better outcomes, fewer side effects, and expansion of the therapeutic window, resulting in significantly larger numbers of patients that benefit from this form of therapy [1,2].

Although several neuroprotection compounds show efficacy in animal models of stroke, no drug shows clinical efficacy in humans [3]. Failure to demonstrate a beneficial clinical effect of neuroprotection in human stroke trials is attributed more to flaws in trial design and less to drug inadequacy. Nevertheless, it is widely believed that clinical benefit from neuroprotectants in humans will be shown in the future, especially if neuroprotection is applied to patients who have acute stroke based on physiology, rather than time, and is combined with other recanalization strategies.

Since the publication of the NINDS (National Institute of Neurological Disorders and Stroke) trial showing benefit of intravenous tissue-type plasminogen activator (tPA) administered within 3 hours of symptom onset, several clinical trials have attempted unsuccessfully to show benefit from intravenous thrombolysis beyond this time window. Similar to current clinical practice, these trials based selection of patients for thrombolytic therapy on time from symptom onset and a noncontrast head CT showing absence of hemorrhage [1]. This approach may not be ideal, as a wide spectrum of clinical outcomes are observed when thrombolytics are administered according to chronologic criteria [4], suggesting that the amount of salvageable brain tissue within the same time window varies from individual to individual. A fixed therapeutic time window in acute stroke is questioned by some investigators [5,6] and, increasingly, selection of patients undergoing acute stroke therapy based on physiologic criteria and on knowledge of the vascular occlusion site is deemed more appropriate [7]. Neuroimaging is the main tool available for assessing cerebral pathophysiology and the site of vascular occlusion. The major aim of assessing cerebral pathophysiology is to distinguish reversible areas of injury from irreversible damage, which constitutes the fundamental principle in selecting patients for acute stroke interventions.

The information obtained from imaging must be sufficiently valuable to offset the possibility of increasing the area of irreversible damage during the time needed to perform the study. CT and MRI technologies used individually or in combination are the

* Corresponding author. Department of Neurology, Stroke Institute, University of Pittsburgh Medical Center, 200 Lothrop Street, Suite C-400, Pittsburgh, PA 15213.

  E-mail address: colejl2@upmc.edu (T.G. Jovin).

imaging modalities that currently are suited best for these purposes.

Recently published clinical trials show that use of MR-based imaging modalities, such as mismatch between perfusion-weighted imaging (PWI) and diffusion-weighted imaging (DWI), can help select patients for acute stroke therapies [7,8]. Because the diffusion abnormality is presumed to represent an approximation of the irreversible ischemic lesion and the perfusion abnormality is believed to represent the brain territory at risk, the area of mismatch between DWI and PWI is considered the territory still viable but at risk for undergoing infarction and corresponds theoretically to the concept of ischemic penumbra.

The major shortcoming of this concept derives from the lack of quantitative data provided by MRI. It is shown that the DWI lesion is not precise in distinguishing irreversible and reversible ischemia [9–11]. It incorporates both types of ischemia and, therefore, cannot be considered equivalent to the ischemic core. Additionally, the PWI lesion is shown to incorporate imminently threatened brain and brain that does not undergo infarction as a consequence of persistent vessel occlusion [12]. This is confirmed in recent positron emission tomography (PET) studies, showing that the size of the PWI abnormality generally exceeds the size of penumbra determined by PET [13]. Because, by definition, penumbra represents tissue that undergoes infarction with continuous vessel occlusion, assessment of penumbral extent based on perfusion MR (PWI MR imaging) is not precise.

Nevertheless, when patients are selected based on these "operationally" derived MR physiologic concepts rather than on time, benefit from acute stroke interventions can be extended up to 9 hours from symptom onset [7,8]. Furthermore, there are reasons to believe that in selected patients, benefit from acute stroke intervention can extend beyond this time frame.

MRI is feasible in acute stroke, but in addition to the shortcomings discussed previously, it may be limited by longer times needed to obtain the scan [14] and by motion artifact. MRI also requires a sophisticated infrastructure for its performance, which greatly limits the number of centers with the capability of providing around-the-clock services.

CT-based perfusion studies and CT angiography are believed to be at least equivalent in providing the type of physiologic data needed to select patients for acute stroke therapy [15]. Given that CT is more widespread and easier to obtain at most hospitals, using CT parameters to select patients who have acute stroke for treatment may lead to an increase in the number of patients eligible for acute stroke therapy.

Stable xenon gas can be used in conjunction with CT imaging to define the pathophysiologic constellation favorable for acute stroke intervention. Its major advantage over other imaging modalities is that by virtue of the quantitative cerebral blood flow (CBF) data provided by this technology, it allows an accurate assessment of brain tissue at risk (penumbra) in relation to infarcted tissue (core) in a relatively fast and cost-efficient manner. This review discusses the clinical applications of xenon CT in acute ischemic stroke.

Acute stroke pathophysiology: ischemic penumbra

Fundamental to understanding patient selection for acute stroke therapies is the relationship between core, penumbra, and oligemia distal to the occluded vessel. After cerebral vessel occlusion, the fate of the brain tissue supplied by the occluded vessel depends on regional CBF and duration of occlusion. A decrease in regional CBF leads to diminished tissue perfusion. Local perfusion pressure, the main determinant of tissue outcome after cerebral vessel occlusion [16], is dependent on the presence and extent of collaterals and systemic arterial pressure (the ischemic brain has lost its autoregulatory capacity); tissue outcome is inversely dependent on local tissue pressure (which is increased by ischemic edema).

Differences in tissue outcome after arterial occlusion are based on the concept of CBF thresholds below which neuronal integrity and function are affected differentially. Astrup and colleagues suggest that brain tissue distal to an arterial occlusion is compartmentalized into ischemic core (irreversibly damaged tissue) and penumbra (reversibly injured tissue) [17]. PET studies in humans suggest that the ischemic core corresponds to CBF values less then 7 mL/100 g/min to 12 mL/100 g/min [18–22]. The ischemic penumbra represents tissue that functionally is impaired but structurally intact and, as such, potentially salvageable. It corresponds to a high CBF limit of 17 mL/100 g/min to 22 mL/100 g/min and a low CBF limit of 7 mL/100 g/min to 12 mL/100 g/min [16]. Salvaging this tissue by restoring its flow to nonischemic levels is the aim of acute stroke therapy.

Evidence suggests that there is temporal evolution of the core, which grows at the expense of penumbra [23–25]. Given the same vascular occlusion site, the speed with which this process is completed varies from individual to individual. This may explain the great variability in outcomes observed with recanalization therapy for the same vascular occlusion site.

Christou and coworkers report that in middle cerebral artery (MCA) occlusion treated with intravenous tPA, even when recanalization occurs within 2 hours post symptom onset, only 50% of patients achieve excellent outcomes [26]. In contrast, excellent outcomes are achieved in selected patients who have acute stroke resulting from MCA occlusion revascularized with extracranial-intracranial bypass as far out as 48 hours post symptoms onset [27].

One of the proposed mechanisms for growth of the ischemic core is progressive recruitment of penumbral areas into the core caused by ischemic edema [23]. The ischemic penumbra represents a dynamic phenomenon. If vessel occlusion persists, the penumbra may shrink because of progressive recruitment into the core. Alternatively, it may return to a normal state after vessel recanalization or possibly neuroprotectant interventions. Restriction of acute stroke therapy aimed at vessel recanalization to 3 hours from onset of symptoms for intravenous thrombolysis and 6 hours for intra-arterial thrombolysis is based on the concept that the ischemic penumbra has a short lifespan, being rapidly incorporated into the core within hours of the ictus. Recent evidence suggests, however, that penumbral brain tissue of significant extent is present beyond 6 hours of stroke onset in a large proportion of patients [28]. PET studies using quantitative CBF assessment or markers of tissue hypoxia, such as fluorine-18–fluoroimidosonidazole, to assess penumbra include patients studied within 6 to as late as 51 hours after stroke onset and report the existence of penumbra comprising 30% to 45% of the total ischemic tissue at risk [29].

Another compartment, termed by Symon and colleagues, "oligemia," represents mildly hypoperfused tissue from the normal range down to approximately 20 mL/100 g/min to 22 mL/100 g/min [30]. It is believed that under normal circumstances, this tissue is not at risk for infarction in humans [16]. Although this compartment is known to survive in the hyperacute stage of arterial occlusion (first 6–12 hours), little is known about its fate if vessel occlusion persists.

It is likely that this compartment is subcompartmentalized further into a more benign range of values (from normal CBF to 30 mL/100 g/min), which is unlikely to undergo infarction even with continuous vessel occlusion. This contention is supported by the work of Linskey and colleagues, showing that, in patients who have a mean ipsilateral hemispheric CBF of 30 mL/100 g/min or above during balloon test occlusion (BTO) of the internal carotid artery (ICA), subsequent vessel sacrifice carries a very small risk for subsequent stroke [31].

In contrast, a range of 20 mL/100 g/min to 30 mL/100 g/min may not portend a good prognosis. Marshall and colleagues show that the only variable that predicts the risk for stroke after ICA sacrifice accurately is the presence of hemispheric CBF under 30 mL/100 g/min on prior BTO [32]. Although this compartment may not be imminently threatened to undergo infarction, as found in landmark experiments conducted by Symon and coworkers [30], it is conceivable that ongoing vessel occlusion, possibly in conjunction with aggravating factors, such as fever, hyperglycemia, hypotension, acidosis, and hypercarbia, may lead to a slow progression toward infarction.

Analyzing different CBF thresholds as predictors of infarction, Jovin and coworkers [33] find that regions of interest with CBF values of 20 mL/100 g/min on xenon CT CBF scans in patients who have acute MCA occlusion are 70% sensitive and 70% specific for predicting final infarction, whereas the sensitivity/specificity of CBF values of 30 mL/100 g/min change to 95% and 35%, respectively (Fig. 1). This dataset includes patients who had early recanalization and those who did not. Therefore, the fate of this CBF compartment under circumstances of continuous vessel occlusion is unknown, but some brain with perfusion in this CBF range eventually will undergo infarction.

Establishing the natural history of this flow compartment in the presence of continuous vessel occlusion is an important task for the future that will clarify the indication and timing of revascularization therapy in patients who have large vessel occlusive disease and who present with hemispheric CBF values in this range.

The xenon CT cerebral blood flow technique

Xenon-133 has been used since the 1960s to calculate CBF. Xenon is a diffusible tracer, as opposed to MR and CT contrast, which use tracer kinetic models to compute CBF. The initial administration was via intracarotid injection [34], but that has been replaced with noninvasive methods through either intravenous administration [35] or stable gas inhalation [36]. The latter method of administration can be used in conjunction with CT imaging, which increases the resolution and applicability of this technique greatly.

This method requires simple calculations to account for the distribution of the inert gas within the brain. Several variables must be accounted for

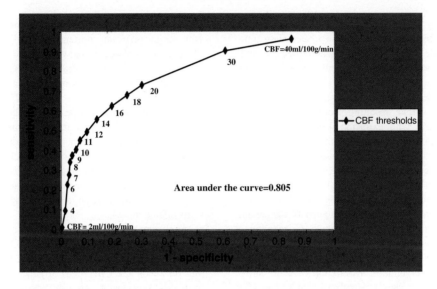

Fig. 1. A receiver-operating characteristic curve shows the sensitivity and specificity of xenon CT CBF for prediction of infarction in patients who have acute stroke as a result of MCA occlusion, studied within 6 hours of symptoms onset.

to obtain reliable CBF values. These variables are related mathematically and can be expressed by the Kety-Schmidt equations (Eqs. 1 and 2):

$$C_{Xebr}(T) = \lambda k \int C_{Xeart}(t) e^{-k(T-t)dt} \qquad (1)$$

$$CBF = \lambda k \qquad (2)$$

$C_{Xebr}(T)$ is the concentration of xenon in the brain, λ is the blood-brain partition coefficient, k is the flow rate constant, and $C_{Xeart}(t)$ is the arterial concentration of xenon, which can be expressed as Eq. 3 [37]:

$$C_{Xeart}(t) = CXe_{max}\left(1 - e^{-bt}\right) \qquad (3)$$

CXe_{max} is the maximum arterial xenon concentration in mL/g and b is the arterial uptake rate constant. CXe_{max} is related to the solubility of xenon gas (S_{Xe}) in blood and the percent uptake of the gas $C(\%)_{max}$ as follows (Eq. 4):

$$CXe_{max} = C(\%)_{max}(5.15)(S_{Xe})(0.01) \qquad (4)$$

The solubility of xenon is related to the hematocrit (Hct) as follows (Eq. 5):

$$S_{Xe} = 0.1 + 0.0011(\%Hct) \qquad (5)$$

Once these equations are solved, the Hounsfield unit enhancement (HE) on CT can be obtained in

relation to the mass attenuation coefficients of water (U_p^w) and xenon (U_p^{Xe}) as in Eq. 6:

$$HE = C_{Xebr}/\left(U_p^w/U_p^{Xe}\right) \qquad (6)$$

Two unenhanced CT images of the brain are obtained before the administration of xenon. The gas then is inhaled and six xenon-enhanced images are obtained at predetermined levels. The unenhanced images are averaged and then subtracted from the enhanced images, yielding a C_{Xebr} for several thousand voxels at each level studied.

This quantification method has been validated previously and shown to be an accurate technique for obtaining CBF values [38]. Normal values for CBF are 80 ± 20 mL/100 g/min in the cortical gray matter and 20 ± 2 mL/100 g/min for white matter [39]. These values decline with advancing age, especially in patients who have cerebrovascular disease [40].

Administration of xenon has few side effects and was found safe in a large cohort of patients studied at the University of Pittsburgh. The most common side effects noted were headaches (0.4%), nausea or vomiting (0.2%), and seizures (0.2%), based on a cohort of 1830 patients [41].

Xenon CT for acute ischemic stroke

Because of its ability to quantify ischemia, xenon CT CBF has several clinical applications in acute ischemic stroke, making it a powerful tool for guiding acute stroke treatment. Although a plain, noncontrast head CT, when interpreted by highly trained physicians, is capable of delineating the extent of critical ischemia with high specificity, it lacks sensitivity. Studies show that extent of early CT changes in the hyperacute stage correlate to poor outcome and increased likelihood of hemorrhage after administration of thrombolytics [42,43]. Although plain CT imaging is rapid and timely for acute stroke, it does not accurately delineate the severity of tissue irreversibly compromised in relationship to the tissue at risk. This information is vital to deciding on patients who may benefit from acute stroke interventions.

The average time to obtain a CT, CT angiogram (CTA), and xenon CT in the emergency room in one study was 44 minutes [44]. This study was conducted before the advent of ultrafast helical CT scanners. In the authors' experience with helical CT technology, images can be obtained and processed in less than 30 minutes. Adding a xenon CT CBF study to a standard head CT protocol requires approximately 15 minutes (4.5 minutes for inhalation of xenon and 10 minutes for computer calculations) [45]. Although this seems lengthy, it likely is shorter than MRI sequences that include transportation out of the emergency department, clearance of patients for metal objects, acquisition and interpretation of images, and transport back to the emergency department for therapeutic intervention.

There are several indications for using xenon CT in acute ischemic stroke: (1) selection of patients for reperfusion therapies beyond currently used time windows based on patient specific pathophysiology; (2) assessment of likelihood of recanalization with revascularization therapy, which allows for better preprocedure planning and determination of degrees of aggressiveness in using pharmacologic versus mechanical methods to recanalize arteries; (3) assessment of likelihood of development of hemorrhage or malignant edema with or without the administration of thrombolytics allowing, in appropriate cases, institution of early decompressive surgery; and (4) manipulation of physiologic parameters (blood pressure, carbon dioxide levels, and so forth) to allow improvement of blood flow in the ischemic area.

Selection of patients

Clinical trials studying thrombolytic therapy for ischemic stroke have focused on chronology-based therapy, usually in heterogeneous groups of patients who have stroke with respect to vascular occlusion site [1,2]. More recently, a significant proportion of patients who have unknown time of onset (wake-up strokes) do not have pathophysiologic characteristics much different from those who present within a 6-hour time window [46]. When patients are selected for acute stroke therapy based on these pathophysiologic characteristics (MRI-based PWI-DWI mismatch), benefit from thrombolysis is shown within a much extended therapeutic window [7,8].

Time-based selection of patients has proved beneficial very early after onset of symptoms, when the majority of patients have a favorable pathophysiologic constellation and more sophisticated imaging tests may not be justified. The next step is to identify patients beyond this ultra-early window who may benefit from revascularization or neuroprotective therapies. In a retrospective case series from the authors' institution, Iacob and colleagues [47] report that of 184 consecutive patients who had acute ischemic stroke, 45 patients (24%) had evidence of persistent large vessel occlusion (ICA, MCA, or tandem lesions). Of these 45 patients, 14 (31%) experienced significant clinical progression evidenced by an increase in their National Institutes of Health Stroke Scale by 4 points, in a delayed fashion beyond 24 hours from symptoms onset. The other 31 patients had a more rapid course of neurologic deterioration without clinical fluctuation. On presentation, all patients who had a delayed deterioration had evidence of large areas of hyperperfusion, far exceeding the areas of infarction. Clinical deterioration was paralleled by imaging evidence of stroke progression (347% increase in infarction volume at 48 to 96 hours). This study indicates that a significant proportion of patients who have large vessel occlusion have large penumbral areas at presentation. Moreover, as many as one third of these patients experience growth of core slowly over days rather than rapidly over hours [47]. These patients may be prime targets for revascularization therapy within time frames that greatly exceed currently used time windows.

The value of xenon CT CBF in identifying these patients was demonstrated by Kilpatrick and colleagues [44], who studied 51 patients who had acute ischemic stroke and underwent a CT/CTA and xenon CT CBF study on admission. This study showed that patients who had occluded vessels and CBFs in the penumbral range were highly likely to have a new infarction on a subsequent CT scan. Conversely, if a patient had a patent vessel or normal CBF values, the likelihood of a new infarction on subsequent head CTs was low.

Jovin and coworkers [48] performed assessment of core and penumbra within time frames currently used for thrombolytic therapy in a retrospective case series of 36 patients who had proven MCA occlusion and were studied with xenon CT CBF within 6 hours of symptoms onset [48]. Twenty-three of these patients underwent intra-arterial thrombolysis, making possible an accurate determination of recanalization status at 2 hours. The cortical core and penumbra were assessed based on previously established perfusion thresholds using a voxel-based method. Voxels in the ipsilateral MCA territory corresponding to CBF ranges of 0 to 8 mL/100 g/min were expressed as percent core relative to ipsilateral MCA territory. Voxels corresponding to CBF ranges of 8 mL/100 g/min to 20 mL/100 g/min were expressed as percent penumbra relative to ipsilateral MCA territory. A third compartment, CBF values above 20 mL/100 g/min are termed noncore, nonpenumbra, comprised voxels with perfusion of 20 mL/100 g/min and above. This study found that penumbra was present in all patients studied and was relatively constant in size, comprising approximately 30% of the cortical MCA territory. In contrast, the core was highly variable, ranging from 7% to 70% cortical MCA territory. Despite similar penumbral volumes, patients who had small core were more likely to have a favorable outcome than patients who had large core. This applied to patients who recanalized at 2 hour, and to those who did not.

It thus seems that although significant penumbral volumes are present in the majority of patients presenting with MCA occlusion within 6 hours from symptoms onset, patients who are unlikely to benefit from revascularization therapy are those who have large core volumes. In those patients, the theoretic benefit derived from preventing penumbral volumes from undergoing infarction through revascularization is offset by the detrimental effect of reperfusing large areas of "dead" brain. Based on their findings, the investigators conclude that the extent of core and not that of penumbra primarily should guide revascularization therapy in patients who have acute stroke.

These findings are validated by several other studies. Hill and coworkers [49] report that the ASPECTS (Alberta Stroke Program Early CT Score) on plain CT is correlated to outcome after intra-arterial thrombolysis in the PROACT II (Prolyse in Acute Cerebral Thromboembolism II) trial. The ASPECTS quantifies the degree of early ischemic changes on head CT based on a 10-point scale [50]. Because early ischemic changes were found highly correlated with regional CBF [33] and, thus, extent of core [48], Hill and coworkers' findings provide indirect support to the concept that the extent of ischemic core drives outcomes in acute stroke. Similarly, Lev and colleagues [51] find that in patients who have acute

stroke, the extent of diminished cerebral blood volume on perfusion studies (believed to represent irreversible ischemia) determines outcome in stroke [51].

Patients undergoing stroke intervention with large areas of ischemic core tissue are at a higher risk for hemorrhage and cerebral edema. Patients who have mean CBFs of the ipsilateral MCA territory in the 9 mL/100 g/min to 13 mL/100 g/min range are at significantly higher risk for developing symptomatic hemorrhage and malignant edema [52,53]. In a small series of 23 patients studied with xenon CT, of the 13 patients who had recanalization, hemorrhage was significantly more common in those who had a higher percent of core. In this series, those who had hemorrhage had twice the volume of ischemic core, in comparison to patients who did not have hemorrhage ($40 \pm 0\%$ versus $20 \pm 11\%$). The association between hemorrhage/malignant edema and large core also was seen in nonrecanalized patients [54]. Determining the extent of core beyond which reperfusion becomes detrimental or futile has not been accomplished and constitutes a major challenge for the future of acute stroke therapy.

Appropriate selection of patients for reperfusion therapy involves not only excluding patients from treatment who will not benefit from recanalization because of large areas of irreversible ischemia but also exclusion of those patients who will have a favorable clinical outcome without interventions. Defining the CBF values that will have a benign natural history aids in this endeavor.

Firlik and colleagues [52] show that xenon CT may help to predict a subgroup of patients who show neurologic improvement when studied within 8 hours of stroke onset [52]. Of the 53 patients studied, eight (15%) improved to normal within 24 hours. The mean CBFs of these eight patients was 35 mL/100 g/min versus 17 mL/100 g/min in patients who continued to decline. Thus, patients who have CBFs greater than 30 mL/100 g/min may not require interventions. This corroborates with BTO studies performed before sacrifice of the ICA (discussed previously). Fig. 2 demonstrates an example of a patient at the authors' institution who presented with a terminal left ICA occlusion 8 hours from symptom onset with CBFs above 30 mL/100 g/min in the affected hemisphere who did well without any acute intervention.

On the basis of these data, the authors propose that patients who have large vessel occlusion in the anterior circulation (MCA/ICA) should be revascularized regardless of the time from symptoms onset, if no or little hypodensity is present on CT (ASPECTS >7) and if CBF values are higher than 15 mL/100 g/min (to minimize the risk for hemorrhage and edema)

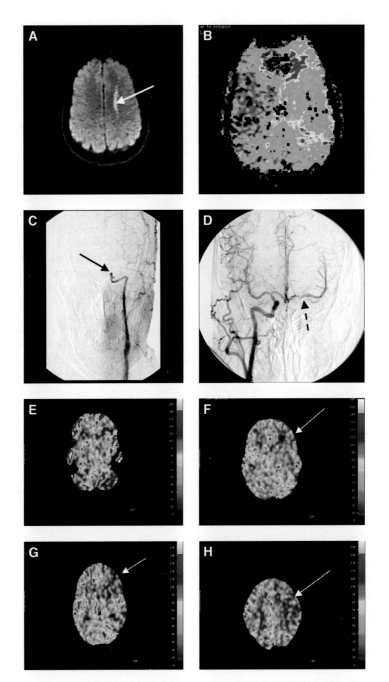

Fig. 2. A 30-year-old man presented with a right hemiparesis 8 hours from symptom onset with subtle clinical fluctuations, and was found to have a (*A*) watershed distribution infarction between the left MCA and anterior cerebral artery territories on DWI (*white arrow*). (*B*) MRI PWI revealed PWI/DWI mismatch with increased mean transit time in the left hemisphere. The patient was taken to cerebral angiography, where he was shown to have (*C*) left internal carotid artery occlusion in the cavernous segment (*solid black arrow*), with (*D*) crossfilling of the left MCA via the anterior communicating artery (*dashed black arrow*). The patient was studied with (*E–H*) xenon CT, which revealed mean cortical CBFs in the left hemisphere of 30 mL/100 g/min (*white arrows*). No intervention was deemed necessary. The patient was placed on intravenous fluids and anticoagulation. He was discharged to rehabilitation after 3 days, without further decline in neurologic function.

and lower than 30 mL/100 g/min (CBF values higher than this portend an excellent prognosis without any aggressive therapies).

Manipulation of blood pressure

Blood pressure management in patients who have large vessel occlusion is an area fraught with major uncertainties, mainly because of lack of adequate technologies that allow precise measurement of the effect of this intervention. Owing to the quantitative information it provides, xenon CT can be useful particularly in this area. Certain patients who have large vessel occlusion may benefit from a double level xenon study, allowing assessment of cerebrovascular reserve with intravenous administration of acetazolamide or assessment of regional CBF changes with change in systemic blood pressure before readministration of xenon gas. Patients may improve neurologically with induced hypertension using vasopressor agents [55]. Through quantitative data, xenon CT allows clinicians to titrate vasopressor agents to optimal CBF values. Fig. 3 shows an example of a double level xenon study, where blood pressure is manipulated to maintain CBF values above penumbral thresholds.

Pharmacologic induction of hypertension is not without risk, as patients may experience cardiac dysrhythmias, myocardial infarction, or other end-organ ischemia. Moreover, optimization of physiologic parameters, such as temperature, blood pressure, pH, and carbon dioxide, may be difficult to sustain even in the intensive care unit. Thus, revascularization may provide more consistent benefit in these patients and, in the authors' opinion, should be attempted whenever possible in preference to hypertensive therapy.

Loss of cerebral vasoreactivity after acetazolamide administration also is associated with higher rates of stroke, especially if there is a greater than 5% reduction of CBF [56,57]. Acetazolamide thus may be of added benefit in patients who have clinical fluctuations believed to be the result of hemodynamic compromise in a vascular territory. Demonstration of loss of vasoreactivity may be a predictor of higher stroke risk and, thereby, justify more aggressive revascularization therapies.

Predictors of vessel recanalization

Recanalization of vessels in acute ischemic stroke is linked to improved clinical outcomes [58]. Xenon

CT might be used to predict which patients are more likely to recanalize after thrombolytic therapy. In a small study of 21 patients who underwent thrombolysis for MCA occlusion at the authors' institution, higher pretreatment mean CBFs were associated significantly with vessel recanalization. Patients who recanalized had CBFs of 20 ± 6 mL/100 g/min versus 13 ± 5 mL/100 g/min in patients who did not ($P < 0.02$) [59].

Similar findings are noted with continuous transcranial Doppler studies performed in the emergency room during administration of thrombolytics. Labiche and colleagues show that as flow partially is established through a thrombus, it has a greater chance of complete recanalization [60]. Hermier and colleagues [61] find that pretreatment PWI parameters on MRI correlate with a higher chance of recanalization.

A possible explanation for this phenomenon is that milder hemispheric hypoperfusion likely is the consequence of a lower clot burden that in turn is less resilient to thrombolysis. Thus, in patients who have pretreatment CBF values greater than 20 mL/100 g/min, the likelihood of recanalization with pharmacologic lysis may be high, justifying a first-line use of this lower risk method. Conversely, in more severely affected hemispheres (mean MCA CBF in the 15–20 mL/100 g/min range), not only is progression to infarction more imminent but also the chance of recanalization is lower. In those situations, more aggressive interventions (angioplasty, mechanical embolectomy, and stenting), which are believed to have faster and higher recanalization rates, may be more appropriate as first-line treatment.

Predictors of malignant edema after middle cerebral artery occlusion

Malignant cerebral edema after MCA occlusion is linked to high mortality or devastating neurologic outcome. Some institutions advocate the use of decompressive craniectomy to allow more space for the brain to swell and prevent herniation [62]. To date, no randomized controlled studies show the benefit of this therapy. Selection of patients for this surgical procedure is a subject of debate, but many agree that criteria are required to predict which patients will develop malignant edema, as timing of the procedure is an issue of critical importance. Currently, this life-saving procedure is performed when patients develop clinical signs of herniation. Several investigators, however, show that early intervention, be-

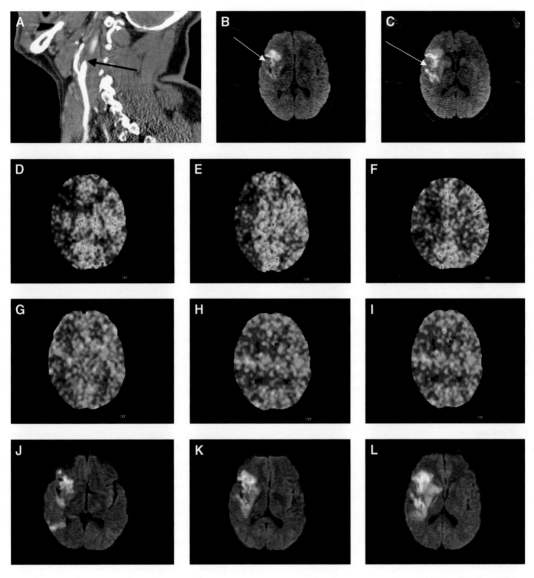

Fig. 3. A 45-year-old man 12-hours after onset of left hemiparesis and right gaze preference. (*A*) CTA reveals a right ICA (RICA) occlusion (*solid black arrow*). (*B* and *C*) DWI-MRI reveals acute infarction in the right insular region (*white arrow*). He was noted to have neurologic fluctuations with changes in blood pressure. A double-level xenon CT was ordered to determine the degree of hemodynamic impairment in the affected hemisphere. (*D–F*) The first xenon scan was performed with the patient's mean arterial blood pressure at 75 mm Hg and shows that the right hemisphere has CBFs in the $17-22$ mL/100 g/min range. With pharmacologic elevation of the mean arterial blood pressure to 100 mm Hg (*G–I*), repeat xenon was performed and demonstrated regional CBFs in the affected hemisphere in the high 20s range. These findings are consistent with severe hemodynamic impairment of the affected hemisphere, and the patient was considered at high risk for further progression. (*J–L*) Follow-up DWI showed growth of the infarction compared with admission. The patient was treated by revascularization of the RICA occlusion with stent placement.

fore herniation, may improve neurologic outcomes significantly [63].

Predicting which patients will develop edema continues to represent a major challenge. Some advocate the use of early MRI DWI volumes [64], whereas others advocate serial CTs to assess for tissue shift in determining patients at highest risk for herniation. Xenon CT is useful in this situation.

Firlik and coworkers show that a mean hemispheric CBF of 9 mL/100 g/min in acute stroke portends a significant risk for developing malignant edema [52]. Similarly, MCA CBF values, predictive of malignant edema/symptomatic hemorrhage, were described by Jovin and colleagues in patients who did not recanalize [54]. The number of patients in these retrospective studies was small. As such, these findings await confirmation from prospective data that should provide quantitative information on the extent of irreversible ischemia that is highly predictive of malignant edema.

Summary

Acute stroke therapy rapidly is evolving as research moves toward extending time windows to treat more patients who have acute stroke. As physiology-based imaging modalities increasingly are used in selecting patients for therapy, it is becoming evident that rigid time windows are not applicable to individual patients. Xenon CT has an important role in acute stroke therapeutic interventions, as it is quantitative, reproducible, and can be obtained safely within a relevant time window. Thus, it can provide valuable physiologic data that can optimize patient selection and aid in acute stroke management.

References

[1] The National Institute of Neurological Disorders and Stroke rt-PA Stroke Study Group. Tissue plasminogen activator for acute ischemic stroke. N Engl J Med 1995;333:1581–7.

[2] Furlan A, Higashida R, Wechsler L, et al. Intra-arterial prourokinase for acute ischemic stroke. The PROACT II study: a randomized controlled trial. Prolyse in acute stroke thromboembolism. JAMA 1999;282:2003–11.

[3] DeGraba TJ, Pettigrew LC. Why do neuroprotective drugs work in animals but not humans? Neurol Clin 2000;18:180–2.

[4] Hacke W, Donnan G, Fieschi C, et al. Association of outcome with early stroke treatment: pooled analysis of ATLANTIS, ECASS, and NINDS rt-PA stroke trials. Lancet 2004;363:768–74.

[5] Baron JC, von Kummer R, del Zoppo GJ. Treatment of acute ischemic stroke. Challenging the concept of a rigid and universal time window. Stroke 1995;26: 2219–21.

[6] Von Kummer R. The time concept in ischemic stroke: misleading. Stroke 2000;31:2523–5.

[7] Hacke W, Albers G, Al-Rawi Y, et al. The desmoteplase in acute ischemic stroke trial (DIAS): a phase II MRI-based-9-hour window acute stroke thrombolysis trial with intravenous desmoteplase. Stroke 2005;36: 66–73.

[8] Gobin YP, Starkman S, Duckwiler GR, et al. MERCI 1: a phase 1 study of mechanical embolus removal in cerebral ischemia. Stroke 2004;35:2848–54.

[9] Marx JJ, Mika-Gruettner A, Thoemke F, et al. Diffusion weighted magnetic resonance imaging in the diagnosis of reversible ischaemic deficits of the brainstem. J Neurol Neurosurg Psychiatry 2002;72: 572–5.

[10] Guadagno JV, Warburton EA, Aigbirhio FI, et al. Does the acute diffusion-weighted imaging lesion represent penumbra as well as core? A combined quantitative PET/MRI voxel-based study. J Cereb Blood Flow Metab 2004;24:1249–54.

[11] Guadagno JV, Wartburton EA, Aigbirhio FI, et al. Does the acute diffusion-weighted imaging lesion represent penumbra as well as core? A combined quantitative PET/MRI voxel-based study. J Cereb Blood Flow Metab 2004;24:1249–54.

[12] Kajimoto K, Moriwaki H, Yamada N, et al. Cerebral hemodynamic evaluation using perfusion-weighted magnetic resonance imaging: comparison with positron emission tomography values in chronic occlusive carotid disease. Stroke 2003;34:1662–6.

[13] Sobesky J, Zaro Weber O, Lehnhardt FG, et al. Does the mismatch match the penumbra? Magnetic resonance imaging and positron emission tomography in early ischemic stroke. Stroke 2005;36(5):980–5.

[14] Sunshine JL, Tarr RW, Lanzieri CF, et al. Hyperacute stroke: ultrafast MR imaging to triage patients prior to therapy. Radiology 1999;212:325–32.

[15] Wintermark M, Reichhart M, Cuisenaire O, et al. Comparison of admission perfusion computed tomography and qualitative diffusion- and perfusion-weighted magnetic resonance imaging in acute stroke patients. Stroke 2002;33:2025–31.

[16] Baron JC. Perfusion thresholds in human cerebral ischemia: historical perspective and therapeutic implications. Cerebrovasc Dis 2001;11(Suppl 1):2–8.

[17] Astrup J, Siesjo BK, Symon L. Thresholds in cerebral ischemia—the ischemic penumbra. Stroke 1981;12: 723–5.

[18] Marchal G, Beaudouin V, Rioux P, et al. Prolonged persistence of substantial volumes of potentially viable brain tissue after stroke: a correlative PET-CT study with voxel-based data analysis. Stroke 1996;27: 599–606.

[19] Marchal G, Benali K, Iglesias S, et al. Voxel-based mapping of irreversible ischaemic damage with PET in acute stroke. Brain 1999;122:2387–400.

[20] Furlan M, Marchal G, Viader F, et al. Spontaneous neurological recovery after stroke and the fate of the ischemic penumbra. Ann Neurol 1996;40:216–26.

[21] Heiss WD. Ischemic penumbra: evidence from functional imaging in man. J Cereb Blood Flow Metab 2000;20:1276–93.

[22] Heiss WD, Kracht LW, Thiel A, et al. Penumbral probability thresholds of cortical flumazenil binding and blood flow predicting tissue outcome in patients with cerebral ischaemia. Brain 2001;124:20–9.

[23] Raichle ME. The pathophysiology of brain ischemia and infarction. Clin Neurosurg 1982;29:379–89.

[24] Heiss WD, Forsting M, Diener HC. Imaging in cerebrovascular disease. Curr Opin Neurol 2001;14:67–75.

[25] Ginsberg MD. Adventures in the pathophysiology of brain ischemia: penumbra, gene expression, neuroprotection: the 2002 Thomas Willis Lecture. Stroke 2003;34:214–23.

[26] Christou I, Alexandrov AV, Burgin WS, et al. Timing of recanalization after tissue plasminogen activator therapy determined by transcranial Doppler correlates with clinical recovery from ischemic stroke. Stroke 2000;31:1812–6.

[27] Jovin T, Yonas H, Hammer M, et al. Extracranial-intracranial bypass for evolving cerebral ischemia in patients selected by neuroimaging: a novel indication for an old operation. J Neurosurg 2004;100:A192.

[28] Marchal G, Beaudouin V, Rioux P, et al. Prolonged persistence of substantial volumes of potentially viable brain tissue after stroke: a correlative PET-CT study with voxel-based data analysis. Stroke 1996;27:599–606.

[29] Read SJ, Hirano T, Abbott DF, et al. The fate of hypoxic tissue on 18F-fluoromisonidazole positron emission tomography after ischemic stroke. Ann Neurol 2000;48:228–35.

[30] Symon L, Branston NM, Strong AJ, et al. The concepts of thresholds of ischaemia in relation to brain structure and function. J Clin Pathol Suppl (R Coll Pathol) 1977;11:149–54.

[31] Linskey ME, Jungreis CA, Yonas H, et al. Stroke risk after abrupt internal carotid artery sacrifice: accuracy of preoperative assessment with balloon test occlusion and stable xenon-enhanced CT. AJNR Am J Neuroradiol 1994;15:829–43.

[32] Marshall RS, Lazar RM, Young WL, et al. Clinical utility of quantitative cerebral blood flow measurements during internal carotid artery test occlusions. Neurosurgery 2002;50:996–1004.

[33] Jovin TG, Grahovac S, Kanal E, et al. Early ischemic changes on head CT in acute stroke: predictive value for infarction and correlation with regional cerebral blood flow. Stroke 2003;34:254.

[34] Lassen NA, Ingvar DH. Radioisotopic assessment of regional cerebral blood flow. Prog Nucl Med 1972;1:376–409.

[35] Austin G, Horn N, Rouhe S, et al. Description and early results of an intravenous radioisotope technique for measuring regional cerebral blood flow in man. Eur Neurol 1972;8:43–51.

[36] Veall N, Mallett BL. Regional cerebral blood flow determination by ^{133}Xe inhalation and external recording: the effect of arterial recirculation. Clin Sci 1966;30:353–69.

[37] Gur D, Good WF, Wolfson Jr SK, et al. In vivo mapping of local cerebral blood flow by xenon-enhanced computed tomography. Science 1982;215:1267–8.

[38] Fatouros PP, Wist AO, Kishore PR, et al. Xenon/computed tomography cerebral blood flow measurements. Methods and accuracy. Invest Radiol 1987;22:705–12.

[39] Yonas H, Darby JM, Marks EC, et al. CBF measured by Xe-CT: approach to analysis and normal values. J Cereb Blood Flow Metab 1991;11:716–25.

[40] Shaw TG, Mortel KF, Meyer JS, et al. Cerebral blood flow changes in benign aging and cerebrovascular disease. Neurology 1984;34:855–62.

[41] Latchaw RE, Yonas H, Pentheny SL, et al. Adverse reactions to xenon-enhanced CT cerebral blood flow determination. Radiology 1987;163:251–4.

[42] Von Kummer R, Meyding-Lamadé U, Forsting M, et al. Sensitivity and prognostic value of early CT in occlusion of the middle cerebral artery trunk. AJNR Am J Neuroradiol 1994;15:9–15.

[43] Levy DE, Brott TG, Haley EC, et al. Factors related to intracranial hematoma formation in patients receiving tissue-type plasminogen activator for acute ischemic stroke. Stroke 1994;25:291–7.

[44] Kilpatrick MM, Yonas H, Goldstein S, et al. CT-based assessment of acute stroke CT, CT angiography, and Xenon-enhanced CT cerebral blood flow. Stroke 2001;32:2543–9.

[45] Firlik AD, Kaufmann AM, Wechsler LR, et al. Quantitative cerebral blood flow determinations in acute ischemic stroke. Relationship to computed tomography and angiography. Stroke 1997;28:2208–13.

[46] Fink JN, Kumar S, Horkan C, et al. The stroke patient who woke up: clinical and radiological features, including diffusion and perfusion MRI. Stroke 2002;33:988–93.

[47] Iacob T, Jovin TG, Mendez OE, et al. Gradual neurological deterioration due to slow progression of cerebral ischemia is prevalent in stroke due to large vessel occlusion. Stroke 2004;35:339.

[48] Jovin TG, Yonas H, Gebel JM, et al. The cortical ischemic core and not the consistently present penumbra is a determinant of clinical outcome in acute middle cerebral artery occlusion. Stroke 2003;34:5426–33.

[49] Hill MD, Rowley HA, Adler F, et al. Selection of acute ischemic stroke patients for intra-arterial thrombolysis with pro-urokinase using ASPECTS. Stroke 2003;34:1925–31.

[50] Barber PA, Demchuk AM, Zhang J, et al. Validity and reliability of a quantitative computed tomography score in predicting outcome of hyperacute stroke before thrombolytic therapy. ASPECTS Study Group. Alberta Stroke Programme Early CT Score. Lancet 2000;355:1670–4.

[51] Lev MH, Segal AZ, Farkas J, et al. Utility of perfusion-weighted CT imaging in acute middle cerebral artery stroke treated with intra-arterial thrombolysis: prediction of final infarct volume and clinical outcome. Stroke 2001;32:2021–8.

[52] Firlik AD, Rubin G, Yonas H, et al. Relation between cerebral blood flow and neurologic deficit resolution in acute ischemic stroke. Neurology 1998;51:177–82.

[53] Goldstein S, Yonas H, Gebel J, et al. Acute cerebral blood flow as a predictive physiologic marker for

symptomatic hemorrhage conversion and clinical herniation after thrombolytic therapy. Stroke 2000;31:275.

[54] Jovin T, Yonas H, Gebel JM, et al. In thrombolysis
treated MCA occlusion, the extent of ischemic core
predicts the development of life-threatening hemorrhage or edema in conjunction with vessel recanalization. Neurology 2002;58(Suppl):A76.

[55] Rordorf G, Koroshetz WJ, Ezzeddine MA, et al. A
pilot study of drug-induced hypertension for treatment
of acute stroke. Neurology 2001;56:1210–3.

[56] Webster MW, Makaroun MS, Steed DL, et al. Compromised cerebral blood flow reactivity is a predictor
of stroke in patients with symptomatic carotid artery
occlusive disease. J Vasc Surg 1995;21:338–44.

[57] Yonas H, Smith HA, Durham SR, et al. Increased
stroke risk predicted by compromised cerebral blood
flow reactivity. J Neurosurg 1993;79:483–9.

[58] Demchuk AM, Burgin WS, Christou I, et al. Thrombolysis in brain ischemia (TIBI) transcranial Doppler
flow grades predict clinical severity, early recovery and
mortality in patients treated with intravenous tissue
plasminogen activator. Stroke 2001;32:89–93.

[59] Jovin T, Gebel J, Yonas H, et al. Pretreatment ipsilateral regional cortical blood flow influences vessel
recanalization in intra-arterial thrombolysis for MCA
occlusion. Stroke 2003;34:280.

[60] Labiche LA, Malkoff M, Alexandrov AV. Residual
flow signal predict complete recnalization in stroke
patients treated with tpa. J Neuroimaging 2003;13:
28–33.

[61] Hermier M, Nighoghossian N, Adeline P, et al. Early
magnetic resonance imaging prediction of arterial
recanalization and late infarct volume in acute carotid
artery stroke. J Cereb Blood Flow Metab 2003;23:
240–8.

[62] Rieke K, Schwab S, Krieger D, et al. Decompressive
surgery in space-occupying hemispheric infarction:
results of an open, prospective trial. Crit Care Med
1995;23:1576–87.

[63] Schwab S, Steiner T, Aschoff A, et al. Early hemicraniectomy in patients with complete middle cerebral
artery infarction. Stroke 1998;29:1888–93.

[64] Thomalla GJ, Kucinski T, Schoder V, et al. Prediction
of malignant middle cerebral artery infarction by early
perfusion- and diffusion-weighted magnetic resonance
imaging. Stroke 2003;34:1892–9.

NEUROIMAGING
CLINICS OF
NORTH AMERICA

ELSEVIER
SAUNDERS

Neuroimag Clin N Am 15 (2005) 543–551

Single-Photon Emission CT Imaging in Acute Stroke

Toshihiro Ueda, MD, PhD[a], William T.C. Yuh, MD, MSEE[b],*

[a]Division of Stroke Diagnostics and Therapeutics, Yokohama Stroke and Brain Center, Takigashira, Yokohama, Japan
[b]Department of Radiology, Ohio State University Medical Center, Columbus, OH, USA

One of the major reasons for interest in using single-photon emission CT (SPECT) for managing ischemia is that it is a reliable and inexpensive functional neuroimaging modality. The technique is safe and can be repeated easily for serial measurements. Unlike positron emission tomography (PET), SPECT cannot measure absolute cerebral blood flow (CBF) values or cerebral metabolism of oxygen. SPECT can be applied routinely in clinical practice, however, and can rapidly provide functional data that are not available by conventional CT, MR imaging, or PET. SPECT therefore is potentially useful for the diagnosis of acute or chronic ischemia (Figs. 1–6), assessment of ischemic tissue viability and reversibility of acute ischemia (Fig. 3), for the evaluation of cerebrovascular reserve in chronic ischemia (Figs. 4–6), and in posttreatment follow-up (Figs. 1–4).

Radiopharmaceutical agents

SPECT imaging requires radiotracers, including xenon-133 (^{133}Xe), the radioiodine-labeled amine N-isopropyl-[^{123}I] iodoamphetamine (IMP), Technetium-99m (^{99m}Tc), hexamnethyl-propyleneamine-oxime (HMPAO), and ^{99m}Tc-ethyl cysteinate dimmer (ECD).

^{133}Xe-SPECT can measure quantitative CBF with the inert gas clearance technique and—importantly—without arterial sampling. ^{133}Xe-SPECT is well suited for repeated studies within a short time in the same patients. The limitations of ^{133}Xe-SPECT include poor spatial resolution because of its low energy and rapid clearance from brain [1]. This technique is relatively expensive and is difficult to apply as an emergency examination.

IMP crosses the blood–brain barrier easily and is extracted almost completely during a single passage through the cerebral circulation [2]. It remains trapped in brain tissue in proportion to CBF and has a short brain-retention time. It tracks high CBF levels more accurately than either ^{99m}Tc- HMPAO or ^{99m}Tc-ECD. It is not consistently available, however, limiting its use in acute stroke and other emergencies.

^{99m}Tc- HMPAO is a lipid-solute, macrocyclic amine that is available for routine clinical use. HMPAO has a high first-pass extraction fraction; its brain uptake reaches maximum within 5 minutes after intravenous injection [3]. The initial distribution of this tracer remains constant for several hours [4]. In contrast to ^{133}Xe-SPECT, it is not possible to quantify CBF with ^{99m}Tc- HMPAO. A nonlinear relationship has been noted between the retention of HMPAO and CBF measured by PET because of flow-dependent back diffusion. To compensate for this nonlinearity, Lassen and colleagues [5] have proposed a correction algorithm for HMPAO SPECT.

ECD has rapid uptake and very slow clearance from the brain. ECD level; stabilize 7 to 20 minutes after intravenous injection. Blood clearance is rapid, resulting in a higher brain-to-background activity ratio than with HMPAO [6]. Therefore, the image quality of ECD is slightly better than that of HMPAO. In addition, and importantly, a "hypofixation" of ECD was described by Lassen and colleagues [7] in

---

* Corresponding author. Department of Radiology, Ohio State University Medical Center, 1654 Upham Drive, 663 Means Hall, Columbus, OH 43210.
 E-mail address: yuh.6@osu.edu (W.T.C. Yuh).

neuroimaging.theclinics.com

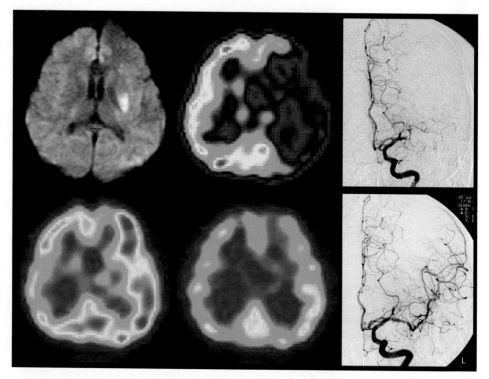

Fig. 1. A 46-year-old man with acute ischemic stroke caused by left middle cerebral artery occlusion. (*Upper left*) Diffusion MR imaging 6 hours after onset shows small focus of high signal intensity in left basal ganglia. (*Upper middle*) Pretreatment SPECT demonstrates perfusion deficit in the area of the left middle cerebral artery. (*Upper right*) Pretreatment cerebral angiography shows occlusion of the distal M1 portion of the left middle cerebral artery. (*Lower left*) Posttreatment SPECT 24 hours after recanalization demonstrates mild hyperperfusion in the area of the left middle cerebra artery. (*Lower middle*) Follow-up SPECT 1 week later shows improvement of hyperperfusion and almost normal perfusion in the area of the left middle cerebral artery. (*Lower right*) Posttreatment cerebral angiography shows complete recanalization of the M1 portion of the left middle cerebral artery, accomplished by intra-arterial administration of urokinase with balloon angioplasty.

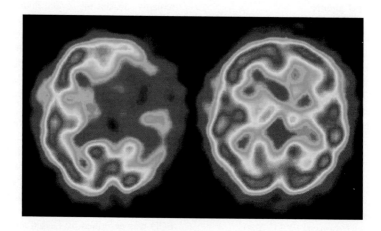

Fig. 2. A 48-year-old woman with cardiac embolic infaretion caused by left middle cerebral artery occlusion at 4 hours after onset. (*Left*) Pretreatment SPECT demonstrates perfusion deficit in the area of the left middle cerebral artery. (*Right*) Second SPECT after successful intra-arterial thrombolysis shows resolution of perfusion deficit.

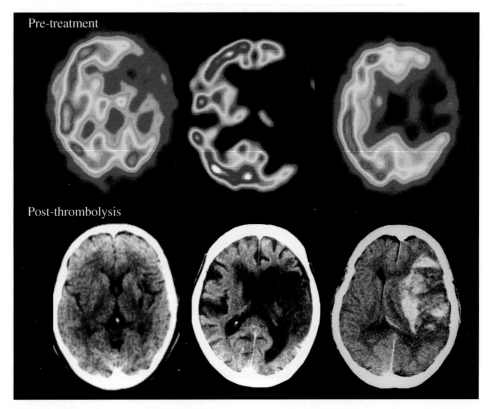

Fig. 3. (*Top left*) Pretreatment SPECT in a patient who had complete recanalization of a left middle cerebral artery occlusion 4 hours after onset of symptoms shows left fronto-temporo-parietal perfusion deficit. The ischemic region to cerebellar flow (R/CE) ratio was 0.5. (*Bottom left*) Posttreatment CT scan 1 month later shows no new apparent infarction. (*Top middle*) Pretreatment SPECT in a patient who had complete recanalization of a left middle cerebral artery occlusion 6 hours after onset of symptoms shows left fronto-temporo-parietal perfusion deficit. The R/CE ratio was 0.45. (*Bottom middle*) Posttreatment CT scan 1 month later shows a large infarction in the territory of the left middle cerebral artery. (*Top right*) Pretreatment SPECT in a patient who had nearly complete recanalization of the left middle cerebral artery occlusion 4 hours after onset of symptoms shows left fronto-temporo-parietal perfusion deficit. The R/CE ratio was 0.21. (*Bottom right*) Posttreatment CT scan shows hemorrhagic transformation in the territory of the left middle cerebral artery.

patients who had subacute stroke; because of this hypofixation, reperfusion of infarcted areas was not detected. This phenomenon results from a slow de-esterification of the compound, with consequent low conversion to the trapped hydrophilic form.

Acute ischemic stroke

Numerous reports describe the usefulness of SPECT in the management of acute stroke. Perfusion status as evaluated by SPECT can be important for differential diagnosis, early detection, assessment of viability, and assessment of potential reversibility of ischemic tissue—all of which can aid in decision

making. Hypoperfusion on SPECT images indicates cerebral ischemia and suggests hemodynamically significant arterial stenosis in chronically diseased patients or large vessel occlusion in acutely diseased patients within minutes after stroke onset [8].

Unenhanced CT scanning is positive in the early hours after stroke onset in as few as 20% of patients, but SPECT scan can be positive in up to 90% of these patients [9,10]. Two large, prospective, blinded trials tested the ability of SPECT to localize acute ischemic stroke. Sensitivities of 61% to 74% (85% for nonlacunar strokes) and specificities of 88% to 98% were reported [11]. SPECT findings have been reported to correlate with both the severity of the admission neurologic deficit and the clinical outcome in

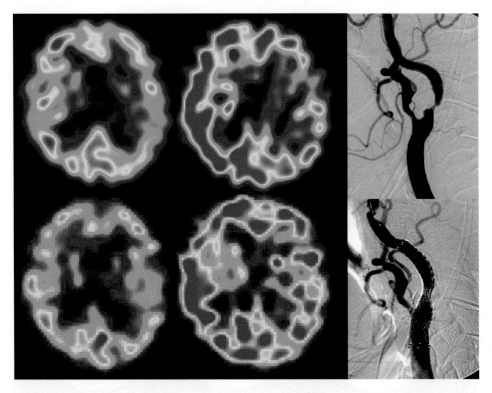

Fig. 4. A 64-year-old woman with severe left carotid stenosis who was treated by carotid stenting. (*Upper left*) The resting ^{99m}Tc-ethyl cysteinate dimmer SPECT image shows mild hypoperfusion in left cerebral hemisphere. (*Upper middle*) Acetazolamide-challenge SPECT demonstrates an increase of CBF in the right cerebral hemisphere and a decrease of CBF in left cerebral hemisphere. (*Upper right*) Pretreatment angiography shows severe left carotid stenosis. (*Lower left*) Posttreatment resting SPECT show no significant change compared with pretreatment SPECT. (*Lower middle*) Posttreatment acetazolamide-challenge SPECT demonstrates increased CBF in the left cerebral hemisphere and improvement of cerebrovascular reserve. (*Lower right*) Posttreatment angiography shows improvement of severe left carotid stenosis.

acute stroke patients. Early, severe hypoperfusion on SPECT during the first 6 hours after ictus was highly predictive (92%) of poor neurologic outcome [11]. Alexandrov and colleagues [12] indicated that SPECT, when performed within 72 hours of stroke onset, was statistically better than the clinical neurologic-deficit scores (National Institutes of Health stroke scale score) in predicting the short-term outcome of ischemic stroke onset. Moreover, SPECT before and after intravenous thrombolysis has been reported to correlate well with outcome and treatment response [13].

Differential diagnosis of stroke subtype is important for therapeutic decision-making and prediction of recovery. SPECT is useful in localizing stroke and in differentiating stroke subtypes. Brass and colleagues [14] indicated that SPECT demonstrated a specificity of 98% and a sensitivity of 86% for localization of strokes.

Endovascular recanalization, thrombolysis, and single-proton emission computed tomography

The advent of effective therapies, such as endovascular recanalization using mechanical disruption or thrombolysis, has made the treatment of acute ischemic stroke possible. The major considerations in selecting patients for acute treatment are twofold: (1) salvaging reversible ischemic tissue, and (2) avoiding reperfusion of dead (nonviable) tissue. The target therapy should be the ischemic tissue that can benefit from reperfusion [15]. Diagnostic modalities that can rapidly distinguish reversibly from irreversibly damaged ischemic tissues are needed because of the high risk for reperfusion injury and hemorrhagic transformation with early intervention in already irreversibly infarcted brain.

Although the window for acute stroke treatment in humans is generally considered to be within the first

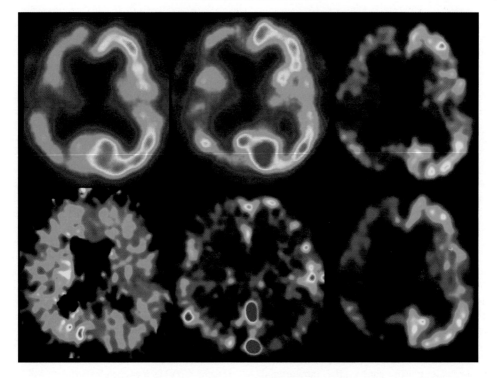

Fig. 5. A 68-year-old man with severe right internal carotid artery stenosis. (*Upper left*) The resting ^{99m}Tc-ethyl cysteinate dimmer SPECT image shows hypoperfusion in the right cerebral hemisphere. (*Upper middle*) Acetazolamide-challenge SPECT demonstrates no increase of CBF in the bilateral cerebral hemispheres. (*Upper right*) Correlative CBF image from PET scan demonstrates marked reduction of CBF in right cerebral hemisphere. (*Lower left*) Oxygen extraction fraction image shows elevation in right cerebral hemisphere. (*Lower middle*) Cerebral blood volume image shows no significant changes. (*Lower right*) Cerebral metabolic rate of oxygen metabolism image demonstrates marked reduction of oxygen use in right cerebral hemisphere.

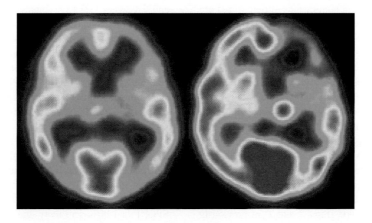

Fig. 6. A 46-year-old woman with Moyamoya disease and a left border-zone infarction. (*Right*) The resting ^{99m}Tc-ethyl cysteinate dimmer SPECT image shows hypoperfusion in left frontal lobe. (*Left*) Acetazolamide-challenge SPECT demonstrates global increase of CBF except in the left frontal lobe.

3 to 6 hours after onset, the therapeutic window for the potentially salvageable ischemic tissue is probably more complex and dependent on factors other than simply time, including the degree of collateral flow and the tissue metabolic status [16]. Rapid assessment of the status of the collateral circulation and associated tissue reversibility before treatment has not been emphasized or considered in most clinical trials of thrombolytic therapy, however.

SPECT has advantages for such rapid functional imaging because it is readily available and can be performed quickly in emergency cases. Laloux and associates [17] found a strong correlation between CBF, as measured by the degree and size of the hypoperfusion lesion, and clinical outcome. Although SPECT cannot measure an absolute value of regional CBF, semiquantitative analysis of CBF may provide important information that identifies threshold values for the severity of ischemia. Shimosegawa and colleagues [18] suggested that in patients who have acute stroke, the lesion-to-contralateral radioactivity ratio for infarction threshold is 0.48 within 6 hours of onset.

SPECT has also been useful in evaluating the risk of hemorrhagic transformation after intra-arterial thrombolysis. Ueda and colleagues [19] suggested that patients who had residual CBF and an ischemic regional activity-to-cerebellar activity (R/CE) ratio of less than 0.35 had a significant risk of hemorrhagic transformation after successful IA-lysis. This semiquantitative analysis of residual CBF in ischemic tissue is quite simple and prompt and can be implemented readily in any institution without using a special computer setting or protocol. In addition, Ueda and associates [19] showed that outcomes of acute ischemia with early and successful recanalization after IA-lysis are significantly different and are significantly influenced by pretreatment CBF as assessed by HMPAO-SPECT (Fig. 3). Thus, CBF thresholds evaluated by SPECT may provide important data that can be useful in the management of patients who have acute stroke. Specifically, they reported that ischemic tissue with a flow index greater than 0.55 is likely to be salvageable, even if treatment is initiated 6 hours after the onset [20]. This observation is further supported by Sasaki and colleagues [21], who reported significant reduction of infarct extent for reperfused ischemic tissue with R/CE ratios between 0.55 and 0.75 recanalized within 7.25 hours of stroke onset.

Marked reperfusion (Figs. 1 and 2) of previously hypoperfused ischemic tissue within 24 to 36 hours, as detected by SPECT, was associated with better-than-expected outcomes [22–24]. Early hyperperfu-

sion, which indicates recanalization of the occluded artery [25], has been observed in up to one third of cases studied by PET between 15 and 18 hours after stroke onset [26]. HMPAO-SPECT is relatively insensitive to focal hyperperfusion [27], and some cases of mild hyperperfusion may be overlooked. HMPAO measures may overestimate hyperemia, especially in the subacute phase of stroke. Hyperfixation of HMPAO in patients who have subacute stroke does not reflect hyperperfusion but rather indicates abnormal penetration of the brain parenchyma by tracer, caused by an altered blood–brain barrier of irreversibly necrotic tissue [28].

Diffusion and perfusion MR imaging may be another potentially useful means to assess tissue viability and reversibility in acute ischemia. Karonen and associates [29,30] reported that a clinically relevant ischemic penumbra, estimated by diffusion–perfusion mismatch, can be detected in most patients who have acute stroke by using the combination of SPECT and diffusion MR imaging. Hatazawa and colleagues [31] found that, for distinguishing between infarction and noninfarction in untreated acute stroke cases, the cut-off ratio for CBF as measured by SPECT was 0.52, and the cut-off ratio for cerebrovascular reserve (CBV) as measured by perfusion MR imaging was 0.85.

Chronic ischemia and cerebrovascular reserve

Evaluation of cardiovascular reserve can be accomplished using vasodilators, such as intravenous administration of acetazolamide or inhalation of CO_2 [32]. The mechanism of acetazolamide-induced increase in CBF increase has not been fully elucidated. Ringelstein and colleagues [33] have suggested that the effects of acetazolamide and CO_2 on CBF augmentation are equally suited for the assessment of vasoreactivity.

Acetazolamide administration resulted in a 13% to 46% (mean 31%) increase in CBF in normal elderly controls as measured by ^{133}Xe-SPECT [34,35]. Leinsinger and colleagues [36] found a positive correlation between basal CBF and vasoreactivity in response to acetazolamide. In a PET study of acetazolamide-induced changes in CBF, Hirano and coworkers [37] found that, in patients who had impaired vasoreactivity, the best correlation was between the percentage change of an asymmetry index and oxygen extraction fraction. Ogasawara and associates [38] found that ^{123}I-IMP SPECT had 90% sensitivity and 92% specificity for detecting patients who had reduced regional cerebrovascular reactivity. They validated the accuracy of IMP for quantifying regional cardiovascular reserve with acetazolamide challenge by comparing it with a PET reference standard.

Two prospective studies have indicated that regional cerebrovascular reactivity to acetazolamide challenge, as measured by quantitative ^{133}Xe-SPECT, can predict outcome in patients who have major cerebral arterial occlusive disease [39,40]. Yokota and others [41], however, failed to find an association between hemodynamic failure and stroke risk in a prospective study performed by measuring regional cerebrovascular reactivity to acetazolamide challenge using qualitative ^{123}I-IMP SPECT.

SPECT studies performed before and after acetazolamide administration, with adjunctive radionuclide angiography (which requires 2 minutes), make it possible for baseline and postacetazolamide CBF to be quantified without blood sampling (Figs. 4–6), using the rectangular gamma camera of the two-head SPECT. This method has been reported to be easy to implement in routine clinical studies and quite useful for the evaluation of vascular reserve, improving sensitivity for detection of regional hemodynamic abnormalities [42].

SPECT has been used mainly to assess regional cardiovascular reserve in an attempt to identify patients who are at high risk of stroke because of pre-existing vascular insufficiency and who might benefit from surgical treatment. This method has been considered a suitable means of evaluating the adequacy of collateral circulation and provides data that supplement CT angiography, catheter angiography, and transcranial Doppler sonography [43]. Recently, Imaizumi and colleagues [44] determined that acetazolamide-challenge SPECT can be applied clinically to detect misery perfusion in a manner analogous to that of acetazolamide H_2O and CO/CO_2-PET. Extracranial/intracranial (EC-IC) bypass surgery and carotid endarterectomy in patients who have severe stenotic or occluded carotid arteries have been shown to increase cerebrovascular reserve postoperatively [45,46]. The efficacy of EC-IC bypass can be assessed by SPECT [47]. Furthermore, acetazolamide-challenge SPECT can be used to guide surgical intervention in Moyamoya disease (Fig. 6); EC-IC bypass may be of some benefit in selected patients who have Moyamoya disease [48,49].

Finally, the sensitivity of SPECT for the detection of vascular insufficiency in patients who have transient ischemic attacks can be improved with the addition of acetazolamide challenge, which may also provide data on the mechanism of ischemia and stroke subtype. Multiple administrations of isotopes and subtraction techniques can increase the sensitivity for detecting failure of perfusion augmentation after acetazolamide challenge. These techniques may have predictive value for early recurrent stroke or for first stroke in asymptomatic patients.

References

[1] Holman BL, Devous MD. Functional brain SPECT: the emergence of a powerful clinical method. J Nucl Med 1992;33:1888–904.

[2] Winchell HS, Baldwin RM, Lin TH. Development of ^{123}I-labeled amines for brain studies: localization of ^{123}I iodophenyllalkylamines in rat brain. J Nucl Med 1980;21:940–6.

[3] Neirinckx RD, Canning LR, Piper IM, et al. Technetium-99m d, l -HM-PAO: a new radiopharmaceutical for SPECT imaging of regional cerebral blood perfusion. J Nucl Med 1987;28:191–202.

[4] Devous MD. SPECT instrumentation, radiopharmaceuticals, and technical factors. In: Van Heertum RL, Tikofsky RS, editors. Functional cerebral SPECT and PET imaging. 3rd edition. Philadelphia: Lippincott Williams & Wilkins; 2000. p. 3–22.

[5] Lassen N, Anderson A, Friberg L, et al. The retention of [99mTc]-d,l-HM-PAO in the human brain after intracarotid bolus injection: a kinetic analysis. J Cereb Blood Flow Metab 1988;8:S13–22.

[6] Leveille J, Demonceau G, Walovitch RC. Intrasubject comparison between technitium-99m-ECD and technetium-99m-HMPAO in healthy human subjects. J Nucl Med 1992;33:480–4.

[7] Lassen NA, Sperling B. ^{99m}Tc-bicisate reliably images CBF in chronic brain diseases but fails to show reflow hyperemia in subacute stroke: report of a multicenter trial of 105 cases comparing ^{133}Xe and ^{99m}Tc-biciste (ECD, Neurolite) measured by SPECT on same day. J Cereb Blood Flow Metab 1994;14(Suppl):44–8.

[8] Raynaud C, Rancurel G, Tzourio N, et al. SPECT analysis of recent cerebral infarction. Stroke 1989;20: 192–204.

[9] Fieschi C, Argentino C, Lenzi GL, et al. Clinical and instrumental evaluation of patients with ischemic stroke within the first six hours. J Neurol Sci 1989; 91:311–21.

[10] De Roo M, Mortelmans L, Devos P, et al. Clinical experience with Tc-99m HMPAO high resolution SPECT of the brain in patients with cerebrovascular accidents. Eur J Nucl Med 1989;15:9–15.

[11] Brass LM, Walvitch RC. Two prospective, blinded, controlled trials of Tc99m bicisate brain SPECT and standard neurological evaluation for identifying and localizing and ischemic strokes. J Stroke Cerebrovasc Diseases 1992;1(Suppl 1):S59.

[12] Alexandrov AV, Black SE, Ehrlich LE, et al. Simple visual analysis of brain perfusion on HMPAO SPECT predicts early outcome in acute stroke. Stroke 1996; 27:1537–42.

[13] Grotta JC, Alexandrov AV. t-PA-associated reperfusion after acute stroke demonstrated by SPECT. Stroke 1998;29:429–32.

[14] Brass LM, Walovitch RC, Joseph JL, et al. The role of single photon emission computed tomography brain imaging with 99mTc-bicisate in the localization and definition of mechanism of ischemic stroke. J Cereb Blood Flow Metab 1994;14:S91–8.

[15] Yuh WTC, Maeda M, Wang A, et al. Fibrinolytic treatment of acute stroke: are we treating reversible cerebral ischemia? AJNR Am J Neuroradiol 1995;16: 1994–2000.

[16] Fisher M. Characterizing the target of acute stroke therapy. Stroke 1997;28:866–72.

[17] Laloux P, Richelle F, Jamart J, et al. Comparative correlations of HMPAO SPECT indices, neurological score, and stroke subtypes with clinical outcome in acute carotid infarcts. Stroke 1995;26:816–21.

[18] Shimosegawa E, Hatazawa J, Inugami A, et al. Cerebral infarction within six hours of onset: prediction of completed infarction with technetium-99m-HMPAO SPECT. J Nucl Med 1994;35:1097–103.

[19] Ueda T, Hatakeyama T, Kumon Y, et al. Evaluation of risk of hemorrhagic transformation in local intra-arterial thrombolysis in acute ischemic stroke by initial SPECT. Stroke 1994;25:298–303.

[20] Ueda T, Sakaki S, Yuh WTC, et al. Outcome in acute stroke with successful intra-arterial thrombolysis and predictive value of initial single-photon emission-computed tomography. J Cereb Blood Flow Metab 1999;19:99–108.

[21] Sasaki O, Takeuchi S, Koizumi T, et al. Complete recanalization via fibrinolytic therapy can reduce the number of ischemic territories that progress to infarction. AJNR Am J Neuroradiol 1996;17:1661–8.

[22] Baird AE, Donnan GA, Austin MC. Early reperfusion in the spectacular shrinking deficits demonstrated by single-photon emission computed tomography. Neurology 1995;45:1335–9.

[23] Herderschee D, Limburg M, van Royen EA, et al. Thrombolysis with recombinant tissue plasminogen activator in acute ischemic stroke: evaluation with rCBF-SPECT. Acta Neurol Scand 1991;83:317–22.

[24] Overgaard K, Sperling B, Boysen G, et al. Thrombolytic therapy in acute ischemic stroke. A Danish pilot study. Stroke 1993;24:1439–46.

[25] Lassen NA. The luxury perfusion syndrome and its possible relation to acute metabolic acidosis localized within the brain. Lancet 1966;2:1113–5.

[26] Marchal G, Rioux R, Serrati C, et al. Value of acute-stage PET in predicting neurological outcome after ischemic stroke: further assessment. Stroke 1995;26: 524–5.

[27] Gartshore G, Bannan P, Patterson J, et al. Evaluation of technetium-99m exametazime stabilized with cobalt chloride as a blood flow tracer in focal cerebral ischemia. Eur J Nucl Med 1994;21:913–23.

[28] Sperling B, Lassen LA. Hyperfixation of HMPAO in subacute ischemic stroke leading to spuriously high estimates of cerebral blood flow by SPECT. Stroke 1993;24:193–4.

[29] Karonen JO, Vanninen RL, Liu Y, et al. Combined diffusion and perfusion MRI with correlation to single-photon emission CT in acute ischemic stroke: ischemic penumbra predicts infarct growth. Stroke 1999;30: 1583–90.

[30] Karonen JO, Nuutinen J, Kuikkla JT, et al. Combined SPECT and diffusion-weighted MRI as a predictor of infarct growth in acute ischemic stroke. J Nucl Med 2000;41:788–94.

[31] Hatazawa J, Shimosegawa E, Toyoshima H, et al. Cerebral blood volume in acute brain infarction: a combined study with dynamic susceptibility contrast MRI and ^{99m}Tc-HMPAO-SPECT. Stroke 1999;30:800–6.

[32] Vorstrup S, Henriksen L, Paulson OB. Effects of acetazolamide on cerebral blood flow and cerebral metabolic rate for oxygen. J Clin Invest 1884;74: 1634–9.

[33] Ringelstein EB, Van Eyck S, Mertens I. Evaluation of cerebral vasomotor reactivity by various vasodilating stimuli: comparison of CO_2 to acetazolamide. J Cereb Blood Flow Metab 1992;12:162–8.

[34] Vorstrup S, Brun B, Lassen NA. Evaluation of the cerebral vasodilatory capacity by the acetazolamide test before EC-IC bypass surgery in patients with occlusion of the internal carotid artery. Stroke 1986; 17:1291–8.

[35] Kreisig T, Schmiedek P, Leinsinger G, et al. ^{133}Xe-DSPECT: normal values of cerebral blood flow at rest and of reserve capacity. Nucl Med (Stuttg) 1897;26: 192–7.

[36] Leinsinger G, Piepgras A, Einhaupl K, et al. Normal values of cerebrovascular reserve capacity after stimulation with acetazolamide measured by xenon-133 single-photon emission CT. AJNR AmJ Neuroradiol 1994;15:1327–32.

[37] Hirano T, Minematsu K, Hasegawa Y, et al. Acetazolamide reactivity on ^{123}I-IMP single-photon emission computed tomography in patients with major cerebral artery occlusive disease: correlation with positron emission tomography parameters. J Cereb Blood Flow Metab 1994;14:763–70.

[38] Ogasawara K, Ito H, Sasoh M, et al. Quantitative measurement of regional cerebrovascular reactivity to acetazolamide using iodine-123-IMP autoradiography with SPECT: validation study using oxygen-15-water with PET. J Nucl Med 2003;44:520–5.

[39] Kuroda S, Houkin K, Kamiyama H, et al. Long-term prognosis of medically treated patients with internal carotid or middle cerebral artery occlusion: can acetazolamide test predict it? Stroke 2001;32:2110–6.

[40] Ogasawara K, Ogawa A, Yoshimoto T. Cerebrovascular reactivity to acetazolamide and outcome in patients with symptomatic internal carotid or middle cerebral artery occlusion: a xenon-133 single-photon emission computed tomography study. Stroke 2002;33: 1857–62.

[41] Yokota C, Hasegawa Y, Minematsu K, et al. Effect of acetazolamide reactivity and long-term outcome in patients with major cerebral artery occlusive disease. Stroke 1998;29:640–4.

[42] Takeuchi R, Matsuda H, Yonekura Y, et al. Non-invasive quantitative measurements of regional cerebral blood flow using technetium-99m-L,L-ECD SPECT activated with acetazolamide: quantification analysis by equal-volume-split ^{99m}Tc-ECD consecutive SPECT method. J Cereb Blood Flow Metab 1997;17:1020–32.

[43] Knop J, Thie A, Fuchs C, et al. ^{99m}Tc-HMPAO SPECT with acetazolamide challenging to detect hemodynamic compromise in occlusive cerebrovascular disease. Stroke 1992;23:1733–42.

[44] Imaizumi M, Kitagawa K, Oku N, et al. Clinical significance of cerebrovascular reserve in acetazolamide challenge: comparison with acetazolamide challenge H$_2$O-PET and Gas-PET. Ann Nucl Med 2004;18:369–74.

[45] Ramsay SC, Yeates MG, Lord RS, et al. Use of technetium-HMPAO to demonstrate changes in cerebral blood flow reserve following carotid endarterectomy. J Nucl Med 1991;32:1382–6.

[46] Cikrit DF, Burt RW, Dalsing MC, et al. Acetazolamide enhanced single photon emission computed tomography (SPECT) evaluation of cerebral perfusion before and after carotid endarterectomy. J Vasc Surg 1992;15:747–53.

[47] Lee HY, Paeng JC, Lee DS, et al. Efficacy assessment of cerebral arterial bypass surgery using statistical parametric mapping and probabilistic brain atlas on basal/acetazolamide brain perfusion SPECT. J Nucl Med 2004;45:202–6.

[48] Kobayashi H, Hayashi M, Handa Y, et al. EC-IC bypass for adult patients with moyamoya disease. Neurol Res 1991;13:113–6.

[49] Hoshi H, Ohnishi T, Jinnouchi S, et al. Cerebral blood flow study in patients with moyamoya disease evaluated by IMP SPECT. J Nucl Med 1994;35:44–50.

**NEUROIMAGING
CLINICS OF
NORTH AMERICA**

ELSEVIER
SAUNDERS

Neuroimag Clin N Am 15 (2005) 553 – 573

Collaterals in Acute Stroke: Beyond the Clot

David S. Liebeskind, MD*

*University of California at Los Angeles Stroke Center, University of California at Los Angeles Medical Center,
Los Angeles, CA, USA*

Collateral circulation

Reduction of cerebral blood flow (CBF) as a result of proximal lumenal obstruction may be offset promptly and adequately by collateral flow [1]. Effective perfusion results from the net balance between residual anterograde flow across the obstructive lesion and circuitous collateral routes—often using retrograde flow via auxiliary vessels. These ubiquitous collateral routes may diminish the impact of a potentially devastating vascular event, such as carotid occlusion, substantially.

Progressive obliteration of flow in the internal carotid artery resulting from atherosclerotic plaque, for example, often is asymptomatic and clinically irrelevant. Alternatively, the same degree of internal carotid artery obstruction, if compensated for ineffectually by collateral flow, can result in loss of cerebrovascular reserve or even extensive "low flow" (also known as borderzone) stroke. Although the rapidity of occlusive onset may be acute with thromboembolic lesions, the ensuing events similarly are dictated by collateral sufficiency.

Collateral routes are not simply vascular channels that may or may not be evident at the time of stroke diagnosis. *Collaterals essentially determine whether or not and when stroke occurs,* in association with proximal vascular compromise caused by either arteriopathic or thromboembolic phenomena. *Collaterals also may influence the nature of the proximal vascular lesion.* For instance, nominal collateral flow

beyond an atherosclerotic lesion may induce or hasten stasis-related thrombosis, thereby promoting occlusion or distal embolization (Fig. 1). The extent and composition of the occlusive lesion itself—clot or plaque with superimposed thrombus—theoretically may influence the therapeutic efficacy of revascularization techniques, yet clot location may be equally important because of the nature and degree of collateral compensation beyond the occlusion.

Temporal and spatial features characterize the dynamic balance between the proximal occlusive lesion and compensatory collateral circulation. *Time is a critical variable* in the development of collateral circulation. Sudden vascular events, such as thrombotic occlusion, may impose dramatic demands for collateral circulation via established conduits, whereas progressive or chronic obstruction of arterial flow may allow for more extensive development of auxiliary channels. Similarly, the location of the occlusive lesion and potential collateral flow may vary with anatomic sites at different branches or bifurcations across the arterial tree [1,2].

Proximal arterial occlusion may threaten extensive brain regions, yet many established arterial routes may compensate rapidly as a result of the considerable network of collaterals inherent in human arterial anatomy [1]. At distal aspects of the arterial tree, in end arteries or perforators of the basal ganglia or cortical surface, the potential for collateral compensation may be seemingly negligible. For instance, collateral flow may play a trivial role in lacunar infarction or cortical branch occlusion (Figs. 2 and 3) [3]. The dynamics and impact of collateral flow, therefore, most commonly are accentuated with occlusive lesions at intermediate points between proximal and distal sites, such as in occlusion of the distal internal carotid or proximal middle cerebral arteries

---

* University of California at Los Angeles Stroke Center, UCLA Medical Center, 710 Westwood Plaza, Los Angeles, CA 90095.

E-mail address: davidliebeskind@yahoo.com

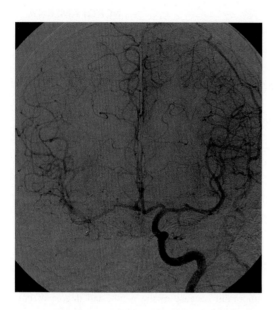

Fig. 1. Arteriography of thromboembolism distal to a severe right extracranial carotid stenosis, with relatively diminished intracranial collateral flow. (© David S. Liebeskind, MD.)

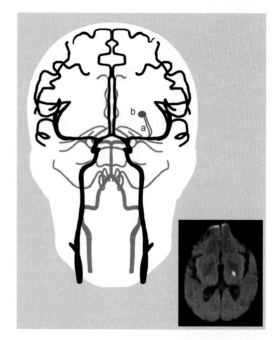

Fig. 2. Schematic of collaterals associated with lenticulo-striate involvement (a) in lacunar infarction (b). (*From* Liebeskind DS. Neuroprotection from the collateral perspective IDrugs 2005; with permission.)

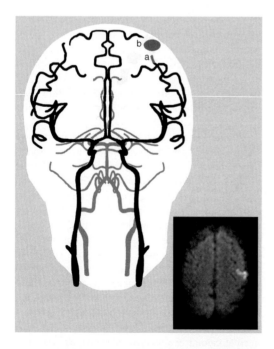

Fig. 3. Schematic of collaterals in branch occlusion (a) with cortical infarction (b). (*From* Liebeskind DS. Neuroprotection from the collateral perspective. IDrugs 2005; with permission.)

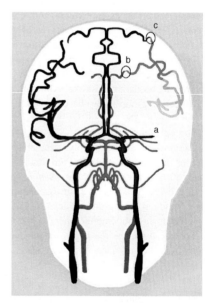

Fig. 4. Schematic of MCA occlusion (a) with collateral flow from the PCA (b) and ACA (c). (© David S. Liebeskind, MD.)

Box 1. American Society of Interventional and Therapeutic Neuroradiology/Society of Interventional Radiology collateral flow grading system

0 — No collaterals visible to the ischemic site
1 — Slow collaterals to the periphery of the ischemic site, with persistence of some of the defect
2 — Rapid collaterals to the periphery of the ischemic site, with persistence of some of the defect, but only to a portion of the ischemic territory
3 — Collaterals with slow but complete angiographic blood flow of the ischemic bed occurring by the late venous phase
4 — Complete and rapid collateral blood flow to the vascular bed of the entire ischemic territory, by retrograde perfusion

(MCAs) (Fig. 4). Moyamoya syndrome serves as the clinical prototype for chronic collaterals [1].

Imaging plays a pivotal role in the characterization of collateral flow. As collaterals sustain blood flow to potentially ischemic regions, the presence of collateral flow may mask an otherwise expected clinical deficit. Such "negative" clinical observations may be difficult to discern, especially in the acute setting. For instance, collateral sparing of the posterior

division of the left MCA may be unapparent on clinical examination because of concomitant aphasia.

The presence and extent of collateral circulation may be depicted with arteriographic imaging (Box 1) or with perfusion imaging based on the associated distribution of ischemic lesions. Such characterization of collateral flow is described best for a particular vascular lesion or site of arterial occlusion. A detailed discussion on imaging of collaterals in acute ischemic stroke, therefore, requires consideration of the standard arterial anatomy of the cerebral circulation.

Arterial collaterals

The anatomy of the cerebral collateral circulation differs extensively in individuals and with varying degrees of disease, although certain patterns are encountered commonly [1]. Cerebral arterial collaterals are dissimilar from collateral routes in the coronary or peripheral arterial beds [4]. Cerebral collaterals typically are elongated, circuitous channels—unlike the shorter, segmental collateral segments that bypass occlusive lesions of the coronary arteries [4].

In contrast to peripheral collaterals, cerebral collaterals rarely disrupt or invade functional tissue. Cerebral collaterals typically exhibit a complex configuration that may be subdivided into: (1) the short bypass segments at the circle of Willis (Fig. 5) and (2) the markedly elongated leptomeningeal anastomotic routes that deliver retrograde perfusion to adjacent vascular territories (Fig. 6).

Reversal of ophthalmic arterial flow may compensate for insufficiency in the anterior portion of the circle of Willis [5]. The anterior communicating artery and reversal of flow in the proximal anterior

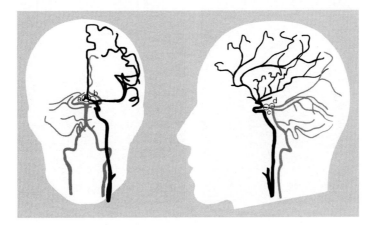

Fig. 5. Schematic of Willisian collaterals, including anterior communicating artery (a), proximal ACA (b), posterior communicating artery (c), and proximal PCA (d). (© David S. Liebeskind, MD.)

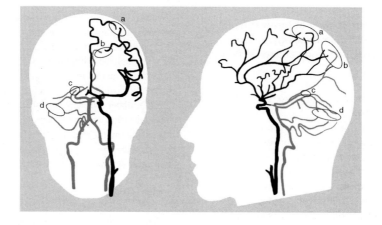

Fig. 6. Schematic of leptomeningeal collaterals, bridging ACA and MCA (a), PCA and MCA (b), superior cerebellar artery and PCA (c), and major cerebellar hemispheric arteries (d). (© David S. Liebeskind, MD.)

cerebral artery also provide collateral support in anterior regions [2]. The posterior communicating arteries may supply collateral flow in either direction between the anterior and posterior circulations. Circle of Willis anatomy varies considerably, with frequent asymmetry and an ideal or complete configuration in only a minority of cases [1]. *Moreover, circle of Willis collaterals may exhibit dynamic behavior, with previously hypoplastic segments enlarging progressively or involuting occasionally as a result of fluctuating demands* (Fig. 7) [6].

Leptomeningeal (pial) anastomoses provide collateral flow to adjacent cerebral and cerebellar arterial territories. Diversion of flow through these diminutive structures allows for retrograde perfusion of the collapsed arterial bed distal to the clot. Atypical col-

lateral routes may use vascular anomalies, including persistent embryologic remnants, such as the trigeminal artery (Fig. 8).

Vascular anatomy and pathophysiology redefined

Occlusion of a proximal arterial segment rapidly transforms the cerebrovascular anatomy and associated physiology [7]. Cerebral circulation is diverted through ancillary channels, redefining the course of arterial flow. The presence of multifocal occlusive lesions may lead to a complex pattern of arterial perfusion. The location of the occlusions dictates the recruitment of specific collateral routes. Such transformation redefines the primary vascular territories and relocates borderzone regions. The borderzone

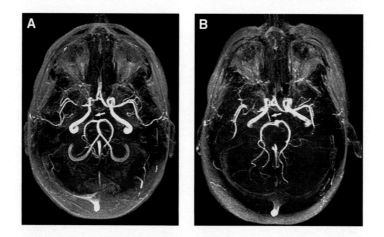

Fig. 7. Serial MRA scans (*A* and *B*) of MCA stenosis, demonstrating progressive changes in the apparent caliber of the posterior communicating artery (*arrows*). (*From* Liebeskind DS, Sansing LH. Willisian collateralization. Neurology 2004;63(2):344; with permission.)

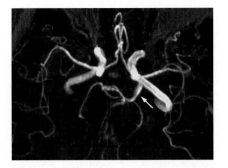

Fig. 8. TOF MRA illustrating collateral flow to the distal basilar artery, via a persistent trigeminal artery (*arrow*). (© David S. Liebeskind, MD.)

between the major cerebral arteries functions as the primary site of collateral flow diversion because of the high density of leptomeningeal anastomoses in these regions [8]. Previously well-perfused regions of the MCA, such as the insular cortex, are transformed instantaneously into borderzone territory after proximal occlusion.

Such anatomic changes may elicit secondary pathophysiologic alterations. Circle of Willis diversion of arterial flow may or may not induce dramatic changes. For instance, internal carotid artery occlusion may be associated with prompt diversion of blood flow from the contralateral carotid distribution or vertebral artery via Willisian collaterals. Such diversion uses short arterial circuits that supply minimal blood flow to regions adjacent to this bypass. In contrast, leptomeningeal collateral flow via retrograde perfusion of the major cerebral or cerebellar territories likely induces prominent alterations as a result of intravascular deoxygenation [8]. The diminutive caliber of leptomeningeal anastomoses may slow flow entering distal reaches of the occluded vascular territory considerably. Vascular collapse distal to an occlusion may act as a pressure sink, allowing blood flow to extend throughout the arterial tree, coursing in retrograde fashion past bifurcations into adjacent branches.

Further slowing of retrograde collateral perfusion may be accentuated by the excessive length and tortuosity of such arterial routes. As leptomeningeal arterial collaterals flow in reverse direction, oxygen is extracted continually to supply adjacent brain tissue (Fig. 9) [8]. Such precapillary oxygen loss may be exaggerated by excessive slowing of flow [8]. Although standard perfusion imaging methods may characterize the delay and dispersion of intravascular contrast, reflecting the complex nature of leptomeningeal collateral flow, current imaging modalities do not account for the quality or oxygen status

of such collateral perfusion [9]. These pathophysiologic events—related to the quantity and quality of collateral perfusion—also may evolve as a result of secondary collateralization commencing within hours or days of stroke onset [1].

Primary collateral diversion of blood flow is driven largely by hemodynamic factors, including the large pressure gradient associated with maximal vasodilatation and vascular collapse within the ischemic territory. Secondary collateral recruitment, however, may rely on alteration of the blood-brain barrier and vascular remodeling associated with the upregulation and local increase of arteriogenic factors. Collateral perfusion resulting from primary and secondary recruitment defines the ischemic penumbra and surrounding regions of benign oligemia. Within the penumbra, the metabolic demands of dysfunctional tissue may not be addressed adequately with collateral perfusion, hastening evolution toward infarction [10]. Alternatively, collateral perfusion may sustain ischemic regions sufficiently and indefinitely or until revascularization is achieved. Oligemic regions may demonstrate only modest reductions in CBF associated with collateral perfusion, without substantial risk of infarction. These seemingly distinct regions, characterized by the nature of collateral perfusion and metabolic status of underlying tissue, stabilize over time, leading to demarcated regions of infarction and complementary areas of salvaged tissue. Certain patterns of infarction, such as deep cerebral lesions associated with transient MCA occlusion, reflect the net result of this dynamic process, balancing flow and metabolism (Fig. 10) [10,11].

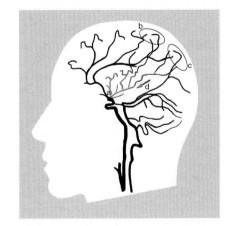

Fig. 9. Schematic of arterial deoxygenation in leptomeningeal collaterals. Proximal MCA occlusion (a) induces recruitment of collaterals from the ACA (b) and PCA (c) with concomitant intravascular deoxygenation of retrograde MCA flow (d). (© David S. Liebeskind, MD.)

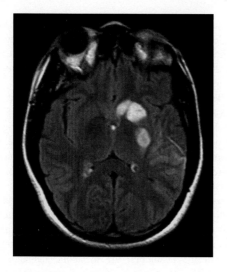

Fig. 10. MR FLAIR image of deep subcortical infarction associated with acute MCA occlusion. (© David S. Liebeskind, MD.)

Clinical correlates: manifestations of collateral sustenance and failure

Collateral sustenance of potentially ischemic regions may mask symptoms or neurologic findings transiently or permanently [7]. This paradoxic relationship makes it difficult to define the clinical correlates of collateral flow. Such clinical correlates may be deduced by recognizing that certain elements of the clinical examination are unexpectedly normal. For instance, collateral sparing may be evident as preservation of sensory function despite complete occlusion of the MCA. During early stages after stroke onset, dramatic changes in clinical examination may be observed with alterations in head positioning [7,9,12]. Simply placing patients in the supine position may lessen the degree of neurologic impairment evident on examination [7]. Such repositioning of patients or candidates for thrombolysis may cause reductions in the National Institutes of Health stroke scale score by several points.

This clinical observation may be interpreted as rapidly improving symptoms, thereby convincing treating physicians to defer thrombolysis. In unusual cases, placing the head in upright position may exacerbate neurologic findings, presumably as a result of attenuation of collateral blood flow distal to an occlusion. Such changes in head positioning and dramatic alterations in neurologic status are observed most frequently at early time points after stroke onset [12]. On occasion, such clinical observations may be noted during the first few days in the intensive care unit in patients who have persistent large vessel occlusion.

Although such seemingly trivial aspects of supportive care, such as head positioning, may influence clinical deficits, most diagnostic modalities other than transcranial Doppler ultrasound (TCD) fail to detect collateral dependency. Most perfusion modalities used in acute ischemic stroke, including CT, MR imaging, and angiography, provide information regarding perfusion solely in the dependent position—failing to reflect the nature of blood flow when patients assume normal head position. Collateral dependency and susceptibility to neurologic deterioration with upright positioning may evade detection until patients are transferred from an intensive care unit to a floor.

Collateral failure or delayed deterioration of collateral perfusion after initial recruitment remains of unclear etiology [7]. It is unknown whether or not such changes are the result of hemodynamic events that precipitate dropout of auxiliary blood flow routes or if the nature of collateral blood supply is insufficient to sustain ischemic tissue indefinitely.

Retrograde perfusion, if significantly deoxygenated because of local tissue demands, may not be adequate in supporting the territory at risk [8]. The concept of collateral failure is invoked frequently when patients deteriorate [13], yet serial evaluation of cerebral perfusion or angiography almost never is pursued. Typically, repeat imaging shows enlarged regions of infarction compared with baseline. Maturation or the expected evolution of the initial ischemic injury also may lead to subsequent reductions in collateral flow, as such perfusion no longer may be required.

In most cases, the ability of retrograde collateral perfusion to compensate for proximal occlusion is determined strongly by the time course of the ischemic event. In acute ischemic stroke, even a short delay in collateral failure may extend the opportunity for revascularization. The endurance of collateral perfusion may determine individual differences in the degree of mismatch and potential response to thrombolysis [14]. Moreover, the degree of initial collateral support may promote collateral endurance through secondary collateralization. For example, initial brisk flow via leptomeningeal anastomoses may stimulate these channels to remain patent, and even to dilate, to accommodate further increases in collateral perfusion.

As time proceeds from the onset of arterial occlusion, the balance between tissue demands and collateral support stabilizes, determining the extent of final infarction. Certain infarction patterns, such as deep subcortical infarctions, reflect the history of this precarious balance between demand and collateral perfusion supply [11,15]. Imaging plays a critical role in characterizing these events, as the clinical correlates may be fairly obscure. Serial imaging is required to demonstrate early collateral sustenance and subsequent diminution.

Therapeutic implications

The development of collateral therapeutics will depend on accurate diagnostic imaging techniques for characterization of collateral flow [7]. Objective tools or scales also will be needed to grade or describe the degree of collateral perfusion for a given site of arterial occlusion [16,17]. Collateral therapeutics may entail simple interventions, such as head positioning, intravenous fluid support, pressure augmentation, or improvements in oxygenation [7]. Collateral augmentation may be used to prolong the time window for revascularization and to improve vascular integrity before reperfusion. Whether or not these interventions are used initially to extend the time window for revascularization or to reduce the extent of ultimate infarction resulting from collateral failure, imaging will play a central role.

Imaging of collateral circulation may be used to identify optimal candidates for intervention. Previous reports note the influential role of collaterals in determining the outcome of thrombolysis [14,18–20]. The presence of vigorous leptomeningeal collaterals is a major predictor of recanalization response to intravenous and intra-arterial thrombolytic therapies [18–20]. Collateral flow also may be an influential factor in the ultimate fate of neuroprotective therapy [3]. *Collaterals are the sole route for delivery of intravenous neuroprotective agents in proximal arterial occlusion* (Fig. 11) [3].

Even aside from influencing therapeutic efficacy of alternative interventions, the mere extent of collateral sustenance may have important prognostic implications. Collateral circulation is a fundamental determinant of stroke outcome in untreated patients [1,21,22]. Further research and increased knowledge of collateral circulation in acute ischemic stroke thus will improve therapeutic options and disclose novel opportunities for intervention [7]. Therapeutic manipulation of collateral blood flow, however, is critically dependent on understanding the status, normal evolution, and detailed pathophysiology of collaterals.

Imaging of collateral circulation: angiography, perfusion, and infarction

Collaterals may be characterized with angiography or described in terms of resultant perfusion or patterns of infarction. The imaging correlates of collaterals parallel the basic four Ps of stroke imaging— *p*ipes, *p*erfusion, *p*enumbra, and *p*arenchyma [23]. From almost all perspectives, the correlates of collateral flow typically are subtle findings that require concerted attention [1]. Such findings also most commonly are located adjacent to, not directly in the area of, ischemic change.

For instance, collateral vessels may be seen at the periphery of the ischemic territory or at more remote

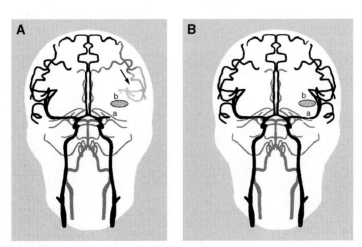

Fig. 11. Schematics illustrating penumbral neuroprotection (*A*), and neuroprotective strategies related to reperfusion (*B*). Direction of flow beyond proximal MCA occlusion (a) may influence delivery to the ischemic bed (b). (*Modified from* Liebeskind DS. Neuroprotection from the collateral perspective. IDrugs 2005;8(3):222–8; with permission.)

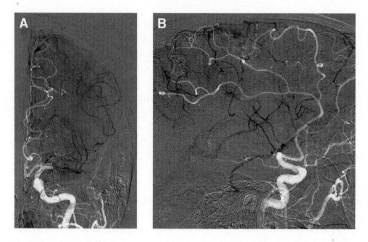

Fig. 12. Conventional subtraction arteriography (*A*, frontal projection and *B*, lateral projection) illustrating antegrade flow in proximal arteries at early phases (*white*), superimposed on retrograde leptomeningeal collateral flow (*dark*), associated with MCA occlusion. (© David S. Liebeskind, MD.)

sites, channeling blood flow to adjacent vascular territories. Proximal diversion of flow at the Circle of Willis may be difficult to detect on noninvasive imaging modalities, often requiring serial evaluation to demonstrate subtle patterns of recruitment. Dynamic behavior of Willisian collaterals may be evident, depending on tissue demands and corresponding supply [6]. Although collateral sources are well recognized as the basis for residual perfusion and the extent of penumbra, perfusion imaging rarely is analyzed from this perspective.

Indeed, the characteristic features of collateral perfusion, delay and dispersion, are paradoxically treated as a nuisance in the calculation of accurate perfusion measures [9]. Delay and dispersion may be

the most accurate measures of collateral function and determinants of tissue outcome in the absence of revascularization. Heterogeneity in collateral perfusion likely accounts for at least some of the variability observed in the pattern of infarction for a given vascular territory.

The resultant perfusion patterns and follow-up infarction topography are understood poorly, likely because of the limited use of conventional angiography in acute stroke. Angiographic studies are ideal for defining collateral flow patterns but typically are not obtained in stroke patients, except late in the decision-making pathway for patients undergoing endovascular therapy. Correlative studies linking conventional angiography with advanced multimodal CT

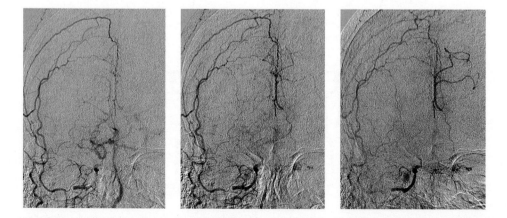

Fig. 13. Dural arteriolar collateral flow from the extracranial to intracranial circulations, seen on conventional arteriography in acute on chronic ischemia, associated with right carotid occlusion. (© David S. Liebeskind, MD.)

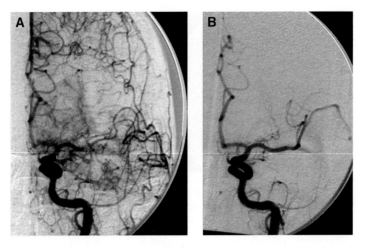

Fig. 14. Angiographic views of retrograde collateral flow (*A*), with restoration of antegrade MCA flow (*B*) associated with clot retrieval from an MCA occlusion. (© David S. Liebeskind, MD.)

or MR imaging techniques in cases of endovascular therapy, therefore, likely will enrich the current understanding of collateral imaging correlates [9].

Angiography

Although potential collateral routes are surmised from classic anatomy and pathology studies conducted centuries ago, the introduction of angiography provided the first depiction of collateral flow. Historical descriptions of angiography emphasize the features of collateral circulation in various types of acute occlusive lesions. The depiction of arterial collaterals on angiography in acute ischemic stroke is almost universal (Fig. 12), yet characterization of collateral findings is unsystematic and nonstandardized [16,17].

There is great variability in individuals with regard to collateral flow, including extracranial-to-intracranial shunting and various intracranial routes (Fig. 13). In most acute stroke cases, however, such information is deferred to implement rapid treatment strategies, such as thrombolysis. When collaterals are assessed before and after revascularization procedures, dramatic changes also may be noted with disappearance of previously illustrated routes (Fig. 14). Unusual filling patterns may be demonstrated using vascular anomalies (Fig. 15) or more subtle cerebral arterial anastomoses. Conventional angiography is critical for evaluation of leptomeningeal anastomoses, as other angiographic modalities lack the exquisite combination of spatial (Fig. 16) and temporal resolution (Fig. 17). In fact, conventional angiography is the only modality that illustrates ret-

rograde leptomeningeal collateral flow reliably and in detailed fashion. Variation in filling patterns and critical temporal information may be assessed crudely on review of source image data from CT and MR imaging perfusion techniques, yet conventional angiography is required to evaluate leptomeningeal collateral flow adequately.

Angiographic technique also is important, as variation in contrast volume and pressure during injection may distort the appearance of distal vessels. Careful review of acquired images may reveal subtle differences in filling with respect to angiographic phase or timing of the injection. Despite the wealth of information regarding collateral flow provided by

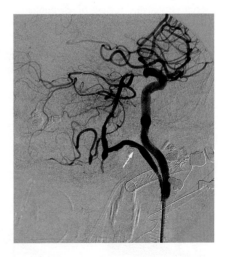

Fig. 15. Collateral flow to the posterior circulation via a persistent hypoglossal artery (*arrow*), demonstrated on conventional arteriography. (© David S. Liebeskind, MD.)

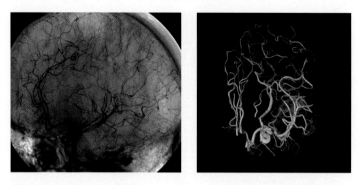

Fig. 16. 3D-rotational angiography of a nearly occluded left MCA, demonstrating distal perfusion arising from a combination of antegrade and retrograde flow. (© David S. Liebeskind, MD.)

angiography, use of this modality increasingly is reserved for potential cases of thrombolysis or thrombectomy. As a result, incomplete or limited studies often are obtained in a highly selected set of cases, limiting knowledge of collateral function in acute ischemic stroke in a larger cohort of patients. As many endovascular procedures for acute ischemic stroke remain investigational, further selection bias regarding collateral flow is imparted by detailed trial inclusion and exclusion criteria.

Prior descriptions of collateral flow used subjective and simplistic schemes to characterize the presence, type, and degree of collaterals [17]. Although various forms of collateral flow may be evident with proximal arterial occlusion, leptomeningeal collaterals play a pivotal role in the pathophysiology of acute ischemic stroke. Characterization of leptomeningeal collaterals often employs vague descriptors, such as good or poor.

A recent systematic review of all published angiographic scales incorporating some rating of collateral flow includes nineteen proposed but unvalidated scales [17]. Multiple flaws in the great preponderance of available scales are identified. For each type of vascular occlusive lesion (eg, M1 occlusion), only a subset of angiographic scales is applicable. Many scales fail to account for important variations in collateral features that depend on the specific site of the occlusive lesion.

For instance, occlusion of the proximal segment of the anterior MCA division typically elicits different collateral patterns from a similar occlusion within the posterior division. The distribution of ratings also is limited with some scales. Objective definitions are omitted frequently, thereby exaggerating inter-rater reliability. Composite scales that combined proximal arterial patency status and collateral flow status into conflated unitary variables obscure, rather than enhance, collateral condition [17].

The development of a reliable and validated angiographic scale for leptomeningeal collaterals would facilitate analyses of ongoing and future trials

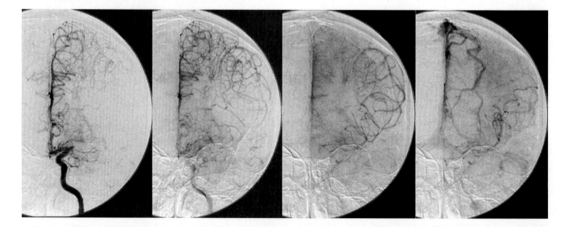

Fig. 17. Serial arteriographic images from a selective left internal carotid artery injection in a patient who has MCA occlusion, illustrating retrograde collateral flow. (© David S. Liebeskind, MD.)

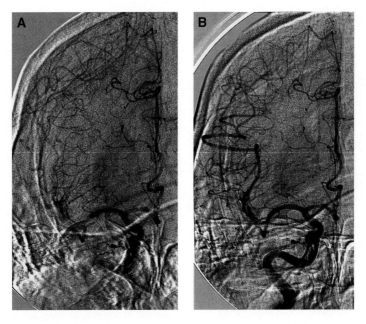

Fig. 18. (*A* and *B*) Diagnostic arteriogram revealing recanalization after administration of intravenous tPA. (© David S. Liebeskind, MD.)

of endovascular therapy. A standardized classification scheme for leptomeningeal collaterals would allow comparisons between studies and permit evaluation of therapeutic interventions mediated principally via collaterals. The need for such a scale is recognized widely [16]. As a result, the Technology Assessment Committees of the American Society of Interventional and Therapeutic Neuroradiology and the Society of Interventional Radiology recently proposed a novel collateral scale, for advancing new trial design and reporting standards for intra-arterial thrombolysis [16]. This scale grades collaterals on an ordinal scale with five strata (see Box 1) [16].

Angiographic studies of collaterals confirm the central role of these ancillary blood flow routes. Systematic angiographic evaluation of collaterals before thrombolysis has important prognostic implications, as the absence of significant collateralization in various types of occlusive lesions is associated with increased mortality [1,20]. In basilar artery occlusion, the degree of collateralization is an important predictor of survival [20]. Clinical outcome also is associated strongly with the extent of collateral flow [1,14,19,24,25]. The degree of collaterals may be inconsequential, however, if initial stroke severity is profound with persistent arterial occlusion [24].

Although collaterals theoretically may influence recanalization efficacy, they also may improve clinical outcome by sustaining ischemic tissue and limiting the extent of parenchymal infarction. In some cases, the extent of collaterals may be unrelated to recanalization [20]. For instance, extensive collaterals may be evident with atherothrombotic basilar occlusion, yet thrombolysis may have limited success in restoring lumenal patency.

In MCA occlusion treated with intravenous thrombolysis, collateral flow may augment recanalization by delivering drug to the distal end of the clot (Fig. 18). Collaterals do not exhibit any influence on the efficacy of recanalization with mechanical

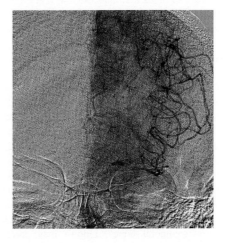

Fig. 19. Exuberant collateral flow to the left MCA territory in acute stroke caused by atrial fibrillation. (© David S. Liebeskind, MD.)

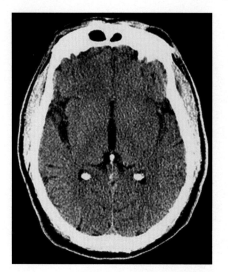

Fig. 20. Noncontrast CT illustrating isolated loss of the left insular ribbon, with relative preservation of adjacent cortex supplied by collaterals. (© David S. Liebeskind, MD.)

thrombectomy, however [24]. Collaterals simply may sustain tissue until recanalization is achieved, allowing for early spontaneous improvement [22].

Predicting who has robust collaterals at angiography is a difficult endeavor. In the Mechanical Embolus Removal in Cerebral Ischemia (MERCI) trial, age, gender, and ethnicity demonstrate no correlation with the extent of angiographic collaterals [26]. Various comorbidities also are unrelated to collateral grade. The results of this study suggest that angiographic collaterals in acute ischemic stroke may not be predicted by most clinical variables [26]. Furthermore, traditional teachings, such as that there is a relative lack of collateral flow with acute cardioembolic events, often are unsubstantiated (Fig. 19).

Transcranial Doppler ultrasonography

TCD and transcranial color-coded Duplex may provide information rapidly regarding collateral flow patterns at the Circle of Willis [27–32]. Diversion of flow in Willisian segments and corresponding velocity information may be assessed readily with these techniques [29]. Careful attention to insonation depths and detailed studies also may reveal retrograde collateral flow distal to the clot. Recent studies demonstrate the dual diagnostic and potential therapeutic roles of TCD in acute ischemic stroke [33]. Inadequate transtemporal bone windows may preclude insonation in a considerable portion of acute stroke cases and TCD often is not acquired until after the acute period. Dilatation of collateral routes associated

with secondary collateralization, commencing within hours of stroke onset, also may lead to normalization of flow velocities. Cerebral vasomotor reactivity testing with TCD during the early subacute phase may provide information on autoregulation and collateral status, using serial evaluation of blood flow in response to a vasodilatory stimulus, such as carbon dioxide inhalation, acetazolamide injection, or apnea [1,32].

Multimodal CT

Multimodal noninvasive imaging techniques using CT or MR imaging may provide comprehensive and complementary information on various aspects of acute stroke pathophysiology, including collateral flow patterns and corresponding areas of evolving infarction [9]. Unlike conventional angiography and TCD, extensive perfusion abnormalities and incorporated areas of core infarction may be discerned in addition to imaging of vascular structures. Such depictions of parenchymal perfusion and associated structural changes in brain tissue resulting from ischemia provide the basis for mismatch models. Mismatch paradigms are used with nuclear medicine techniques, MR imaging, and, most recently, CT to estimate or gauge the extent of penumbra. Although the borders or exact delineation of ischemic perfusion abnormalities and more restricted regions of core infarction are difficult to define in detail, in clinical practice the crude extent of mismatch often serves as an imaging parameter for

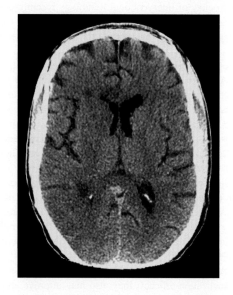

Fig. 21. Deep subcortical infarction on CT associated with transient right MCA occlusion. (© David S. Liebeskind, MD.)

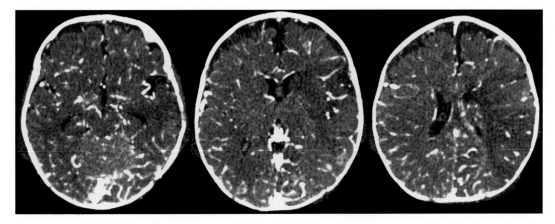

Fig. 22. CTA-SI of collaterals adjacent to evolving infarction in the left MCA territory. (© David S. Liebeskind, MD.)

estimation of risk-benefit ratios with acute therapeutic interventions.

The underlying basis of each mismatch variant differs, yet collateral flow is a principal feature [9]. Collateral perfusion evident on CT or MR imaging may sustain large areas where mismatch is apparent. The advent of helical CT scanners and the concomitant ability to perform CT angiography (CTA) and CT perfusion (CTP) promote CT as a multimodal approach to rival stroke MR imaging [34,35]. A discussion of multimodal CT and comparison with analogous MR imaging techniques must consider the inherent basis and limitations of the underlying technology.

Multimodal CT typically includes noncontrast CT of the head, CTA, and CTP. Modified algorithms may use only isolated components, such as CT and CTA, or alter the amount of contrast volumes for each component. The acquisition of noncontrast CT provides rapid information regarding early patterns of evolving ischemia. As this imaging approach has been used for almost 3 decades, recognition of early CT signs already is well established. The significance of these findings, however, remains controversial. Although specific early CT signs recently are correlated with sites of proximal arterial occlusion on angiography, such regions of restricted hypodensity may reflect patterns of collateral flow more accurately.

For instance, isolated loss of the insular ribbon with hypodensity on CT obscuring the expected architecture of this region may accompany MCA occlusion with extensive collaterals that spare adjacent regions of moderately hypoperfused cortex (Fig. 20). Alternatively, deep subcortical hypodensity restricted to the lenticulostriate distribution may signify exuberant collateral flow with proximal MCA occlusion (Fig. 21) [11]. In other cases, extensive regions of CT hypodensity within the first few hours of symptom onset may be associated with poor collateral flow [36]. CT hypodensity, however, may be subtle or difficult to discern and these ischemic changes may take more time to develop when compared with MR imaging correlates, such as diffusion-weighted imaging (DWI) lesions. Borderzone or watershed patterns on early CT may be particularly difficult to resolve, as such lesions may be small and susceptible to partial volume averaging as a result of adjacent convoluted areas of cortical tissue.

Although CTA may be used primarily to identify proximal arterial occlusion, source images from this approach may be useful in estimating the extent of collateral flow [34,35,37]. CTA source images (CTA-SI) may provide high-resolution depiction of vascular structures opacified during a specific period of contrast arrival in the cerebral vasculature (Fig. 22). The prolonged enhancement phase, compared with that of conventional angiography and MRA, may delineate diminutive vascular structures

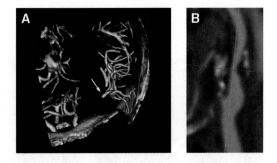

Fig. 23. Volume-rendered CTA of terminal internal carotid artery occlusion (A) with prominent collateral flow beyond the occlusion (arrow). Simultaneous oblique reformatted views of the neck (B) reveal an ulcerative carotid plaque. (© David S. Liebeskind, MD.)

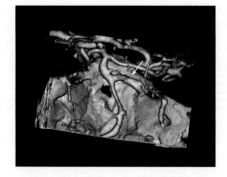

Fig. 24. Volume-rendered CTA views of a persistent trigeminal artery (*arrow*) functioning as a collateral conduit. (© David S. Liebeskind, MD.)

with superb anatomic accuracy. CTA-SI, therefore, may not be able to provide information regarding the temporal profile or chronologic details of contrast arrival via collateral routes, yet this approach identifies vascular structures filled by collaterals at prolonged time points. *In other words, CTA-SI depicts the maximal extent of collateral perfusion.* Such images, therefore, likely overestimate the potential beneficial effects of collateral routes, as even regions with marginal collateral perfusion are demarcated [38].

The use of a standardized scale for delineation of collaterals on CTA-SI may facilitate description and use of these images. A 4-point leptomeningeal collateral scale on CTA demonstrates excellent interrater reliability [37]. Systematic evaluation of CTA-SI with this simple scale may provide reliable and potentially valuable information rapidly regarding the proximal and leptomeningeal collateral circulation [37]. Postprocessing of CTA data may be more informative, but use of these images is less practical, as such reformatting may impart significant delays that are unacceptable in acute ischemic stroke.

At centers with advanced imaging laboratories, CTA data may be reconstructed rapidly to demon-strate remarkable detail of cerebrovascular structures. Causative lesions in stroke etiology, such as ulcerated carotid atherosclerotic plaque, may be identified readily, whereas leptomeningeal collateral flow may be illustrated vividly extending to the distal aspect of the clot lodged in the terminal internal carotid artery (Fig. 23). Collaterals at the circle of Willis or Willisian collaterals may be depicted clearly and even ophthalmic artery patency may be discerned typically [37].

Atypical vascular segments, such as persistent embryonic arteries linking the anterior and posterior circulations, also may be evident on CTA (Fig. 24). Such anatomic detail may suggest the potential for collateral flow, yet actual flow physiology or function remains speculative. Distal collateral routes, such as leptomeningeal anastomoses, may evade detection with CTA. Discontinuous segments may be seen at such anastomoses, as the size of these vessels may surpass the spatial resolution of this technique. As discussed previously, the exquisite anatomic detail in larger segments may establish the presence of collateral flow, yet temporal aspects or delays in contrast arrival may confound even this.

CTP, using an additional contrast bolus after acquisition of CTA, may characterize tissue perfusion and provide estimates of collateral flow (Fig. 25). This technique is similar to dynamic contrast-enhanced perfusion technique with MR imaging (perfusion-weighted imaging [PWI]) and is discussed at length in an article elsewhere in this issue. Dynamic acquisition of serial CT scans after a timed contrast bolus may be performed at several levels to generate perfusion estimates. Inspection of the raw, or source, images may reveal collateral flow patterns. For instance, collateral flow from the posterior cerebral artery (PCA) into the MCA may be evident on review of serial scans (Fig. 26).

Postprocessing of CTP data may seem a formidable obstacle in the setting of acute stroke, yet after prompt transmission of data from the scanner to the

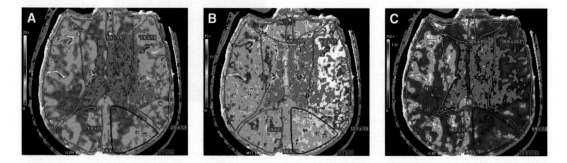

Fig. 25. CTP parameter maps in acute ischemic stroke, including CBV (*A*), MTT (*B*), and CBF (*C*). (© David S. Liebeskind, MD.)

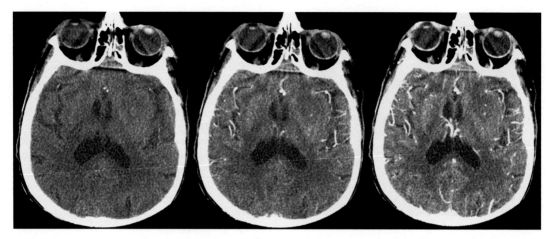

Fig. 26. Serial images of raw CTP data illustrating collateral flow from the PCA to the MCA territories. (© David S. Liebeskind, MD.)

laboratory or workstation, the generation of CTP parameter maps may require only a minute or two. The user selects arterial and venous seed points to define an arterial input function and the postprocessing software constructs perfusion parameter maps rapidly (Fig. 27). The presence of collateral flow typically is evident as preservation of CBF and potential augmentation of cerebral blood volume (CBV), whereas mean transit time (MTT)—a measure of circulation time—is prolonged. As collateral flow dissipates, MTT prolongs even further after CBV is maximized and CBF subsequently declines. Collateral flow may be evident on parameter maps as a result of gradations from adjacent collateral territories. Although

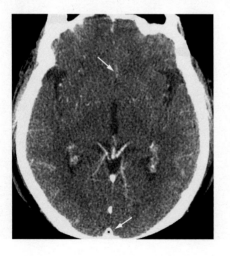

Fig. 27. Arterial and venous seed points (*arrows*), used for processing of CTP data. (© David S. Liebeskind, MD.)

typically not performed in acute stroke, serial CTP with and without diamox may demonstrate the extent of vascular reserve. Tissue perfusion may improve after the injection of diamox as a result of dilatation of either the primary or adjacent collateral territories. Dilatation of adjacent collateral vessels may represent a beneficial form of vascular steal, where blood subsequently is shunted into distal aspects of the occluded vascular territory via anastomoses. Perfusion parameters, such as MTT, may improve with such steal phenomena. The source of arterial flow, via the primary vessel or collateral circuits, also may influence the quality of perfused blood, however, because of degradation in oxygen content.

Multimodal MR imaging

Recent advances in multimodal MR imaging of acute ischemic stroke permit rapid evaluation of occlusive arterial lesions, regional perfusion, and the extent of evolving infarction [9]. Multimodal MR imaging encompasses many aspects analogous to multimodal CT, with even further information regarding vessel and tissue status. Parenchymal structures are characterized exquisitely and in great detail, delineating acute from chronic lesions. Subtle differences in the signal intensity of lesions depicted across several pulse sequences may provide a wealth of information regarding tissue status. Multimodal MR is discussed at length in articles from the previous issue, "Stroke I: Overview and Current Clinical Practice." The artifacts of MR imaging also differ considerably from those of CT. CT artifacts typically detract from image interpretation, whereas MR imaging artifacts may

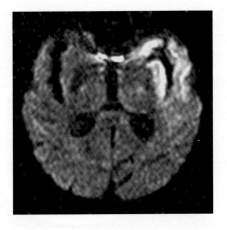

Fig. 28. DWI hyperintensity of the insula resulting from acute left MCA stroke. (© David S. Liebeskind, MD.)

provide useful information, such as flow-related findings. These aspects of stroke MR imaging are germane particularly to imaging of collateral circulation.

The remarkable sensitivity of DWI for the detection of acute ischemia allows for rapid characterization of the ischemic core, with the remainder of the vascular territory sustained by collateral flow. Early DWI lesions may parallel findings on CT [35]. For instance, DWI hyperintensity of the insular cortex may be analogous to loss of the insular ribbon on CT (Fig. 28). The location of the ischemic core within a collateral poor portion of vascular territory,

such as the deep MCA, and the relative sparing of collateral-endowed regions, such as the peripheral cortex, may be mapped.

Current PWI techniques generally provide only indirect or qualitative information regarding collateral pathways. For example, collateral perfusion may be evident as prolongation of time-to-peak (TTP) or MTT with relative preservation of CBV.

Retrograde perfusion in an arterial tree and marked elongation of blood flow routes via circuitous channels also may cause dispersion in the arrival times of blood delivered by collaterals. Such dispersion may be appreciated easily with visual inspection of the arterial input function used in PWI. Some postprocessing software accounts for such delay and dispersion by using an arterial input function from an uninvolved territory, such as the contralateral MCA.

The delay associated with collateral flow may be apparent readily on inspection of TTP maps, reflecting large vessel contrast passage (Fig. 29). Gradations in such parameter maps also may indicate the source of collateral flow and the distal extent of such perfusion. TTP or other time parameters characterizing circulation time may be specific markers for collateral flow, as CBV and CBF may not necessarily be altered. For instance, branch occlusion may not result in significant CBV or CBF alterations, although such regions supplied via collateral perfusion may be recognized by inspection of the TTP maps (Fig. 30).

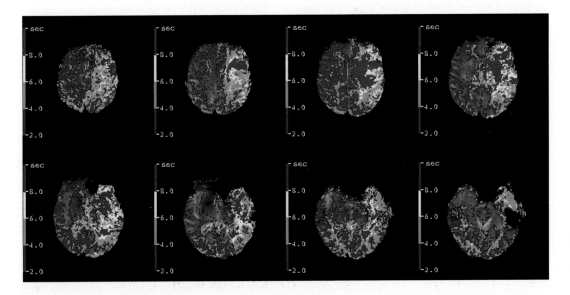

Fig. 29. PWI Tmax image revealing prominent delays in collateral perfusion associated with left MCA occlusion. (© David S. Liebeskind, MD.)

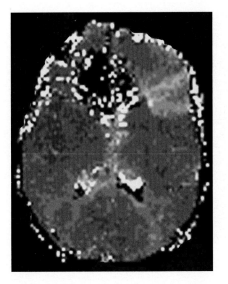

Fig. 30. PWI TTP map reveals hyperintensity resulting from collateral flow distal to a branch artery occlusion. (© David S. Liebeskind, MD.)

Continuous arterial spin-labeled perfusion imaging also may depict delays associated with collateral perfusion. Such flow-related effects correlate with retrograde perfusion, demonstrated on fluid-attenuated inversion recovery (FLAIR) images as FLAIR vascular hyperintensity (FVH) caused by slow leptomeningeal flow distal to an occluded cerebral artery (Fig. 31) [39].

Although FVH may be associated with thrombosis and flow abnormalities proximal to the MCA clot, the hyperintense serpiginous structures extend-ing across the sylvian fissure and the convexities frequently are observed to be patent on angiography (Fig. 32) [40–42]. Such segments typically demonstrate retrograde collateral perfusion from adjacent territories, including the anterior and posterior cerebral arteries. Although leptomeningeal collaterals are difficult to discern with noninvasive angiographic techniques, such as CTA or MRA, FVH may provide detection of these subtle collateral routes.

A correlative study of CTA and FVH demonstrates that distal FVH correlates with either a proximal vessel stenosis or occlusion ($r = 0.52$; $P < 0.001$), although a stronger correlation is noted with occlusion ($r = 0.65$; $P < 0.001$) [41]. The presence of distal FVH shows a strong correlation with the presence of leptomeningeal collaterals on CTA-SI ($r = 0.71$; $P < 0.001$).

Careful inspection of gradient recalled echo (GRE) sequences also may reveal subtle abnormalities that colocalize with FVH. One analysis of patients who had MCA stroke reveals FVH in 49 cases and GRE hypointensity in 40 [8]. Intravascular GRE hypointensity of such leptomeningeal collaterals likely reflects the paramagnetic effects of arterial deoxyhemoglobin (predominating over expected slow flow-related GRE hyperintensity) [8]. Leptomeningeal collateral deoxygenation may be the result of precapillary oxygen loss in arterial blood traversing along extended, tortuous routes through regions with elevated oxygen extraction [8]. Such GRE hypointensity is distinct from the prominent "blooming" frequently seen with intra-arterial thrombus. In cases with only marginal leptomeningeal collateral flow, collapse or disappearance of the expected GRE flow

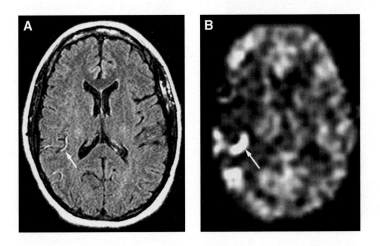

Fig. 31. FVH (*A, arrow*) and corresponding delayed arterial transit effects (*B, arrow*) resulting from slow leptomeningeal collateral flow. (© David S. Liebeskind, MD.)

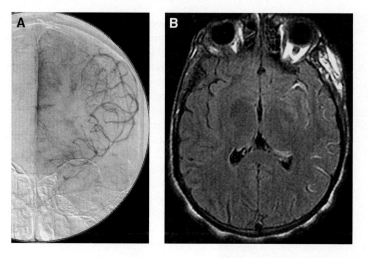

Fig. 32. Conventional angiography reveals retrograde collateral flow (*A*) corresponding to FVH (*B*) in acute stroke. (© David S. Liebeskind, MD.)

void may be seen in distal segments (Fig. 33). This appearance is appreciated best using the contralateral MCA as a reference.

These indirect vascular correlates of collateral flow may escape detection with standard MRA techniques [43,44]. Intracranial MRA is performed routinely using time-of-flight (TOF) techniques susceptible to signal loss in regions of disturbed flow [44]. Diminutive arterial segments and slow flow may

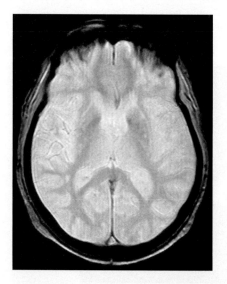

Fig. 33. Asymmetry in the appearance of distal MCA flow voids on GRE suggesting proximal occlusion of the left MCA. (© David S. Liebeskind, MD.)

not be apparent on such images. The compressed axial MIP views of the intracranial circulation on TOF MRA may provide clues to the presence of collateral pathways at the circle of Willis, via ophthalmic arteries, and even at dural arteriolar anastomoses but seldom are able to visualize distal branches—even after gadolinium administration (Fig. 34) [45]. Also, flow direction cannot be assessed.

With arterial occlusion or severe stenosis, collateral compensation may be seen in adjacent arterial segments. For instance, acute MCA occlusion consistently is accompanied by prominence of the ipsilateral PCA on MRA [45–47]. Apparent elongation of the ipsilateral PCA is reported in several cohorts, with a high degree of sensitivity and specificity for MCA occlusion [45–47]. This PCA collateral sign can be assessed rapidly on TOF MRA and manifests as an asymmetric pattern compared with the contralateral PCA, extending posteriorly and laterally (Fig. 35) [45]. The proximal diameter of the involved PCA also may appear greater than that of the contralateral "normal" PCA [45]. This PCA collateralization may be a practical marker of collateral recruitment in the acute and early subacute phases, although this finding dissipates over time [45].

As with perfusion imaging techniques, MRA provides a snapshot or static view of potentially dynamic alterations in cerebral circulatory patterns [48]. Although CTA may be regarded as superior in anatomic accuracy for measurement of lumenal features, the apparent vessel diameter on MRA may reflect more subtle changes in flow. Such subtle changes may require careful visual inspection and even measurement rather than cursory assessment of vascular patency.

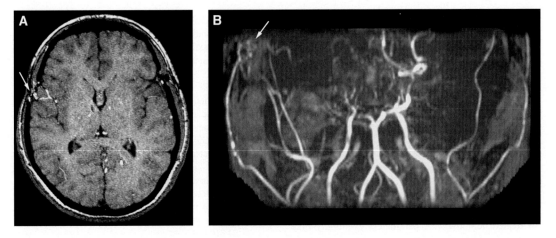

Fig. 34. TOF MRA (*A*, source image; and *B*, maximum intensity projection) exhibiting dural arteriolar collaterals (*arrows*) in acute stroke associated with moyamoya syndrome. (© David S. Liebeskind, MD.)

An analysis of simultaneous MR imaging and MRA in 96 cases of MCA stroke demonstrates that Willisian patterns are not related to infarction volume or infarction topography [48]. This study demonstrates that cortical sparing and the extent of infarction in MCA stroke are determined more strongly by leptomeningeal collaterals than Willisian collaterals and that a single MRA study may not reflect such secondary leptomeningeal collateralization that enlarges over time [48].

Collateral failure is an explanation frequently invoked for stroke progression, but its underlying pathophysiology remains obscure. Preliminary studies suggest that serial MRA may be able to demonstrate and quantify enlargement in apparent vessel diameter of Willisian collaterals over weeks to months in some patients who have ischemic stroke. Conversely, in other patients who have extensive infarctions, Willisian collaterals may diminish.

Novel techniques and approaches

Collateral imaging techniques are lacking [1,9]. Many of the previously described findings of collateral flow on emergent diagnostic studies are overlooked, with the principal focus on identification being proximal arterial occlusion and associated mismatch. Collateral flow is a fundamental determinant of mismatch and the potential for successful clinical outcome after thrombolytic therapy. Angiographic delineation of collateral routes may clarify the dynamic nature of mismatch. Further considerations of the delay and dispersion apparent with perfusion imaging techniques may expand current knowledge of collaterals. The heterogeneity evident within perfusion lesions also may provide clues to the source and endurance of collaterals.

Moreover, the definition of vascular territories may be reassessed with recognition of collateral flow patterns [49]. Selective arterial spin-labeled MR imaging or regional perfusion imaging may delineate more accurately the extent of primary vascular territories [49,50]. Blood oxygen level–dependent studies may be adapted for use in acute stroke, and oxygen sensitive imaging may augment current knowledge regarding the quality, not just the quantity, of collateral perfusion.

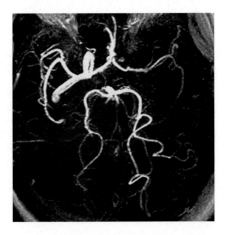

Fig. 35. PCA collateral sign on TOF MRA associated with ipsilateral MCA occlusion. (© David S. Liebeskind, MD.)

Summary

Collateral circulation is a critical, yet unexplored, facet of acute stroke pathophysiology. Diagnostic and therapeutic aspects of collateral flow demand further investigation. Neuroimaging correlates of collateral flow may improve the current approach to the evaluation and management of acute stroke. Elucidation of the clinical correlates, such as collateral dependency and potential collateral failure, will require dedicated imaging strategies that consider not only the inciting proximal occlusion or seemingly autonomous concept of mismatch. Collateral determinants of infarct topography and consideration of related hemodynamic parameters eventually may lead to the development of novel collateral therapeutics, complementing the narrow range of treatment options for acute ischemic stroke.

References

[1] Liebeskind DS. Collateral circulation. Stroke 2003; 34:2279–84.

[2] Bisschops RH, Klijn CJ, Kappelle LJ, et al. Collateral flow and ischemic brain lesions in patients with unilateral carotid artery occlusion. Neurology 2003;60: 1435–41.

[3] Liebeskind DS. Neuroprotection from the collateral perspective. IDrugs 2005;8:222–8.

[4] Liebeskind DS. Anatomic considerations in therapeutic arteriogenesis for cerebral ischemia. Circulation 2004; 109:e4 [author reply: e4].

[5] Saqqur M, Demchuk AM, Hill MD, et al. Bedside emergency transcranial Doppler diagnosis of severe carotid disease using orbital window examination. J Neuroimaging 2005;15:138–43.

[6] Liebeskind DS, Sansing LH. Willisian collateralization. Neurology 2004;63:344.

[7] Liebeskind DS. Collateral therapeutics for cerebral ischemia. Expert Rev Neurother 2004;4:255–65.

[8] Liebeskind DS, Ances BM, Weigele JB, et al. Intravascular deoxygenation of leptomeningeal collaterals detected with gradient-echo MRI [abstract]. Stroke 2004;35:266.

[9] Selco SL, Liebeskind DS. Hyperacute imaging of ischemic stroke: role in therapeutic management. Curr Cardiol Rep 2005;7:10–5.

[10] Hossmann KA. Viability thresholds and the penumbra of focal ischemia. Ann Neurol 1994;36:557–65.

[11] Wong EH, Pullicino PM, Benedict R. Deep cerebral infarcts extending to the subinsular region. Stroke 2001;32:2272–7.

[12] Wojner-Alexander AW, Garami Z, Chernyshev OY, et al. Heads down: flat positioning improves blood flow velocity in acute ischemic stroke. Neurology 2005; 64:1354–7.

[13] Alexandrov AV, Felberg RA, Demchuk AM, et al. Deterioration following spontaneous improvement: sonographic findings in patients with acutely resolving symptoms of cerebral ischemia. Stroke 2000;31: 915–9.

[14] Kucinski T, Koch C, Eckert B, et al. Collateral circulation is an independent radiological predictor of outcome after thrombolysis in acute ischaemic stroke. Neuroradiology 2003;45:11–8.

[15] Yamauchi H, Kudoh T, Sugimoto K, et al. Pattern of collaterals, type of infarcts, and haemodynamic impairment in carotid artery occlusion. J Neurol Neurosurg Psychiatry 2004;75:1697–701.

[16] Higashida RT, Furlan AJ, Roberts H, et al. Trial design and reporting standards for intra-arterial cerebral thrombolysis for acute ischemic stroke. Stroke 2003; 34:e109–37.

[17] Liebeskind DS, Sayre JW, Weigele JB, et al. Angiographic collateral scales for intra-arterial thrombolysis [abstract]. In: Proceedings of the ASNR 42nd Annual Meeting, Seattle, 2004.

[18] Christou I, Felberg RA, Demchuk AM, et al. Intravenous tissue plasminogen activator and flow improvement in acute ischemic stroke patients with internal carotid artery occlusion. J Neuroimaging 2002; 12:119–23.

[19] Bendszus M, Urbach H, Ries F, et al. Outcome after local intra-arterial fibrinolysis compared with the natural course of patients with a dense middle cerebral artery on early CT. Neuroradiology 1998;40:54–8.

[20] Brandt T. Diagnosis and thrombolytic therapy of acute basilar artery occlusion: a review. Clin Exp Hypertens 2002;24:611–22.

[21] Kim HY, Chung CS, Moon SY, et al. Complete nonvisualization of basilar artery on MR angiography in patients with vertebrobasilar ischemic stroke: favorable outcome factors. Cerebrovasc Dis 2004;18: 269–76.

[22] Toni D, Fiorelli M, Bastianello S, et al. Acute ischemic strokes improving during the first 48 hours of onset: predictability, outcome, and possible mechanisms. A comparison with early deteriorating strokes. Stroke 1997;28:10–4.

[23] Rowley HA. The four Ps of acute stroke imaging: parenchyma, pipes, perfusion, and penumbra. AJNR Am J Neuroradiol 2001;22:599–601.

[24] Liebeskind DS, Hurst RW for the MERCI® Investigators. Angiographic collaterals and outcome in mechanical thrombolysis [abstract]. Stroke 2005;36:449.

[25] Kim JJ, Fischbein NJ, Lu Y, et al. Regional angiographic grading system for collateral flow: correlation with cerebral infarction in patients with middle cerebral artert occlusion. Stroke 2004;35:1340–4.

[26] Liebeskind DS, Hurst RW for the MERCI® Investigators. Clinical predictors of angiographic collaterals in acute ischemic stroke [abstract]. Stroke 2005; 36:450.

[27] Wessels T, Bozzato A, Mull M, et al. Intracranial collateral pathways assessed by contrast-enhanced

three-dimensional transcranial color-coded sonography. Ultrasound Med Biol 2004;30:1435–40.

[28] Koga M, Kimura K, Minematsu K, et al. Relationship between findings of conventional and contrast-enhanced transcranial color-coded real-time sonography and angiography in patients with basilar artery occlusion. AJNR Am J Neuroradiol 2002;23:568–71.

[29] Baumgartner RW, Baumgartner I, Mattle HP, et al. Transcranial color-coded duplex sonography in the evaluation of collateral flow through the circle of Willis. AJNR Am J Neuroradiol 1997;18:127–33.

[30] Hoksbergen AW, Majoie CB, Hulsmans FJ, et al. Assessment of the collateral function of the circle of Willis: three-dimensional time-of-flight MR angiography compared with transcranial color-coded duplex sonography. AJNR Am J Neuroradiol 2003;24:456–62.

[31] Krejza J, Baumgartner RW. Clinical applications of transcranial color-coded duplex sonography. J Neuroimaging 2004;14:215–25.

[32] Ringelstein EB, Weiller C, Weckesser M, et al. Cerebral vasomotor reactivity is significantly reduced in low-flow as compared to thromboembolic infarctions: the key role of the circle of Willis. J Neurol Sci 1994;121:103–9.

[33] Alexandrov AV, Molina CA, Grotta JC, et al. Ultrasound-enhanced systemic thrombolysis for acute ischemic stroke. N Engl J Med 2004;351:2170–8.

[34] Knauth M, von Kummer R, Jansen O, et al. Potential of CT angiography in acute ischemic stroke. AJNR Am J Neuroradiol 1997;18:1001–10.

[35] Schramm P, Schellinger PD, Fiebach JB, et al. Comparison of CT and CTA source images with diffusion-weighted imaging in patients with acute stroke within 6 hours after onset. Stroke 2002;33:2426–32.

[36] Roberts HC, Dillon WP, Furlan AJ, et al. Computed tomographic findings in patients undergoing intra-arterial thrombolysis for acute ischemic stroke due to middle cerebral artery occlusion: results from the PROACT II trial. Stroke 2002;33:1557–65.

[37] Liebeskind DS, Messe SR, Luciano JM, et al. A novel CT angiography scale for assessment of collaterals in acute stroke [abstract]. Stroke 2003;34:265.

[38] Grond M, Rudolf J, Schneweis S, et al. Feasibility of source images of computed tomographic angiography to detect the extent of ischemia in hyperacute stroke. Cerebrovasc Dis 2002;13:251–6.

[39] Liebeskind DS, Cucchiara BL, Kasner SE, et al. FLAIR MRI vascular hyperintensity reflects perfusion status in cerebral ischemia [abstract]. Presented at the 53rd Annual Meeting of the American Academy of Neurology. Philadelphia, 2001.

[40] Kamran S, Bates V, Bakshi R, et al. Significance of hyperintense vessels on FLAIR MRI in acute stroke. Neurology 2000;55:265–9.

[41] Liebeskind DS, Bemporad JA, Melhem ER. FLAIR vascular hyperintensity as a marker of leptomeningeal collaterals in subacute stroke [abstract]. In: Proceedings of the ASNR 41st Annual Meeting, Washington, D.C., 2003.

[42] Maeda M, Yamamoto T, Daimon S, et al. Arterial hyperintensity on fast fluid-attenuated inversion recovery images: a subtle finding for hyperacute stroke undetected by diffusion-weighted MR imaging. AJNR Am J Neuroradiol 2001;22:632–6.

[43] Patrick JT, Fritz JV, Adamo JM, et al. Phase-contrast magnetic resonance angiography for the determination of cerebrovascular reserve. J Neuroimaging 1996; 6:137–43.

[44] Liu Y, Karonen JO, Vanninen RL, et al. Acute ischemic stroke: predictive value of 2D phase-contrast MR angiography–serial study with combined diffusion and perfusion MR imaging. Radiology 2004;231:517–27.

[45] Liebeskind DS, Weigele JB, Hurst RW. Collateralization of the posterior cerebral artery. Stroke 2004; 35:266 [abstract].

[46] Uemura A, O'Uchi T, Kikuchi Y, et al. Prominent laterality of the PCA at three-dimensional time-of-flight MR angiography in M1-segment middle cerebral artery occlusion. AJNR Am J Neuroradiol 2004;25: 88–91.

[47] Lee JH, Han SJ, Kang WY, et al. Dominant ipsilateral posterior cerebral artery on magnetic resonance angiography in acute ischemic stroke. Cerebrovasc Dis 2004;18:91–7.

[48] Liebeskind DS, Krejza J, Hurst RW, et al. Willisian collateral circulation is not a determinant of infarct volume or infarct topography in middle cerebral artery stroke [abstract]. Proceedings of the ASNR 42nd Annual Meeting, Seattle, 2004.

[49] Taoka T, Iwasaki S, Nakagawa H, et al. Distinguishing between anterior cerebral artery and middle cerebral artery perfusion by color-coded perfusion direction mapping with arterial spin labeling. AJNR Am J Neuroradiol 2004;25:248–51.

[50] Davies NP, Jezzard P. Selective arterial spin labeling (SASL): perfusion territory mapping of selected feeding arteries tagged using two-dimensional radiofrequency pulses. Magn Reson Med 2003;49:1133–42.

ELSEVIER
SAUNDERS

Neuroimag Clin N Am 15 (2005) 575 – 587

NEUROIMAGING
CLINICS OF
NORTH AMERICA

Extending the Time Window for Thrombolysis: Evidence from Acute Stroke Trials

Howard A. Rowley, MD*

Department of Radiology, University of Wisconsin, Madison, WI, USA

Overview of risk–benefit factors in thrombolysis

The results of the pivotal intravenous tissue plasminogen activator (tPA) trials have been reported and its use approved for acute ischemic stroke treatment for nearly 10 years [1–3]. Although tPA has been clearly shown to improve neurologic outcome, it also has practical limitations when applied according to published guidelines using routine CT within a rigid 3-hour window. Only approximately one fifth of patients arrive within the 3-hour time cutoff, and half of these have other contraindications to tPA [4]. Unfortunately, we cannot help many more patients by simply trying to treat later using the same selection criteria; meta-analysis of large tPA trials has shown rapidly diminishing benefits beyond 3 hours, crossing over to no benefit after approximately 4.5 hours in group statistics [5]. Largely as a result of this brief 3-hour window and physician fear of postthrombolytic bleeding, only approximately 4% of stroke patients receive tPA in the United States today [4]. Clearly, we need better therapeutic strategies to attack a potentially fatal illness in which 96% of cases are left untreated or must be managed off-label.

A welcome trend in recent acute stroke treatment trials is the use of advanced imaging, particularly perfusion assessment, for acute treatment triage and follow-up [6]. Time and plain CT alone cannot predict the status of an individual patient's collateral pathways or ability to autoregulate, yet these are the

crucial determinants of neuronal death or survival in the first hours [7]. Every patient is different from his or her group, and imaging selection can help to distinguish the key individual physiologic features to help inform treatment decisions. Review of current stroke trials with time windows beyond 3 hours shows prominent use of advanced imaging to select patients and to assess intended effects of intervention (Table 1). Use of imaging parameters for patient selection and surrogate outcome measures is increasingly accepted by stroke trialists and regulatory bodies [8].

Imaging triage aims to select all the patients likely to benefit and to turn away those too risky to treat. Imaging therefore has two complementary selection roles: patient exclusion and patient inclusion. Exclusion tends to be more straightforward, with acute hemorrhage, nonstroke lesions (eg, tumor, infection), and, sometimes, extensive infarction usually viewed as standard contraindications to lytic agents. Inclusion criteria are more vigorously debated and, of course, depend on the expected risk–benefit profile of the intended thrombolytic drug or device itself. Nevertheless, many agree that the best target population may be those patients with a penumbral tissue-at-risk pattern identified on perfusion images [9]. In MR imaging, the perfusion-diffusion mismatch (a perfusion defect larger than the diffusion defect within it) helps to identify a logical tissue target for urgent revascularization. CT perfusion parameters have also been shown to provide similar information to help guide therapy [10,11]. Most patients imaged within several hours of stroke onset are found to have a penumbral pattern, and several case series have shown the potential utility of

* Department of Radiology, University of Wisconsin, 600 Highland Avenue, Box 3252, Madison, WI 53792.
  E-mail address: ha.rowley@hosp.wisc.edu

1052-5149/05/$ – see front matter © 2005 Elsevier Inc. All rights reserved.
doi:10.1016/j.nic.2005.08.002

Table 1
Currently active stroke trials beyond 3 hours

Trial acronym	Drug/device	Time range (h)	Imaging modality/selection	Description/comments
AbESTT-II	IV abciximab	<5 and 5–6 arms	Standard CT	Wake-up arm (3 h) stopped early (May 2005) due to safety concerns
DEFUSE	IV tPA (no control arm)	3–6	MR PWI-DWI mismatch	Open-label study
DIAS-2	IV desmoteplase	3–9	MR PWI-DWI or pCT mismatch	First randomized, placebo-controlled trial to use perfusion CT for selection.
EPITHET	IV tPA vs placebo	3–6	CT selection; PWI-DWI also obtained acutely	Treatment is given according to CT criteria, but MR data are also being collected. Will be key data regarding mismatch hypothesis. As of May 2005, 72 of 100 recruited.
IMS II	IV then IA tPA, assisted by EKOS (Bothell, Washington) ultrasound device	3 for IV, followed by IA for 2 h	CT, then conventional angiography	—
IST-3	IV tPA	3–6	CT or MR	Study begun in 2000, with plan to recruit 6000 subjects. As of May 2005, only 352 enrolled.
MR Rescue	IA concentric clot retriever	0–8	MR PWI-DWI mismatch	Early data show benefit for treatment when mismatch is present
ROSIE	IV abciximab and retaplase	3–24	One arm with CT, the other with MR PWI-DWI mismatch	Open label dose escalation design
SaTIS	IV tirofiban + tPA	6–22	Standard	Placebo-controlled, randomized

Abbreviations: AbESTT-II, Abciximab in Emergent Stroke Treatment Trial–II; DEFUSE, Diffusion-weighted imaging Evaluation For Understanding Stroke Evolution; DIAS-2, Desmoteplase in Acute Ischemic Stroke-2; EPITHET, Echoplanar Imaging Thrombolysis Evaluation Trial; IA, intra-arterial; IMS II, Interventional Management of Stroke Study; IST-3; Third International Stroke Trial; IV, intravenous; MR Rescue, MR and Recanalization of Stroke Clots Using Embolectomy; ROSIE, ReoPro Retavase Reperfusion of Stroke Safety Study–Imaging Evaluation; SaTIS, Safety of Tirofiban in Acute Ischemic Stroke.
Data from The Internet Stroke Center. Stroke Trials Directory. Available at: http://www.strokecenter.org/trials. Accessed June 11, 2005. [Supplemented by recent meeting presentations and personal correspondence with several of the trialists.]

imaging-based selection to improve outcomes in thrombolysis [12–14].

The intra-arterial Prolyse in Acute Cerebral Thromboembolism (PROACT) II trial was the first randomized placebo-controlled trial to show benefit for thrombolysis at the 3- to 6-hour time window [15]. Excellent recanalization rates (66% versus 18% control), positive clinical outcomes (40% versus 25% control), and acceptable symptomatic intracranial hemorrhage rates (10% versus 2% control) were observed after intra-arterial therapy. Because of the small sample size and other factors, however, the experimental drug used in the PROACT II trial has not been cleared to the market. Nonetheless, this trial was important in showing the potential to treat severely affected stroke patients successfully at time points beyond 3 hours using advanced imaging selection and effective thrombolysis.

The recently completed sister trials, Desmoteplase in Acute Ischemic Stroke (DIAS) and the Dose Escalation Study of Desmoteplase in Acute Ischemic Stroke (DEDAS), successfully stretched the treatment window to 3 to 9 hours using a novel intravenous thrombolytic drug and MR imaging–based selection [16,17]. The fibrinolytic drug used in these trials, desmoteplase, was originally isolated from vampire bats (who have apparently engineered the compound to their evolutionary advantage). Now made by recombinant techniques, desmoteplase has a number of favorable pharmacologic properties: it is a highly fibrin-specific plasminogen activator, is not activated by β-amyloid, and has a long half-life (~4–5 hours), allowing it to be given by single bolus instead of infusion. Selection in the DIAS and DEDAS trials was based on a perfusion-diffusion mismatch, defined as a perfusion defect visually 20% larger than the diffusion defect. The perfusion defect needed to be at least 2 cm in diameter and to involve cortex. The simplest and most sensitive perfusion metric was used for these trials—the dynamic time course reflected by mean transit time (MTT) or time to peak image (TTP) maps, or even simple visual inspection of the raw dynamic perfusion data set. MR angiography recanalization (Thrombolysis in Myocardial Infarction [TIMI] scale improvement by 2 points) or perfusion parameter improvement (MTT volume reduction by at least 30%) was used to assess reperfusion. High reperfusion rates (46.7%–71.4% versus 19.2% control), positive clinical outcomes (46.7%– 60% versus 22.2% control), and low symptomatic bleeding rates (less than 3%) were found for the weight-adjusted dose tiers at 90- and 125-µg/kg levels in the DIAS trial. Of particular note, the volume of the baseline diffusion lesion partially reversed at follow-up in the 125-µg/kg group [18]. This raises the question of whether even perfusion-diffusion–matched patients might also stand to gain from acute reperfusion. The favorable results from the DIAS and DEDAS trials have led to a new trial, DIAS-2, which is scheduled to start recruiting subjects in the middle of 2005 [19]. The DIAS-2 trial is expected to include centers using either perfusion-weighted imaging (PWI)–diffusion-weighted imaging (DWI) mismatch or perfusion CT mismatch criteria for patient selection.

More details related to patient and imaging factors that need to be taken into account when selecting and following patients for thrombolysis protocols at time points beyond 3 hours are reviewed next. Comprehensive CT and MR imaging protocols can be designed to drive the triage process and measure treatment outcomes. A bird's-eye view of these factors and their imaging implications is given in Fig. 1.

Patient-specific factors

In the emergency stroke triage setting, most of the patient-specific factors are preexisting and cannot be controlled by the treating physician. These factors still need to be considered to understand individual patient risk profiles, particularly at later treatment windows. When only routine CT is used for intravenous tPA screening, duration of symptoms is the key determinant of risk–benefit, with benefit rapidly declining after 3 hours and approaching parity at approximately 4.5 hours [20]. Regardless of the time point or route of drug delivery, older age, more severe baseline stroke deficits (high National Institutes of Health [NIH] Stroke Scale score), and elevated serum

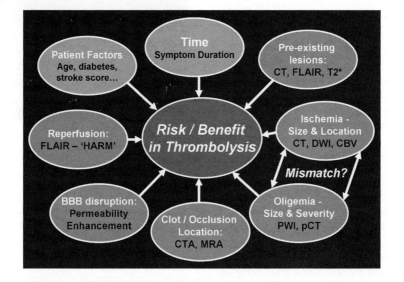

Fig. 1. Overview of risk–benefit considerations in urgent stroke thrombolysis. Primary prevention and stroke awareness can improve some patient-specific risk factors and time to presentation. Most new treatment algorithms beyond 3 hours are driven by individualized physiologic data obtained from comprehensive CT or MR imaging protocols, however. CBV, cerebral blood volume; HARM, hyperacute reperfusion marker; FLAIR, fluid-attenuated inversion recovery; MRA, MR angiography; pCT, perfusion CT.

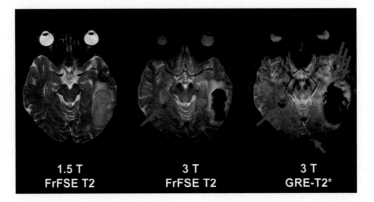

Fig. 2. Amyloid angiopathy and acute and chronic hemorrhage. Detection with T2* sequences. Images done with a fast spin echo (FSE) technique at 1.5 T show an acute isointense left temporal lobar hematoma with scant surrounding edema. At 3 T later the same day, the inherently greater T2* susceptibility effects at higher field strength show more signal dropout within the intracellular deoxyhemoglobin of the clot and also show a second small focus of older blood in the right temporal lobe (*arrow*). At 3 T with a gradient echo–recalled (GRE) T2* sequence, additional lesions are seen (*arrows*), compatible with older microbleeds related to amyloid.

glucose levels have all been found to confer poor outcome or higher risk when thrombolysis is undertaken. Primary prevention, public education about stroke warning signs (brain attack), improved emergency response systems, and stroke teams can all help to improve the profile of the community and individual patient factors over time.

Preexisting lesions

Imaging is required to confirm the diagnosis of ischemic stroke, rule out other lesions, and exclude hemorrhage. One special preexisting lesion of considerable current interest is the amyloid-related cerebral microhemorrhage, or microbleed. These lesions are characterized by amyloid deposition in small arteries. They have been linked to recurrent ischemic stroke, lobar hemorrhage, and advanced white matter disease [21–23]. Incidence and multiplicity increase sharply with each decade after the age of 60 years. CT cannot detect microbleeds, so these were never part of the original selection criteria for tPA. More widespread use of MR imaging for treatment triage has made it possible, even inevitable, that such lesions are seen during thrombolysis triage examinations. Microbleeds contain hemosiderin and are therefore best seen on gradient echo–recalled T2* MR imaging [24] and at higher field strengths (Fig. 2). Anecdotal reports have linked postthrombolytic hemorrhage to preexisting amyloid, but the risk is likely to be low (perhaps < 1%) based on data from large myocardial thrombolysis trials [25]. The risk may also vary according to the method of thromboly-

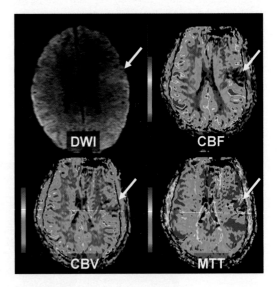

Fig. 3. Early ischemic changes of Broca's aphasia (*arrows*), seen more conspicuously with PWI than with DWI. This 55-year-old man developed sudden expressive aphasia later determined to be from a cardiogenic source. Emergent routine CT at another hospital was normal. On evaluation at our hospital at approximately 3 hours, there was persistent severe aphasia, but symptoms had already improved. MR imaging done at 3.5 hours shows a subtle DWI lesion in the inferior left frontal operculum with a slightly larger PWI defect (long transit times, low blood flow) surrounding it. Cortical cerebral blood volume (CBV) values are at or slightly below those of normal white matter, likely near the threshold for infarction. He was treated with heparin and then abciximab, with further improvement over the next 3 days. At 1 month, he had fully recovered. CBF, cerebral blood flow.

sis and the extent to which the specific lytic agent is activated by amyloid. Whether the size, number, or even presence of microhemorrhages should be taken into account in screening patients for thrombolysis is unclear. Our own approach is to inform the patients that they may possibly be at somewhat higher risk if they have known microbleeds, but we do not exclude them from thrombolysis based on this factor alone.

Characteristics of the ischemic lesion

Size, location, and severity of the ischemic lesion are the key characteristics to determine, whether by CT or MR imaging. CT has the advantage of speed and availability, whereas diffusion MR imaging is more sensitive for detection of acute ischemia and shows higher interobserver agreement (Fig. 3) [26]. On CT, acute ischemia is detected as decreased density or decreased gray-white distinction on CT images, CT angiography (CTA) source data, or other enhanced CT images. On MR imaging, hyperintense DWI signal, decreased apparent diffusion coefficient (ADC) values, and later increased T2/T2 fluid-attenuated inversion recovery (FLAIR) signal all indicate ischemic injury (Figs. 4 and 5). These signs likely reflect shifts of water content attributable to

cytotoxic edema and, possibly, critically low blood volume as well [27–29]. Larger lesions with more severe decreases in CT density or ADC values generally predict poor outcome and also greater likelihood of significant hemorrhage [30–33]. Simple qualitative assessment of DWI and ADC images seems to work as well as more advanced pixel-based analysis, likely because of heterogeneity within the diffusion lesion [34]. The size and severity of the baseline imaging lesion influence outcome, assuming no treatment is given. Location with respect to eloquent areas also clearly influences functional status. Such morphologic and functional features can be combined into multiparametric risk hazard maps to help account for involvement of eloquent territories [35].

Characteristics of the perfusion deficit

Just as for the ischemic lesion discussed previously, the key perfusion characteristics to evaluate are size, location, and severity. Armed with this knowledge, an assessment of the penumbra can then be made (ie, PWI-DWI mismatch). With CT or MR imaging perfusion techniques, ischemic tissue typically shows prolonged MTT or TTP, decreased over-

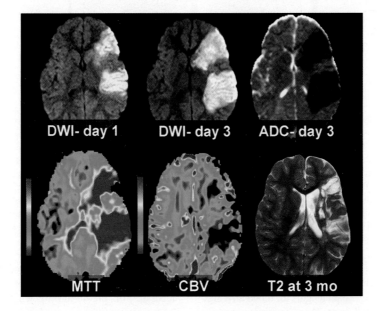

Fig. 4. Prediction of infarction based on acute PWI-DWI features. This 4-year-old girl with moyamoya syndrome suffered acute embolic infarctions related to left supraclinoid carotid artery stenosis. Although qualitative unthresholded MTT maps tend to overestimate tissue at risk, the DWI lesion expands into the MTT abnormality during supportive care on days 1 through 3. Severely decreased ADC and markedly low CBV are good predictors of follow-up infarction territory when no definitive intervention is undertaken. The patient later underwent an encephaloduroarteriosynangiosis bypass procedure. CBV, cerebral blood volume.

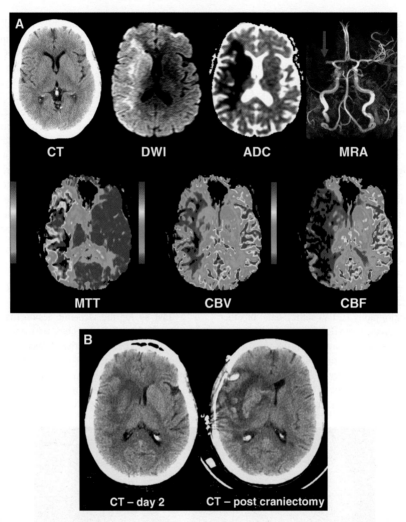

Fig. 5. Natural history of a large cardiac embolism with hemorrhagic transformation. This 55-year-old woman had undergone cardiac transplantation 1 month earlier because of constrictive pericardial disease. (*A*) While still hospitalized, she developed acute left hemiplegia. CT at 1 hour shows subtle fogging of the right lentiform nucleus, confirmed by diffusion at 5 hours. There is proximal M1 middle cerebral artery (MCA) occlusion by MR angiography and severe uncompensated perfusion defects in the entire right MCA territory. Because of the size and matched nature of the DWI-PWI lesion as well as recent cardiac surgery, she was not treated with thrombolytic drugs or heparin. (*B*) Follow-up CT scan at day 2 shows edema and mass effect in the deep right hemisphere, with the morphologic pattern resembling the most severe PWI reductions seen at baseline (*A*). The patient then developed symptomatic hemorrhagic transformation and uncal herniation, prompting an urgent craniectomy later that day. Malignant edema and symptomatic hemorrhage are fairly common in the natural evolution of large embolic strokes and are likely related to recanalization into infarcted tissue.

all cerebral blood flow (CBF), and variable cerebral blood volume (CBV). The dynamic maps (MTT or TTP) reflect the longer path lengths for blood arriving through collateral pathways. These dynamic maps are the most sensitive for detection of tissue being perfused in an abnormal way but tend to overestimate tissue at risk of actual infarction, because some portion may be well compensated [36]. Application of deconvolution techniques and longer time thresh-

olds (eg, MTT or T-max 6–8 seconds longer than that of normal tissue) makes these maps more specific and accurate for prediction of what is destined to infarction. It can be argued that preserved sensitivity is a good feature when detecting abnormal blood delivery, however [37]. Because the explicit intent of acute treatment is to intervene and reverse the defect, a more precise predictive threshold may not be required for routine management. This is an important point—many of us in the field (laudably, we hope) debate the fine details of various dynamic perfusion parameter maps, thresholds, choice of arterial input function, and deconvolution methods, for example, yet the simplest gross dynamic maps or even visual inspection or raw PWI image loops were sufficient in the DIAS and DEDAS trials to select patients with penumbra successfully (Fig. 6). Fast and simple methods are a good choice when they work.

The CBV gives a snapshot of autoregulatory status. Assuming there is still proximal occlusion, the precapillary arterioles dilate to help compensate and preserve CBF (through the central volume principle: CBF = CBV/MTT). Elevated CBV within an area of prolonged MTT thus suggests preserved autoregulation. Once perfusion pressure becomes insufficient to support the elevated volume, however, the vascular bed collapses and CBV falls precipitously. When CBV is severely depressed, it therefore indicates severely ischemic core tissue likely to undergo infarction [38]. Low CBV can predict not only poor outcome for that tissue but higher likelihood of hemorrhagic transformation (HT) if the tissue is reperfused. As a practical matter, low CBV may provide the perfusion CT equivalent of diffusion in MR

imaging. Wintermark and colleagues [39] have shown high correlations between low CBV on perfusion CT and DWI in acute stroke patients imaged in tandem fashion. Wintermark and coworkers [40] have also studied series of acute stroke patients and proposed that CT perfusion parameters, including a long MTT (>1.45 compared with the opposite) and low CBV (<2 mL per 100 g) may predict tissue destined to infarction. Mismatches based on low cortical CBV (approximately less than normal white matter) and larger surrounding CBF or MTT defects may provide the practical CT correlate of PWI-DWI mismatch.

The predictive value of any imaging parameter, of course, depends on whether the study evaluates good or poor outcome or hemorrhage (symptomatic or not) as well as on whether the series is drawn from patients treated with conservative therapy (natural history) versus cases treated with thrombolytic drugs. As a general guideline, MTT tends to overestimate tissue at risk, CBV tends to underestimate risk, and CBF is somewhere in between. Among patients who did not receive thrombolytics, several studies have shown that relative CBF values are good predictors of tissue viability versus infarction [41–43]. Others

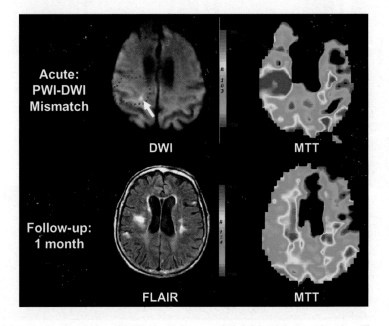

Fig. 6. DEDAS trial patient enrolled with an NIH Stroke Scale score of 13, left hemiplegia, and neglect. The acute scan, done at 5.5 hours, shows a small DWI lesion near the motor strip (*arrow*), surrounded by a larger area of presumed tissue at risk on MTT maps (abnormal perfusion shown on DWI as dotted region for comparison). After randomized treatment (intravenous placebo versus desmoteplase), follow-up images show small areas of ischemic change in the cortical and subcortical regions, with normalization of acute right-sided cortical perfusion defects. Slightly long transit times are still seen in the central white matter, a common finding in patients with chronic gliosis. At 90 days, the patient was doing well, with only minimal residual weakness (NIH Stroke Scale score of 1).

have found that TTP prolongations of approximately 4 to 5 seconds, peak height less than 54% [44], and more severe ADC lesions are predictors of lesion growth or malignant edema [45].

The value of perfusion parameters needs to be reconsidered when dealing with patients treated with thrombolytics or other urgent revascularization. Here, the intent is to interfere with natural history and forestall damage; therefore, predictive models based on conservatively treated patients do not fully apply. The main role may be in selecting patients, with risk prediction considered a secondary but related goal. CT and MR imaging protocols have been used to relate lesion volumes to successful recanalization [46]. Series have shown perfusion parameters to be a strong predictor of late infarct volume (TTP), irreversible core (T-max), and lesion growth (low CBF) [47–49]. These topics have been reviewed recently in an excellent article by Butcher [50] based on the initial 40 patients in the Echoplanar Imaging

Thrombolysis Evaluation Trial (EPITHET) database. A state-of-the-art multicenter review of experience in developing MR imaging criteria for thrombolysis, including site-specific protocols, is available from Hjort [51].

Site of vascular occlusion

CT signs of occlusion include the hyperdense artery sign and truncation of contrast on the CTA source or reconstructed images. MR imaging signs of occlusion include the T2* clot sign, MR angiography occlusion, and stasis on FLAIR or postgadolinium series. The site of occlusion can help to determine the stroke mechanism, influence prognosis, and assist in the decision to treat using an intravenous versus intra-arterial route (Fig. 7). Although routine MR imaging signs related to vessel occlusion are helpful from a diagnostic standpoint, they generally do

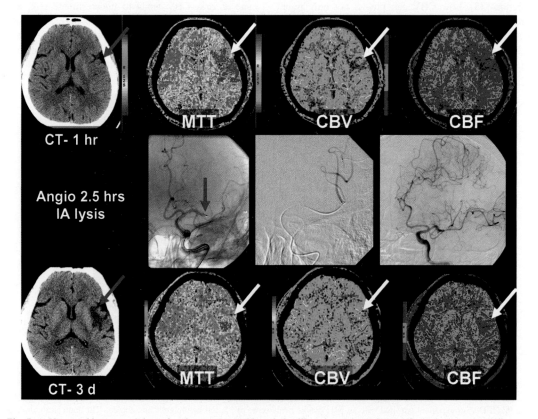

Fig. 7. A 58-year-old woman, 6 days after thoracotomy, with an indwelling chest tube and runs of ventricular tachycardia, now with sudden onset of aphasia and right hemiplegia. Emergent CT shows subtle left opercular edema (*red arrow*) and a much larger middle cerebral artery (MCA) territory perfusion defect (*white arrows*). At angiography, a distal mainstem MCA occlusion was confirmed (*red arrow*) and opened with intra-arterial tPA. At follow-up, there is limited insular infarction (*red arrow*), the perfusion defect has shrunk dramatically (*white arrows*), and the patient has recovered function. IA, intra-arterial; 3 d, three-dimensional. (Case courtesy of Brant-Zawadzki, MD, Newport Beach, CA.)

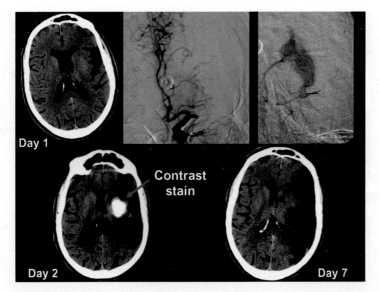

Fig. 8. Post–intra-arterial thrombolytic scans. This patient with acute right hemiparesis and aphasia was found to have a large MCA embolism in the proximal M1 segment. During attempted but unsuccessful thrombolysis, a prominent contrast blush is seen in the lenticulostriate territory. At follow-up, a dense lesion is seen in the lentiform nucleus in the midst of evolving total MCA infarction. This marked density reflects BBB disruption, with retention of contrast (staining) in the ischemic parenchyma (*arrow*). Although hemorrhage can also occur, this confluent marked density should not be confused with blood. Follow-up at 7 days shows resolution of the contrast stain, with only scant HT (HT1).

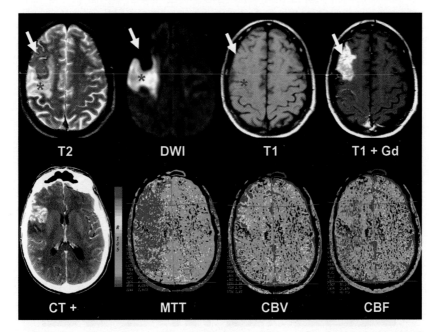

Fig. 9. Recurrent infarction, with baseline parenchymal enhancement. This man first developed symptoms 3 weeks before presentation but did not seek attention until progressive left hemiparesis developed 2 days before admission. (*Top row*) MR imaging findings at admission: an acute nonenhancing infarction (*) that borders a subacute enhancing infarction. Gd, gadolinium. (*Lower row*) CT the following day confirms enhancing and nonenhancing components within an even larger area of prolonged MTT. The acute infarction shows low blood flow and volumes that are matched or smaller than the new infarction. This patient is not a good candidate for thrombolysis because of the late presentation and enhancing parenchyma, both of which increase the risk of post-tPA hemorrhage.

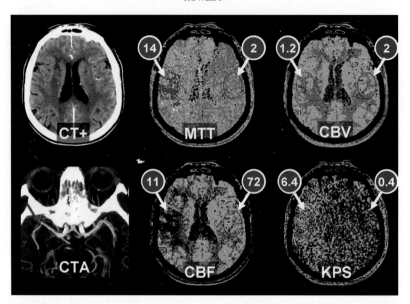

Fig. 10. CT characterization of ischemia, including BBB permeability assessment. This 86-year-old woman had a stroke with residual left hand numbness 3 months earlier. She was referred for CT because of intermittent worsening in left-sided symptoms. There are ischemic white matter changes in the right frontal white matter but no large infarction or parenchymal enhancement. CTA shows tight stenosis of the distal right M1 to M2 MCA junction (*arrows*). Routine perfusion maps show significant resting oligemia, with a long MTT (seconds), slightly low CBV (mL per 100 g), and low CBF (mL per 100 g/min). Even though there is no parenchymal enhancement, the estimated permeability capillary surface product map (mL per 100 g/min) shows striking focal elevation of permeability in the same territory. Such maps indicate a damaged BBB, and thus a possibly higher risk of hemorrhage or edema after revascularization. The patient has been maintained on medical therapy without symptomatic infarct extension or bleeding.

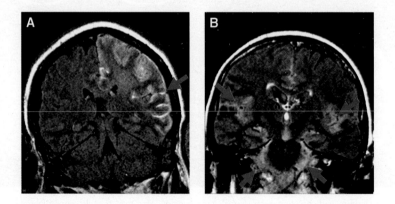

Fig. 11. Retention of gadolinium within subarachnoid spaces. (*A*) Postthrombolysis HARM pattern showing high signal confined to the subarachnoid spaces of the recently ischemic territory. This should be distinguished from many other causes of high FLAIR sulcal signal, such as slow flow, meningitis, vasculitis, high protein content, supplemental oxygen, subarachnoid hemorrhage, and delayed clearance of contrast in the setting of renal failure. (*B*) Retained contrast in a patient with renal insufficiency and history of high-dose gadolinium MR angiography the day before his brain MR imaging. Note the more diffuse pattern throughout the cisterns and ventricles.

not have useful prognostic value for patients treated with tPA [52]. Patients with carotid "T" occlusions tend to do poorly even with aggressive thrombolysis. Proximal middle cerebral artery (MCA) occlusions may only show sustained recanalization in 13% of intravenous tPA-treated subjects [53], prompting some centers to pursue intra-arterial treatment or serial intravenous–intra-arterial combination protocols.

Status of the blood-brain barrier

Although the primary focus of imaging has been directed to the brain parenchyma and perfusion, the status of the blood-brain barrier (BBB) is critical to consider in controlling the risk of late thrombolysis. As reviewed by del Zoppo and his colleagues [54,55], cerebral microvessels undergo progressive ischemic injury in the minutes and hours after occlusion or reperfusion. This may contribute to no reflow phenomena as well as to a variety of manifestations of BBB disruption. Manifestations of BBB dysfunction depend on the severity of injury and status of reperfusion. The injured BBB can leak fluid, contrast material, or blood (Figs. 5, 8, and 9). Perfusion studies may also indicate loss of vasomotor tone and autoregulation, such as luxury perfusion patterns, as would be expected from animal data [56,57].

The finding of parenchymal enhancement at pretreatment baseline seems to be a particularly strong predictor of subsequent hemorrhage after thrombolysis [58–60]. This makes intuitive sense: an already leaky BBB likely indicates severe ischemic endothelial and tight junction damage, a substrate for reperfusion bleeding. Whether this finding should become an exclusion criterion for thrombolysis trials awaits further study.

Kassner and colleagues [61] have recently reported a series of patients in whom MR imaging–based permeability measurements were obtained in the triage of acute stroke patients who later received intravenous tPA. They were able to demonstrate focal elevations of permeability within the centers of the diffusion defects, and abnormal permeability changes were correlated with later HT. Roberts and coworkers [61] have suggested that this may be the core of the core—the most ischemic part of the diffusion lesion. Of note, tPA itself has been linked to neuronal injury and endothelial damage, so it may paradoxically contribute to this change [62].

Permeability maps can also be obtained with dynamic CT methods [63]. Our early experience has shown that some patients demonstrate abnormal permeability patterns related to ischemia (Fig. 10). These results are quite preliminary but suggest a potential role for permeability assessment in the assessment of the BBB and potential risk after thrombolysis.

Vessel recanalization and tissue reperfusion

Vessel recanalization can be judged by CTA or MR angiography, whereas related tissue reperfusion is judged by follow-up perfusion studies. Such metrics are highly correlated with recovery: among the possible parenchymal and perfusion parameters, MTT improvements after thrombolysis are the best imaging predictors of good outcome [8]. HT is common after tPA, but is usually petechial and asymptomatic. In fact, some series have shown that HT in the setting of tPA is actually a favorable prognostic sign and is linked to early recanalization [64]. The key morphologic-functional point to consider is whether the hemorrhage is petechial and confined to the ischemic territory (likely of no consequence) versus the rarer occurrence of a parenchymal hematoma with mass effect and neurologic decline.

One recently reported sign related to reperfusion and BBB disruption has been dubbed HARM— hyperintense acute reperfusion marker (Fig. 11) [65,66]. This consists of hyperintense signal on T2 FLAIR images after thrombolysis. It is only seen when gadolinium has been given but is not detected on routine T1-weighted images. In analysis of small case series, HARM was associated with HT and worse clinical outcomes. These findings suggest that the HARM pattern is caused by leakage of gadolinium from injured vascular beds. Although HARM is seen after the fact, when detected, it could potentially help to guide closer surveillance for blood pressure management.

References

[1] Hacke W, Kaste M, Fieschi C, et al. Intravenous thrombolysis with recombinant tissue plasminogen activator for acute hemispheric stroke. The European Cooperative Acute Stroke Study (ECASS). JAMA 1995;274(13):1017–25.

[2] Hacke W, Kaste M, Fieschi C, et al. Randomised double-blind placebo-controlled trial of thrombolytic therapy with intravenous alteplase in acute ischaemic stroke (ECASS II). Second European-Australasian Acute Stroke Study Investigators. Lancet 1998;352(9136): 1245–51.

[3] Group NS. Tissue plasminogen activator for acute

ischemic stroke. The National Institute of Neurological Disorders and Stroke rt-PA Stroke Study Group. N Engl J Med 1995;333(24):1581–7.

[4] Kleindorfer D, Kissela B, Schneider A, et al. Eligibility for recombinant tissue plasminogen activator in acute ischemic stroke: a population-based study. Stroke 2004;35(2):E27–9.

[5] Hacke W, Donnan G, Fieschi C, et al. Association of outcome with early stroke treatment: pooled analysis of ATLANTIS, ECASS, and NINDS rt-PA stroke trials. Lancet 2004;363(9411):768–74.

[6] Warach S. Thrombolysis in stroke beyond three hours: targeting patients with diffusion and perfusion MRI. Ann Neurol 2002;51(1):11–3.

[7] Liebeskind DS. Collateral circulation. Stroke 2003; 34(9):2279–84.

[8] Chalela JA, Kang DW, Luby M, et al. Early magnetic resonance imaging findings in patients receiving tissue plasminogen activator predict outcome: insights into the pathophysiology of acute stroke in the thrombolysis era. Ann Neurol 2004;55(1):105–12.

[9] Warach S. Measurement of the ischemic penumbra with MRI: it's about time. Stroke 2003;34(10):2533–4.

[10] Lev MH, Koroshetz WJ, Schwamm LH, et al. CT or MRI for imaging patients with acute stroke: visualization of "tissue at risk"? Stroke 2002;33(12):2736–7.

[11] Wintermark M, Bogousslavsky J. Imaging of acute ischemic brain injury: the return of computed tomography. Curr Opin Neurol 2003;16(1):59–63.

[12] Parsons MW, Barber PA, Chalk J, et al. Diffusion- and perfusion-weighted MRI response to thrombolysis in stroke. Ann Neurol 2002;51(1):28–37.

[13] Butcher KS. Perfusion thresholds in acute stroke thrombolysis. Stroke 2003;34:2159–64.

[14] Rother J. Effect of intravenous thrombolysis on MRI parameters and functional outcome in acute stroke <6 hours. Stroke 2002;33:2438–45.

[15] Furlan A, Higashida R, Wechsler L, et al. Intra-arterial prourokinase for acute ischemic stroke. The PROACT II study: a randomized controlled trial. Prolyse in Acute Cerebral Thromboembolism. JAMA 1999; 282(21):2003–11.

[16] Hacke W, Albers G, Al-Rawi Y, et al. The Desmoteplase in Acute Ischemic Stroke Trial (DIAS): a phase II MRI-based 9-hour window acute stroke thrombolysis trial with intravenous desmoteplase. Stroke 2005; 36(1):66–73.

[17] Rowley H. Successful patient selection with DWPW-MRI for IV treatment with desmoteplase at 3–9 hours: DIAS and DEDAS trial results. Presented at the American Society of Neuroradiology Meeting. Toronto, Ontario, Canada, May 21–27, 2005.

[18] Warach S. Early reperfusion related to clinical response in DIAS: phase II, randomized, placebo-controlled dose finding trial of IV desmoteplase 3–9 hours from onset in patients with diffusion-perfusion mismatch. Presented at the American Stroke Association Meeting. San Diego, California, February 5–7, 2004.

[19] The Internet Stroke Center. Stroke Trials Directory. Available at: http://www.strokecenter.org/trials. Accessed June 11, 2005.

[20] Hacke W. Association of outcome with early stroke treatment: pooled analysis of ATLANTIS, ECASS, and NINDS rt-PA stroke trials. Lancet 2004;363:768–74.

[21] Naka H, Nomura E, Wakabayashi S, et al. Frequency of asymptomatic microbleeds on T2*-weighted MR images of patients with recurrent stroke: association with combination of stroke subtypes and leukoariosis. AJNR Am J Neuroradiol 2004;25(5):714–9.

[22] Fan YH, Zhang L, Lam WWM, et al. Cerebral microbleeds as a risk factor for subsequent intracerebral hemorrhages among patients with acute ischemic stroke. Stroke 2003;34(10):2459–62.

[23] Nighoghossian N, Hermier M, Adeleine P, et al. Old microbleeds are a potential risk factor for cerebral bleeding after ischemic stroke: a gradient-echo T2*-weighted brain MRI study. Stroke 2002;33(3):735–42.

[24] Kidwell CS, Chalela JA, Saver JL, et al. Comparison of MRI and CT for detection of acute intracerebral hemorrhage. JAMA 2004;292(15):1823–30.

[25] McCarron MO, Nicoll JA. Cerebral amyloid angiopathy and thrombolysis related intracerebral haemorrhage. Lancet Neurol 2004;3:484–92.

[26] Fiebach JB, Schellinger PD, Jansen O, et al. CT and diffusion-weighted MR imaging in randomized order. Stroke 2002;33(9):2206–10.

[27] Zimmerman RD. Stroke wars: episode IV CT strikes back. AJNR Am J Neuroradiol 2004;25(8):1304–9.

[28] Grond M, von Kummer R, Sobesky J, et al. Early x-ray hypoattenuation of brain parenchyma indicates extended critical hypoperfusion in acute stroke. Stroke 2000;31(1):133–9.

[29] Dzialowski I, Weber J, Doerfler A, et al. Brain tissue water uptake after middle cerebral artery occlusion assessed with CT. J Neuroimaging 2004;14(1):42–8.

[30] Tong DC, Adami A, Moseley ME, et al. Prediction of hemorrhagic transformation following acute stroke: role of diffusion- and perfusion-weighted magnetic resonance imaging. Arch Neurol 2001;58(4):587–93.

[31] Oppenheim C, Grandin C, Samson Y, et al. Is there an apparent diffusion coefficient threshold in predicting tissue viability in hyperacute stroke? Stroke 2001; 32(11):2486–91.

[32] von Kummer R. Early major ischemic changes on computed tomography should preclude use of tissue plasminogen activator. Stroke 2003;34(3):820–1.

[33] Selim M. Predictors of hemorrhagic transformation after intravenous recombinant tissue plasminogen activator. Stroke 2002;33:2047–52.

[34] Na DG. Diffusion-weighted MR imaging in acute ischemia: value of apparent diffusion coefficient and signal intensity thresholds in predicting tissue at risk and final infarct size. AJNR Am J Neuroradiol 2004; 25:1331–6.

[35] Wu O, Koroshetz WJ, Ostergaard L, et al. Predicting

tissue outcome in acute human cerebral ischemia using combined diffusion- and perfusion-weighted MR imaging. Stroke 2001;32(4):933–42.

[36] Rowley HA, Roberts TP. Clinical perspectives in perfusion: neuroradiologic applications. Top Magn Reson Imaging 2004;15(1):28–40.

[37] Carroll TJ, Rowley HA, Haughton VM. Automatic calculation of the arterial input function for cerebral perfusion imaging with MR imaging. Radiology 2003; 227(2):593–600.

[38] Kucinski T, Naumann D, Knab R, et al. Tissue at risk is overestimated in perfusion-weighted imaging: MR imaging in acute stroke patients without vessel recanalization. AJNR Am J Neuroradiol 2005;26(4):815–9.

[39] Wintermark M, Reichhart M, Cuisenaire O, et al. Comparison of admission perfusion computed tomography and qualitative diffusion- and perfusion-weighted magnetic resonance imaging in acute stroke patients. Stroke 2002;33(8):2025–31.

[40] Wintermark M, Flanders AE, Velthuis B, et al. Perfusion CT evaluation of cerebral vascular autoregulation in a large series of acute stroke patients. Presented at the American Society of Neuroradiology Meeting. Toronto, Ontario, Canada, May 21–27, 2005.

[41] Parsons M. Perfusion magnetic resonance imaging maps in hyperacute stroke. Stroke 2001;32:1581–7.

[42] Rohl L. Viability thresholds of ischemic penumbra of hyperacute stroke defined by perfusion-weighted MRI and apparent diffusion coefficient. Stroke 2001;32: 1140–6.

[43] Schaefer PW. Assessing tissue viability with MR diffusion and perfusion imaging. AJNR Am J Neuroradiol 2003;24:436–43.

[44] Grandlin C. Which MR-derived perfusion parameters are the best predictors of infarct growth in hyperacute stroke? Comparative study between relative and quantitative measurements. Radiology 2002;223:361–70.

[45] Thomalla GJ, Kucinski T, Schoder V, et al. Prediction of malignant middle cerebral artery infarction by early perfusion- and diffusion-weighted magnetic resonance imaging. Stroke 2003;34(8):1892–9.

[46] Lev MH. Utility of perfusion-weighted CT imaging in acute middle cerebral artery stroke treated with intraarterial thrombolysis. Stroke 2001;32:2021–8.

[47] Hermier M. Early magnetic resonance imaging prediction of arterial recanalization and late infarct volume in acute carotid artery stroke. J Cereb Blood Flow Metab 2003;23:240–8.

[48] Shih L. Perfusion-weighted magnetic resonance imaging thresholds identifying core, irreversibly infarcted tissue. Stroke 2003;34:1425–30.

[49] Fiehler J. Cerebral blood flow predicts lesion growth in acute stroke patients. Stroke 2002;33:2421–5.

[50] Butcher KS. Refining the perfusion-diffusion mismatch hypothesis. Stroke 2005;36:1153–9.

[51] Hjort N. Magnetic resonance imaging criteria for thrombolysis in acute cerebral infarct. Stroke 2005; 36:388–97.

[52] Schellinger PD, Chalela JA, Kang DW, et al. Diagnostic and prognostic value of early MR imaging vessel signs in hyperacute stroke patients imaged <3 hours and treated with recombinant tissue plasminogen activator. AJNR Am J Neuroradiol 2005;26(3): 618–24.

[53] Alexandrov A. Ultrasound-enhanced systemic thrombolysis. N Engl J Med 2004;351(21):2170–8.

[54] del Zoppo GJ. Cerebral microvessel response to focal ischemia. J Cereb Blood Flow Metab 2003;23: 879–94.

[55] del Zoppo GJ, von Kummer R, Hamann GF. Ischaemic damage of brain microvessels: inherent risks for thrombolytic treatment in stroke. J Neurol Neurosurg Psychiatry 1998;65(1):1–9.

[56] Cipolla MJ, Curry AB. Middle cerebral artery function after stroke: the threshold duration of reperfusion for myogenic activity. Stroke 2002;33(8):2094–9.

[57] Cipolla MJ, Lessov N, Clark WM, et al. Postischemic attenuation of cerebral artery reactivity is increased in the presence of tissue plasminogen activator [editorial comment]. Stroke 2000;31(4):940–5.

[58] Knight RA. Prediction of impending hemorrhage transformation in ischemic stroke using magnetic resonance imaging in rats. Stroke 1998;29:144–51.

[59] Neumann-Haefelin C. Prediction of hemorrhagic transformation after thrombolytic therapy of clot embolism. Stroke 2002;33:1392–8.

[60] Vo K. MR imaging enhancement patterns as predictors of hemorrhagic transformation in acute ischemia stroke. AJNR Am J Neuroradiol 2003;24:674–9.

[61] Kassner A, Roberts TP, Taylor K, et al. Prediction of hemorrhagic transformation of acute ischemic stroke using dynamic contrast-enhanced permeability MRI. Presented at the International Society for Magnetic Resonance in Medicine Meeting. Miami Beach, Florida, May 7–13, 2005.

[62] Liu D, Cheng T, Guo H, et al. Tissue plasminogen activator neurovascular toxicity is controlled by activated protein C. Nat Med 2004;10(12):1379–83.

[63] Roberts HC, Roberts TP, Lee TY, et al. Dynamic, contrast-enhanced CT of human brain tumors: quantitative assessment of blood volume, blood flow, and microvascular permeability: report of two cases. AJNR Am J Neuroradiol 2002;23(5):828–32.

[64] Molina C. Thrombolysis-related hemorrhagic infarction. Stroke 2002;33:1551–6.

[65] Warach S. Evidence of reperfusion injury, exacerbated by thrombolytic therapy, in human focal brain ischemia using a novel imaging marker of early blood-brain barrier disruption. Stroke 2004;35:2659–61.

[66] Latour LL. Early blood-brain barrier disruption in human focal brain ischemia. Ann Neurol 2004;56: 468–77.

ELSEVIER
SAUNDERS

Neuroimag Clin N Am 15 (2005) 589 – 607

NEUROIMAGING
CLINICS OF
NORTH AMERICA

Pediatric Stroke: The Child Is Not Merely a Small Adult

Brad R. Brobeck, MD, P. Ellen Grant, MD*

Massachusetts General Hospital, Boston, MA, USA

Pediatric stroke is a cerebrovascular event occurring between 14 weeks of gestation and 18 years of life. It occurs in more than eight children per 100,000 per year [1], with 5% to 10% resulting in death, one third having a recurrent episode, and more than 50% developing neurologic or cognitive sequelae [2]. The prevalence of pediatric stroke seems to be on the rise, possibly in part because of increased availability of and access to imaging studies (in particular MR imaging) and improved image quality, leading to an increase in diagnosis [2].

Despite the significant prevalence, morbidity, and mortality of pediatric stroke, treatment often is controversial because of the paucity of randomized trials in the pediatric population. According to the Brain Attack Coalition, at least three fundamental problems arise with pediatric stroke research and clinical care [3]. First, although the incidence is rising, cerebrovascular disease still is less frequent than adult stroke, making it difficult to organize multicenter controlled clinical trials. Second, the causes of childhood stroke are numerous and often overlap, with no single risk factor predominating. Third, many physicians know little about the pediatric disease processes leading to stroke, which may delay diagnosis and hinder treatment options. Finally, no distinct guidelines exist for workup and treatment, as for adult patients. Physicians often rely on modified guidelines for adults or expert opinion, both of which may not be completely accurate. Thus, pediatric stroke research and clinical

care are behind those for adults. Increased awareness leading to early MR imaging and identification as to the likely cause of pediatric stroke will facilitate the development of optimal treatment strategies.

This article reviews the common clinical presentations, causes, and imaging findings of pediatric stroke and discusses other causes of pediatric brain injury that may be confused with cerebrovascular insults. Pediatric stroke is separated into fetal, perinatal, and childhood stroke, and within these age groups, strokes are divided into arterial ischemic strokes and sinovenous thrombosis (SVT).

Fetal and perinatal strokes

Fetal strokes are defined as cerebrovascular insults occurring between 14 weeks of gestation and the onset of labor [4], whereas perinatal strokes are defined as cerebrovascular insults occurring between 28 weeks of gestation and 28 days of postnatal life [2]. Perinatal strokes are identified in at least 1 in 4000 live births per year [2], but the true prevalence of fetal stroke is unknown [5]. For unknown reasons, arterial ischemic stroke and SVT are detected more commonly in boys [6].

Arterial ischemic stroke

Fetal

The literature on fetal stroke can be confusing, as most studies use the term, fetal stroke, to include arterial ischemic stroke, hemorrhagic stroke, and global hypoxia and ischemia. All types of fetal stroke rarely are identified before birth because maternal or fetal symptoms rarely are present. Furthermore, the majority of antenatal ischemia is diagnosed at ultra-

* Corresponding author. Division of Pediatric Radiology, Massachussetts General Hospital, 55 Fruit Street, Boston, MA 02114.

E-mail address: ellen@nmr.mgh.harvard.edu (P.E. Grant).

doi:10.1016/j.nic.2005.08.013

neuroimaging.theclinics.com

sound screening performed in the second trimester, whereas the majority of ischemic events seem to occur between 24 and 34 weeks of gestational age (GA) [4]. In utero detection is reported on fetal MR imaging and, rarely, arterial stroke is identified acutely with positive fetal diffusion-weighted imaging (DWI) [4]. It is likely that fetal arterial ischemic stroke will be recognized increasingly, as fetal MR imaging with DWI becomes more a common modality for the assessment of fetal health.

In fetal arterial ischemic stroke, the middle cerebral artery (MCA) is the most common territory involved [7]. In the second trimester, focal ischemic events can disrupt cortical organization, resulting in polymicrogyria or, if there is a transmantal injury, schizencephaly [8,9]. A porencephalic cyst typically results if the injury occurs between approximately 22 and 27 weeks' GA as a result of the high water content of the unmyelinated brain, the lack of tightly packed white matter bundles, and the lack of astroglial response [10]. After approximately 27 weeks' GA, vascular territory ischemic injuries result in encephalomalacia with gliosis and, often, cystic change.

The risk factors and causes of fetal arterial ischemic injury are unclear [11,12]. All types of fetal strokes can be caused by maternal conditions, pregnancy-related disorders, and fetal conditions. Arterial ischemic causes are not separated from the broader group. Risk factors for the larger category of fetal strokes include maternal conditions, such as alloimmune thrombocytopenia; diabetic ketoacidosis is reported [4]. An association with maternal anticoagulation is noted in women taking warfarin and heparin. In these cases, there is a good chance that an unidentified risk factor is in play, such as thrombophilia, which may necessitate the anticoagulant in the first place. Antiepileptics also play a role in fetal ischemia.

Pregnancy-related causes include placental infarction, thrombosis, and hemorrhage, all of which can bypass the fetal liver and lungs, involving the cerebral circulation [13]. Trauma, placenta previa, and abruption are additional pregnancy-related causes [14], and twin-twin syndrome is a risk factor affecting as many as 30% of monochorionic twins [15,16].

Despite these many potential causes, more than half of all cases of fetal focal ischemia have no identifiable cause [4]. Although outcomes in the combined group of all fetal strokes, including hemorrhagic events and venticulomegaly, reportedly are poor, the subset with injuries that are likely of arterial ischemic origin has better outcomes. In five patients who had clinical follow-up identified in the literature, one was normal at 20 months, two had spastic hemi-

paresis with mild delay, and one had spastic quadraparesis with severe delay.

Neonatal

Unlike in the mature brain, focal arterial ischemic strokes in neonates usually present as unexpected focal seizures within 2 to 3 days of birth. Typically, the neonate is a low-risk term neonate who has normal Apgar scores [10]. Because these lesions are focal arterial events in an otherwise normal brain, encephalopathy is not a typical feature. It is unclear why the seizure seems to occur a few days after the event, but a possibility is secondary swelling and progressive cellular injury with release of excitatory amino acids. The actual timing of the focal stroke often is difficult to determine, but the imaging findings and evolution often suggest the stroke occurred at or near the time of birth. This clinical presentation is different from that in the mature brain, where a focal neurologic defect occurs immediately and seizures are rare.

Although large strokes may be visible by experienced readers on CT or ultrasound, MR imaging with DWI is the study of choice (Fig. 1). DWI is more sensitive at detecting arterial strokes, especially if they are small or within the deep gray nuclei. The authors' MR imaging protocol includes axial T2 fast spin echo (FSE) (with a longer echo time than is used in the mature brain), gradient-echo T2, 3-D spoiled gradient-recalled echo, and DWI. Although magnetic resonance angiography (MRA) may be helpful to exclude large branch occlusions, turbulent flow often results in multiple sites of signal dropout. In addition, the authors use arterial spin labeling (ASL) to determine if the DWI abnormal region has reperfused. The authors find ASL superior to dynamic susceptibility contrast dynamic susceptibility contrast in the neonate, as ASL does not require contrast injection and provides more information on cortical flow. In dynamic susceptibility contrast, the signal seems dominated by large cortical veins, even if spinecho, echoplanar imaging is used.

Ultrasound studies, although less sensitive than MR imaging at detecting focal ischemic injury, are helpful in evaluating regions of signal loss on MRA further. On gray scale imaging, the circle of Willis (COW) often can be identified and, in combination with color flow Doppler and evaluation of Doppler waveforms, residual clot can be detected. Ultrasound also is helpful in screening for thrombus in other major vessels throughout the body and monitoring for interval resolution if a focal complete or partial occlusion is identified.

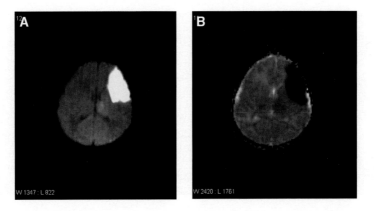

Fig. 1. Focal arterial ischemic stroke: the patient is a 2-day-old GA child of an otherwise healthy mother who had chorioamnionitis. Apgar scores were 9 and 9 at 1 and 5 minutes, respectively. MR imaging demonstrates a well-defined, cortical-based, diffusion-weighted hyperintensity involving the left frontal lobe (*A*) with corresponding decreased ADC values (*B*), consistent with an acute focal arterial embolic event.

When imaging with DWI immediately after detection of a first seizure, lesions with different degrees of apparent diffusion coefficient (ADC) decrease occasionally are identified. In some cases, this is not likely the result of two different events in time but more likely the result of differences in the length of time the vessel was occluded. For example, an M1 embolus may lyse partially and propagate into a distal M2 branch, resulting in a large MCA territory region of moderately decreased ADC and a region of more profoundly decreased ADC in the territory supplied by the distal occlusion. The region of brain with more rapid reperfusion often has a delayed nadir for the ADC decrease and, within a few days, it is markedly decreased also.

Occasionally, clinicians ask if the DWI abnormalities could be secondary to seizure activity. Although DWI abnormalities are described with seizures, it often is after an episode of status epilepticus, which is unusual in these neonates, and the DWI abnormalities typically are not confined to the cortex, as is the case in postictal situations.

There are several risk factors associated with neonatal arterial ischemic stroke described recently [17]; these include prepartum and intrapartum factors, such as primiparity, fetal heart rate abnormality, emergency cesarean delivery, chorioamnionitis, prolonged rupture of membranes, prolonged second stage of labor, vacuum extraction, cord abnormalities, pre-eclampsia, and oligohydramnios [17]. Eighty-eight percent of the lesions are unilateral, with the MCA territory the most commonly affected distribution [18].

The causes of focal neonatal ischemia are many, with thrombotic and embolic sources. Common causes of embolic infarctions include placental thrombosis, placental infarction, placental tissue fragments, and congenital heart disease. Thrombosis often results from trauma, disseminated intravascular coagulation, polycythemia, thrombophilia, dehydration, and infection. Additional causes include vasospasm and vasculopathy. Fifty percent of the cases have no identifiable cause [19].

In all cases, the placenta is examined, an echocardiogram is performed to exclude cardiac abnormalities, and parents are screened for plasma phase risk factors. The screen includes prothrombin gene mutation, hypercoagulability panel (screen for mutant factor V [chiefly factor V Leiden] and levels of the anticlotting proteins, protein S, protein C, and antithrombin III), homocysteine level, lipoprotein (a), and anticardiolipin antibodies. The last can cross the placenta from a mother who has these antibodies and are associated with arterial and venous thrombi in newborns. There are cases reported of newborns who have stroke having inherited a tendency for an elevation in lipoprotein (a) from both parents (homozygous state).

Arterial ischemic strokes often are cavitated, with subsequent development of multicystic encephalomalacia, volume loss, gliosis, or ulegyria, but overall outcomes of isolated cerebral arterial ischemic strokes typically are good compared with those of neonates who have hypoxic ischemic encephalopathy. Hemiplegia occurs in approximately 25% and can be predicted when cortex, basal ganglia, and posterior limb internal capsule are involved [20]. Recurrence is rare (approximately 3.3%), but risk of recurrence increases if there is an underlying disease or prothrombotic risk factors [21].

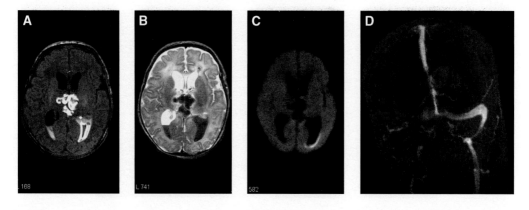

Fig. 2. Neonatal SVT with bilateral thalamic hemorrhage: 3-week-old boy who had fever and septic shock imaged 5 days after presentation. Bithalamic and intraventricular hemorrhage with increased T1 (*A*) and decreased T2 (*B*) signal is consistent with intracellular methemoglobin and, hence, blood products at least a few days old. DWI (*C*) is "negative" because of the markedly decreased T2 signal (susceptibility effect). Although the thalamic hemorrhage likely was the result of straight sinus thrombosis, at the time of the MRV (*D*), only right transverse and sigmoid sinus thrombosis was identified.

Sinovenous thrombosis

Commonly, neonates who have SVT present with seizures [22] and lethargy [23]. Focal neurologic signs are not common in the neonatal period, secondary to the lack of myelination and lack of motor skills, but are common in older children. The incidence of SVT is estimated to be as high as 0.67 per 100,000 children, with more than half of the cases occurring in neonates [23]. Forty percent of neonates who have SVT develop ischemic infarctions, and 70% of those go on to hemorrhage [23].

MR imaging, with gradient-echo T2, DWI, and magnetic resonance venogram (MRV), is the authors' imaging modality of choice for evaluating the venous sinuses and detecting associated cerebral injury (Figs. 2 and 3). Noncontrast CT has a 16% false-negative rate [23]. CT venography probably is the most sensitive and specific study for SVT detection but carries the added risk of ionizing radiation, re-

quires bolus injection of viscous iodinated contrast through what may be a tenuous and solitary intravenous access, and is less sensitive than MR imaging at detecting associated nonhemorrhagic brain injury. Any full-term neonate who has an unexplained intraventricular hemorrhage or deep gray matter hemorrhage should have MR imaging with MRV [22]. The authors also routinely obtain gradient-echo images to detect subtle areas of venous hemorrhage. Duplex Doppler ultrasonography often demonstrates an echogenic sinus clot and can be helpful for interrogating regions of concern on MRV and to monitor clot evolution.

The risk factors for SVT in neonates include maternal complications (most commonly chorioamnionitis, seen in 40% of the mothers in one study), eclampsia, diabetes, perinatal distress (including extracorporeal membrane oxygenation, meconium aspiration, intubation, and low Apgar scores), and neonatal complications (such as coronary heart disease, disseminated

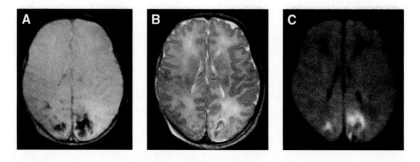

Fig. 3. Neonatal venous infarctions: term neonate presenting with thrombocytopenia and seizures on first day of life. Bilateral parasagittal venous hemorrhages are identified better on gradient-echo T2 (*A*) than on the T2 FSE images (*B*). The ischemic component is identified best on DWI as bright signal (*C*). MRV (not shown) showed partial superior sagittal sinus thrombosis.

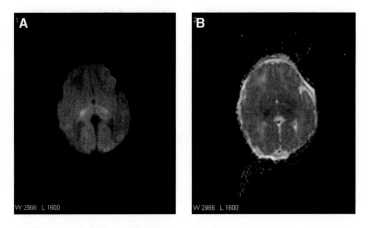

Fig. 4. Profound global hypoxia and ischemia: 35-week-old girl born by emergency cesarean section secondary to fetal bradycardia, with Apgar scores of 2, 3, and 3 at 1, 5, and 10 minutes, respectively. DWI (*A*) and ADC maps (*B*) demonstrate decreased diffusion in the ventrolateral thalamus and corticospinal tracts.

intravascular coagulation, sepsis, polycythemia, severe dehydration, and coagulation disorders). The coagulation disorders associated with venous thrombosis include factor V Leiden, protein C and S, anticardiolipin antibodies, lipoprotein (a), prothrombin G20210A, and methylenetetrahydrofolate dehydrogenase (MTHFR) deficiency.

It is reported that 77% of neonates who have SVT have no neurologic sequelae after 1 year [23]. Bithalamic hemorrhages secondary to straight sinus thrombosis and fourth ventricular dilation secondary to intraventricular hemorrhage are poor prognostic factors [24,25]. Because of the overall good outcomes of isolated VST and concerns for anticoagulation when parenchymal hemorrhages are present, treatment is controversial. Future prospective trials are needed.

Other

Global hypoxia and ischemia

A combination of global hypoxia and hypoperfusion is a common cause of perinatal brain injury. When these decreases are profound, reduced ADCs involve at least the corticospinal tracts and ventrolateral thalamus (Fig. 4). The most severe injuries show DWI abnormalities in the posterior brainstem. Less profound insults spare these regions but involve other areas of cortex and, often, subcortical white matter (Fig. 5). A full discussion of this topic is beyond the scope of this article, but interested readers are referred to other recent reviews [26].

It is important to appreciate the difference between the causes and outcomes of cerebral injuries resulting from global cerebral hypoxia and those

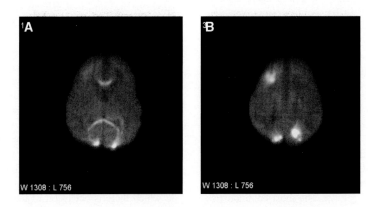

Fig. 5. Partial global hypoxia and ischemia: 38-week-old girl born via cesarean section with Apgar scores 4, 8, and 9 at 1, 5, and 10 minutes, respectively. DWI (*A*) demonstrates multiple foci of decreased (bright DWI signal) diffusion in the frontal subcortical white matter, as well as in the posterior parietal and occipital regions with extension to cortex. Decreased diffusion is also noted in the corpus callossum (*B*).

resulting from hypoperfusion and focal arterial ischemic infarctions.

In hypoxic and ischemic infarctions, there is a
global brain insult, with maximal injury occurring
in regions of maximal vulnerability. In general, the
outcomes are poorer and more difficult to predict in
global insults because of the inability of DWI to
detect and predict areas of injury accurately on long-
term follow-up. In focal arterial ischemic infarctions,
however, the injuries most commonly are local as
a result of arterial occlusions in otherwise normal
brains. In these cases, the regions of cerebral injury
on follow-up are closer in size to the regions of acute
ADC decrease.

Inborn errors of metabolism

Occasionally, an inborn error of metabolism can
mimic an arterial ischemic event and should be considered in the differential diagnosis. The most common inborn errors to present acutely in the neonatal
time period (which can be confused with arterial ischemic injury) are mitochondrial disorders and urea
cycle deficits (which may have regions of bright DWI
signal). These most often are bilaterally symmetric,
have unusual patterns of injury, or have minimal
ADC decrease in the areas of DWI abnormality.

Childhood stroke

Childhood strokes are defined as cerebrovascular
insults occurring between 30 days and 18 years of
life. The incidence ranges from 2 to 6 per 100,000 per
year [27]. Causes of cerebrovascular insults in children include congenital or acquired heart disease,
systemic vascular disease, vasculitis, vasculopathies,
metabolic disorders, vasospastic disorders, hematologic disorders, coagulopathies, congenital cerebrovascular anomalies, trauma, and iatrogenic causes
[28]. The more common etiologies are discussed later
and categorized as arterial ischemic stroke or SVT.

Arterial ischemic stroke

According to the Canadian Pediatric Ischemic
Stroke Registry, 40% of cases of arterial ischemic
stroke are in children less than 1 year old with a male-
to-female ratio of 1.5:1 [2]. The most common risk
factors for childhood arterial ischemic stroke in patients up to 16 years of age reported in the Swiss
Neuropediatric Stroke Registry are infections (40%),
cardiomyopathies (25%), and coagulopathies (25%)

[29]. Although imaging may identify vascular abnormalities in up to 80% of cases, no cause may be
identified in up to 50% of cases [30].

Sickle-cell disease

Sickle-cell disease (SCD) is an autosomal reces-
sive disorder of hemoglobin synthesis found most
commonly in patients of African descent. A substitu-
tion of a valine amino acid in place of a glutamate
amino acid in the sixth position of the beta-globin
chain is the cause of the disease. Sickle-cell trait is
carried in 8% to 10% of African-Americans; one gene
is affected and the other gene is normal. SCD results
from both genes being affected and is seen in 0.15%
of African-American newborns [31].

Many stressors, among a host of factors, such as
fever, pain, hypoxia, infection, and certain medications, result in decreased oxygen tension within
the blood. When SCD is present and red blood cells
(RBCs) are placed under oxidative stress, the defective hemoglobin molecule alters its shape, causing
RBCs to sickle. The sickling results in turbulent
flow, which injures the endothelial lining of the
vessel wall, causing RBC clumping in small vessels
leading to occlusion and infarction.

Stroke is a major cause of morbidity and mortality in SCD. At a mean age of 10 years, the estimated rate of cerebrovascular infarction, ischemia, or
atrophy in children who have SCD is reported to be
as high as 44%, with 55% demonstrating vasculopathy [32]. Of patients homozygous for SCD, 11% have
a clinical event by the age of 20, and 22% of children
have clinically silent events [33,34]. The majority
of patients demonstrate recurrent infarctions. Unlike
adults, children tend to have ischemic rather than
hemorrhagic infarctions [33]. Evidence of a silent
stroke on imaging indicates an increased risk of future silent strokes, which in turn are associated with
cognitive deficits [35,36].

Strokes as a result of SCD are seen in children
as young as 1 year of age, with occlusions occurring
in small and large vessels. In large vessels, intimal
lesions and thrombosis often combine to cause large
vessel occlusion. Distal strokes result from emboli,
capillary sludging, or abnormal vasomotor regulation, which increases the risk for watershed injury
with hypotension or anemia (Fig. 6).

Rarely, probably within subgroups with genetic predisposition, a moyamoya pattern develops,
in which there is occlusion of the distal internal carotid arteries with development of collateral vessels.
Presence of a moyamoya pattern doubles the risk
of stroke and poor cognitive outcome [37]. In some
cases, most often in patients who have silent strokes,

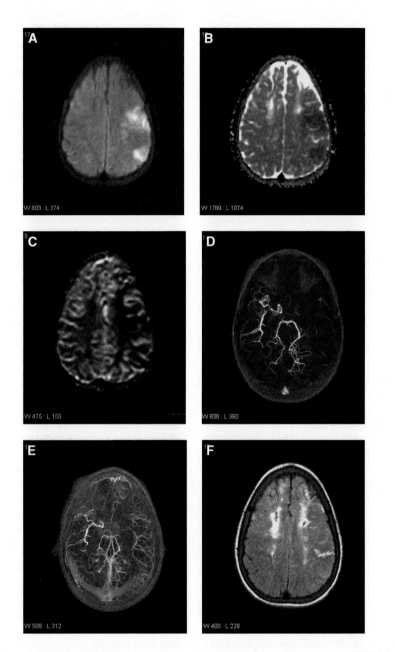

Fig. 6. SCD: 12-year-old boy who had SCD presented with right-sided weakness and speech loss. DWI (*A*) and ADC map (*B*) show decreased diffusion of the left frontal and parietal regions, consistent with evolving ischemic infarction. Perfusion-weighted imaging (*C*) demonstrates decreased cerebral blood volume and cerebral blood flow (not shown) in this area. 2-D time of flight MRA of the COW (*D*) demonstrates lack of flow-related enhancement in the distal left internal carotid artery, left A1 segment, left M1 segment, and left M2 segments. Gadolinium-enhanced MRA demonstrates minimal signal in the left MCA, consistent with slow flow and multiple enlarged collateral vessels (*E*). Chronic areas of ischemia are noted in the bifrontal white matter (*F*).

the major intracranial vessels are normal, but small infarctions—primarily in white matter—are identified, suggesting a. distinct microvascular process [34].

Because of the many contributing factors and different mechanisms contributing to stroke in SCD, strategies for effective treatment likely differ, depending on the site and degree of damage and the acute trigger [38]. The exact role of the sickle erythrocyte is unclear, however, as are the relative roles of other factors, such as the nitric oxide pathway, coagulation system, and inflammatory mechanisms, which limit the development of optimal treatment strategies.

As a result of the Stroke Prevention Trial in Sickle Cell Anemia (STOP), transcranial Doppler ultrasonography (TCD) plays a central role in the management of patients who have SCD [39]. TCDs are performed every 6 months, from 2 to 16 years of age, to determine which patients are at high risk for stroke and, thus, require transfusion for stroke prophylaxis. The protocol for TCD is specific and based on the results of the STOP trial [40]. MR imaging evaluation plays a major role in the detection of infarction and in the evaluation of major vessels. As recommended by Zimmerman [41], the MR imaging evaluation of patients who have SCD should include T1, T2, fluid attenuated inversion recovery (FLAIR), gradient-echo T2, diffusion, and MRA.

Recent reports suggest that a combination of TCD and MRA may help determine which patients may be treated safely with hydroxyurea for prophylaxis. In this initial study, patients who had abnormal TCD but normal MRA were treated with hydroxyurea if velocities normalized after a transfusion program [42]. MR perfusion imaging has the potential to add further relevant information in the triage process, as perfusion abnormalities are identified in symptomatic patients even when other MR sequences and TCD are normal. It also is likely that ASL could replace dynamic susceptibility imaging, as it provides more quantitative data and obviates contrast injection. More detailed reviews on SCD are available elsewhere [43,44].

Cardioembolic stroke

Cardiac disease is the most common cause of cerebrovascular occlusion in young children [45]. Congenital right-to-left shunts have the greatest risk for embolic events, as the lungs are bypassed. Tetralogy of Fallot is the most common right-to-left shunt, with D-transposition of the great vessels, pulmonary atresia, and tricuspid atresia. The mechanism involves chronic hypoxia with a resultant polycythemia that increases the viscosity of the blood, leading to the clumping of RBCs and subsequent clot

formation. The majority of patients who have thromboembolic events are less than 2 years old [46].

Valvular disease, such as mitral valve prolapse, is associated with embolic events. Cardiac tumors, such as rhabdomyomas, often are located in the left atrium or ventricle and are associated with cerebrovascular emboli, as small portions of tumor can break away [47]. Arrhythmias, such as atrial flutter, are shown to promote ventricular stasis, with RBC clumping leading to emboli. Cardiomyopathy and metabolic disease can lead to the thinning of the myocardium with aneurysmal dilatation that promotes stasis and clumping of RBCs, also providing a source of emboli.

Moyamoya syndrome

Moyamoya syndrome is an idiopathic, progressive arterial occlusive vasculopathy resulting in occlusion of the distal internal carotid arteries, with resultant proliferation of the lenticulostriate and thalamoperforating arteries, giving the angiographic appearance of a "puff of smoke." The occlusion of the distal internal carotid arteries is believed secondary to intimal hyperplasia and medial fibrosis. The most common site of involvement is within the supraclinoid segments of the internal carotid arteries, with extension into the proximal anterior and MCAs. Less commonly, occlusion of the basilar artery can occur but usually is less severe.

On CT angiography (CTA), MRA, or conventional angiography, the appearance is that of a chronic occlusive process with collateral arterial development. Associations are documented with the Epstein-Barr virus [48], antiendothelial cell antibodies, and anti-alpha-fodrin antibodies [49]. An associated marker is transforming growth factor-beta 1, which is involved in angiogenesis [50]. Inflammatory changes of the media activate the cyclooxygenase-2 proteins, leading to increased production of prostaglandins, which results in intimal thickening and fibrosis. Additional associated markers include α_1-antitrypsin antibodies [51]. Increased expression of the elastin gene is believed responsible for protein synthesis leading to arterial smooth muscle hyperplasia.

A nonspecific pattern of occlusion can be seen with other diseases, such as Down syndrome [52–54] and neurofibromatosis type 1 [55]; in radiation/chemotherapy [56]; and in hemoglobinopathies, such as SCD [37].

Demographically, moyamoya is most common in Asia, particularly in patients of Japanese descent [57,58]. It is uncertain whether or not the disease is congenital or acquired, although genetic mapping recently has indicated that chromosomal abnormalities play a role [59]. A bimodal age distribution occurs, with the first peak in the first decade of life and a second less common peak in the fourth decade [60]. In the former, the presentation most commonly is of an occlusive process, whereas in the latter, typically it is more likely hemorrhagic (usually intraparenchymal, less commonly intraventricular, and rarely subarachnoid).

Angiographic narrowing of the supraclinoid internal carotid arteries and proximal COW branches is present. Development of a diffuse collateral vascular network occurs, most commonly involving the perforator vessels. Additional collaterals can arise from the ophthalmic, posterior cerebral, transdural leptomeningeal (via pial branches), and external carotid arteries. The different forms of moyamoya are known as ethmoidal, basal, and vault. Staging

of moyamoya can be classified as definite or probable, according to the Guidelines for the diagnosis and treatment of spontaneous occlusion of the circle of Willis [61].

MR imaging demonstrates loss of the normal flow voids in the distal carotid branches on long-echo images, with development of abnormally large and irregular lenticulostriate and thalamoperforating collateral vessels. Commonly, wide perivascular spaces are seen in the basal ganglia, secondary to the collateral vessels that create the characteristic puff of smoke appearance. DWI can demonstrate acute focal or confluent areas strokes, especially in the first decade [62].

Perfusion-weighted images often show peripheral areas of increased mean transit time and decreased

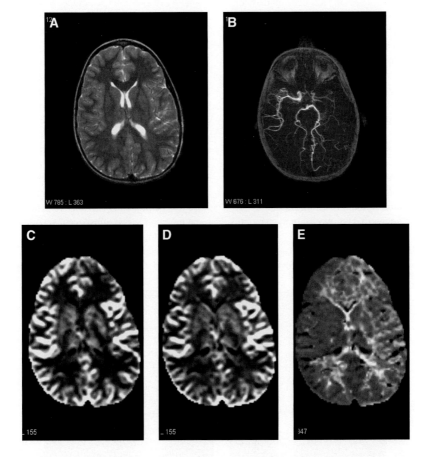

Fig. 7. Moyamoya: 9-year-old girl who had developmental delay and was diagnosed clinically with neurofibromatosis type 1. The T2-weighted images (*A*) demonstrate no T2 abnormalities vacuolization (often seen in neurofibromatosis type 1). MRA of the COW (*B*) demonstrates decreased flow-related enhancement in the intracranial left internal carotid artery, with severe narrowing at the level of the left ophthalmic artery increased relative size and collateral are noted in the patent right MCA and right PCA. The left middle cerebral and anterior cerebral arteries are small, with multiple lenticulostriate collaterals, consistent with moyamoya. Perfusion-weighted images demonstrate normal cerebral blood volume (*C*), normal cerebral blood flow (*D*), and prolonged mean transit time (*E*), suggesting circulatory alterations without ischemia.

cerebral blood flow, corresponding to prolonged transit time but maintained blood volume in regions perfused by collateral flow [63]. Regions of infarction can appear as a small vessel ischemic pattern, an embolic pattern, a low flow pattern involving the watershed distributions, or a large confluent territorial infarction (Fig. 7). MRA demonstrates stenosis of the distal intracranial carotid arteries extending into the proximal M1 and A1 branches, usually bilaterally, but can overestimate severity because of slow or turbulent flow [64]. Performing postcontrast MRA improves accuracy, but CTA provides more accurate assessment of vascular stenoses and enlarged perforating lenticulostriate and thalamoperforating collaterals.

Arterial dissection

Dissection predisposes to lumenal narrowing, with decreased flow or distal embolic events. Fullerton and colleagues reviewed 118 cases and found a male predominance, even in a nontraumatic setting [65]. All presented with signs and symptoms of a focal ischemic event, and just over half reported headaches. Approximately one third were spontaneous, one third the result of trivial trauma, and the remainder the result of trauma or strenuous activity [66].

As distinct from adults, pediatric anterior circulation dissections most commonly are intracranial and spontaneous but, as in adults, vertebral artery dissections occur most commonly at C1-2 [65]. Although presentation often is within hours of the presumed onset, delays of days, weeks, or even months are common [65].

A brain MR imaging with DWI, a head and neck MRA, and an axial T1-weighted fat-saturated image of the neck from the aortic arch to the cavernous sinus are the initial studies of choice. These examinations allow accurate detection of embolic stroke and an initial screen for dissection (Fig. 8). If flow artifacts limit interpretation, CTA can be performed. The presence of a dissection is diagnosed when MRA or CTA demonstrates an abrupt, focal tapering, with segmental stringlike narrowing of the vessel and an occasionally present intimal flap. On MR, crescentic subacute blood (methemoglobin phase) within the dissection wall is T1 hyperintense. This is seen best on the T1-weighted fat-saturated images [67].

Steno-occlusive cerebral arteritis and arteriopathy

Arteritis can result in arterial strokes when there is invasion of the vessel wall or secondary inflammatory response to pathogens. In addition, septic emboli can lead to focal cerebral arteritis and vascular occlusion [68,69]. Meningitis, particularly bacterial, is a common cause of arterial and venous occlusion in children [70–72]. These cases rarely are a diagnostic dilemma, as the patients are quite sick with known bacterial meningitis at the time of the complicating stroke.

An important but less obvious cause of postinfectious vasculopathy in children is varicella infection, with stroke occurring within 12 months of infection in otherwise healthy children [73–75]. In one study, 57% percent of children developed a dense hemiparesis, whereas 26% developed dystonia, 13% had a hemisensory deficit, 13% had a speech impediment, 4% had subsequent seizures, and 31% had no neurologic sequelae [76].

Varicella-zoster virus, chickenpox, is a common childhood disease, rare before 6 months of age but

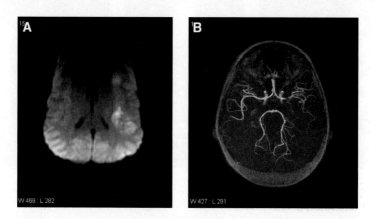

Fig. 8. Left MCA dissection: 12-year-old girl who had 2-day history of right-sided numbness, weakness, and episodic aphasia. DWI (*A*) demonstrates decreased diffusion in the left insula, middle frontal gyrus, and paracentral regions, consistent with acute ischemia. MRA of the COW (*B*) demonstrates focal irregularity with tapering in the midportion of the left M1 segment of the left MCA, consistent with dissection.

seen in up to 90% of children by the age of 12 [77]. Although childhood immunization increasingly is common, the overall effectiveness and the fact that not all children receive the vaccine underscore the need to recognize varicella as a potential cause of childhood arterial ischemia.

The rate of varicella-associated ischemic stroke is 6 times higher in children who have idiopathic arterial ischemia than in the general population [78]. The frequency of varicella with delayed hemiparesis is reported to be 1 in 6500 [79]. The mean time to infarction ranges from 2.6 to 5.7 months after infection, with no age or sex predilection [73].

Autopsies of these children reveal varicella zoster within the media of the walls of the diseased arteries [80]. Several mechanisms of how this might occur are proposed, including intraneuronal migration of the virus from the trigeminal ganglion along the ophthalmic division of the trigeminal nerve, which innervates the commonly affected arterial segments [81–84]. Imaging consists most commonly of MR imaging with MRA, CTA, or catheter angiography, which demonstrates unilateral arterial stenosis involving the distal internal carotid artery, often extending into the proximal A1 and M1 segments and rarely to the M2 segments [85]. Irregular stenosis and beading of the vessels can be seen, with ischemia in the basal ganglia, similar to granulomatous angiitis [82,83]. DWI demonstrates ischemia within the basal ganglia/internal capsule in 96% of subjects in one large study, with cerebral hemispheric ischemia in 43% and thalamic ischemia in 13% [76]. Although the location of vessel occlusion is similar to that of moyamoya, imaging studies fail to demonstrate lenticulostriate collateral vessels, suggesting that occlusion occurs so rapidly that collaterals do not have time to develop.

As further confounding variables, heterozygosity for factor V Leiden and transient protein S deficiency are associated with purpura fulminans, a rapidly progressive hemorrhagic necrosis of the skin associated with viral infections, such as varicella [86]. In general, a monophasic course is demonstrated with occasional progression in the first 6 months, followed by regression for up to 48 months without restenosis [76]. This same study reveals that 52% of children had a single episode of ischemia, 39% had multiple episodes of ischemia, and 9% had a transient ischemic event. In addition they report that after regression, arterial ischemic stroke or transient ischemic attack rarely recurred with antithrombotic prophylaxis.

Other vasculopathies that can cause vaso-occlusive disease in children include neurofibromatosis, Kawa-

saki disease, polyarteritis nodosa, fibromuscular dysplasia, and the phakomatoses. With neurofibromatosis type 1, intimal hyperplasia often results in the development of a moyamoya-type pattern [55]. Kawasaki disease more commonly involves the extracranial circulation but can embolize causing focal ischemia [87,88]. Arterial stenoses may improve over time. Fibromuscular dysplasia is an idiopathic vasculopathy that often affects the carotid arteries bilaterally, giving a string-of-beads appearance on MRA, CTA, and conventional angiography. Fibromuscular dysplasia predisposes to ischemia, transient ischemic attacks, and thromboembolic events.

Plasma-phase risk factors

Plasma-phase risk factors may contribute to childhood arterial ischemic stroke [89]. There are many genetic and acquired disorders that result in thrombophilia. The most common reported disorder is the factor V Leiden mutation (activated protein C resistance). Although associations with factor V Leiden and childhood arterial ischemic stroke are reported, not all studies concur, and its role is controversial.

Other genetic causes of thrombophilia that may play a role in childhood arterial ischemic stroke include increased prothrombin activity (prothrombin G20210A), elevated lipoprotein a:b deficiencies (of antithrombin III, protein C, or protein S), and increased plasminogen activator inhibitor-1.

The role of homozygous or heterozygous MTHFR polymorphism in childhood stroke also is controversial. Of the acquired causes of thrombophilia, some of the more common causes are antiphospholipid syndrome, lupus anticoagulant, and disseminated intravascular coagulation (as a result of cancer). In the majority of individuals who have these deficiencies, clotting problems begin in young adulthood. When thrombophilia results in ischemic stroke in childhood, multiple thrombophilia factors may potentiate one another.

All children who have arterial ischemic infarction (and SVT) should be evaluated for prothrombotic state. The authors' workup includes prothrombin gene mutation, a hypercoagulability panel (screen for mutant factor V [chiefly factor V Leiden levels of the anticlotting proteins], protein S, protein C, and antithrombin III), homocysteine level, lipoprotein (a), and anticardiolipin antibodies. When family history is suggestive, parental testing also may be helpful.

Sinovenous thrombosis

As opposed to neonates, for whom venous thrombosis presents most commonly with seizures or diffuse neurologic deficits, older children typically have symptoms similar to adults, including headaches, lethargy, irritability, papilledema, decreased consciousness, nausea, vomiting, and focal neurologic deficits (including motor or sensory deficits and isolated cranial nerve palsies) [1,90]. In general, when the major venous sinuses are thrombosed, intracranial hypertension occurs, but when cortical veins become occluded, focal injuries, such as edema, parenchymal hemorrhage, or ischemic stroke, occur [91].

As noted previously, noncontrast CT is insensitive for detecting thrombus but may show a hyperdense clot within the sinus. Contrast-enhanced CT may show a filling defect, the empty delta sign, surrounding the thrombosis but may miss as many as 40% of SVTs [23,92]. MR imaging with gradient-echo T1, DWI, and MRV is the authors' initial study of choice for optimal detection of cerebral involvement and for an initial assessment of the degree of venous thrombosis. Thrombus causes the vein or sinus to be isointense or hyperintense on T1-weighted MR imaging, and MRV demonstrates lack of flow-related enhancement.

In some cases, flow artifacts make MRV interpretation complex, and accurate assessment of small veins may be difficult. In these cases, CT venography can be helpful. In the authors' experience, CTV is more sensitive at detecting SVT than MR imaging with MRV, but because of the ionizing radiation and lower sensitivity at detecting cerebral involvement, it is not always the authors' initial study of choice. Associated venous hemorrhages are detected best with gradient-echo T2* susceptibility images. Parenchymal injuries are most common in areas drained by

large cortical veins, such as in the lateral temporal lobe when the Labbé's vein is occluded, and in the parasagittal frontal/parietal region when Trolard's vein is occluded.

The superficial venous system is involved more commonly than the deep venous system, in particular the superior sagittal and transverse sinuses. Approximately half of infants and children have multiple sinuses or veins involved, and 40% have associated parenchymal infarctions [23,92–94]. Hemorrhagic infarctions are seen in 23% of older children as compared with 35% of neonates, with 11% of the children demonstrating parenchymal lesions, such as tumors, arteriovenous malformations, and multifocal white matter lesions [23]. One study shows that iron deficiency, parietal involvement, and lack of caudate involvement independently predicted SVT over arterial ischemic stroke [93].

Risk factors in older children are different from those of neonates. Systemic illness with resultant sepsis and dehydration and head and neck pathology—particularly otitis media, mastoiditis, and sinusitis (Figs. 9 and 10)—are major risk factors for SVT. When transverse sinus thrombosis occurs secondary to otitis media or mastoiditis, increased intracranial pressure with papillary edema may occur as a result of decreased CSF resorption, especially if there is a hypoplastic contralateral transverse sinus. Although this often is referred to as otitic hydrocephalus, ventricular enlargement does not occur [91].

As discussed regarding neonates, prothrombotic risk factors are a major cause of SVT. The risk for SVT is increased when at least one prothrombotic risk factor is present. In particular increased lipo-

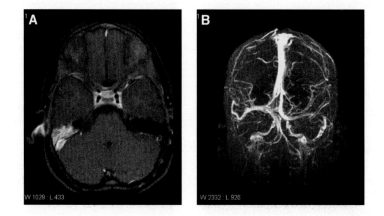

Fig. 9. Otitic hydrocephalus: 6-year-old girl presented with fever resulting from otitis media that progressed to headaches and blurred vision while on antibiotics. Papilledema was noted on fundoscopic examination. Postcontrast T1-weighted images with fat saturation (*A*) showed right mastoiditis and enhancing clot in the right sigmoid sinus. MRV (*B*) confirmed right sigmoid sinus thrombosis.

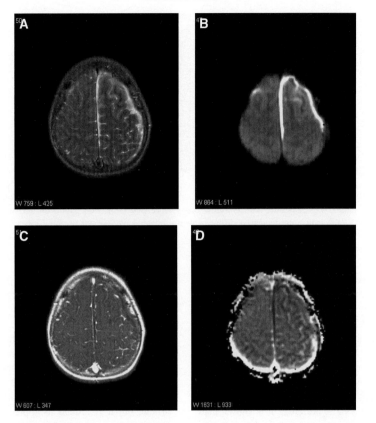

Fig. 10. Frontal sinusitis with an adjacent left frontal empyema and subsequent ischemia: a previously healthy 2-year-old girl had headache for 6 days, with subsequent fever and altered mental status 3 days later. The left frontal sinus, not shown, was opacified, consistent with sinusitis. Bifrontal subdural collections demonstrate T2 prolongation (*A*), with decreased diffusion (*B*). The T1 gadolinium-enhanced images (*C*) demonstrate peripheral enhancement surrounding the collections, consistent with bilateral subdural empyema. T2 prolongation was seen in the frontal lobe cortex, left greater than right (*A*), with bright DWI (*B*) and decreased diffusion (*D*), consistent with focal cortical ischemia.

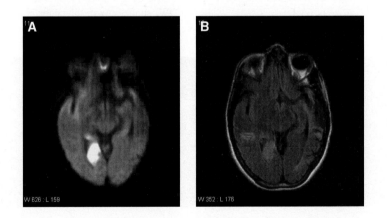

Fig. 11. Lupus: young woman who had a history of two prior cerebrovascular accidents and presented with bilateral vision loss and left lower extremity weakness. DWI (*A*) demonstrates a confluent focus of decreased diffusion in the right occipital lobe with T2 prolongation on the FLAIR images (*B*) consistent with evolving infarction. Encephalomalacia with accompanying laminar necrosis is seen in the left temporal lobe.

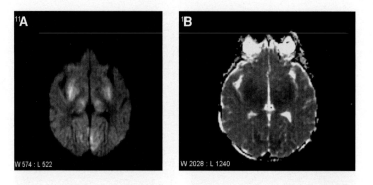

Fig. 12. Drowning: the patient was an 18-month-old boy found face down in a wading pool after several minutes of un-supervised play. The patient was asystolic, with Glasgow coma score (GCS) of 3 on paramedic arrival. DWI (*A*) and cor-responding ADC map (*B*) demonstrate decreased diffusion in the bilateral parasagittal occipital lobes, lentiform nuclei, and thalamic nuclei.

protein (a), followed by decreased protein C type I and an underlying systemic disease, are risk factors of decreasing proportion [90].

Additional risk factors include trauma, steroid treatment with concomitant infection, meningitis, si-nusitis, connective tissue disorders (such as lupus) (Fig. 11), trauma, cardiac surgery, indwelling cathe-ters, obesity, diabetes, nephrotic syndrome, and oral contraceptives. Although the long-term outcome of children who have SVT is not clear, it is shown that older age, lack of parenchymal insult, and thrombosis of the transverse or sigmoid sinus are predictors of better outcome [93]. Although as many as 77% of children may have no long-term sequelae [23], focal and diffuse neurologic insults, seizures, developmen-tal delay, cognitive impairment, speech impairment, visual impairment, increased intracranial pressure, cra-nial nerve palsies, recurrent thrombosis, and even death are potential sequelae of SVT.

Other

Global hypoxia and ischemia

Global hypoxia and hypoperfusion is also a com-mon cause of childhood brain injury; this includes drowning, choking, and suffocation [26]. As in the perinatal population, these injuries often are asso-ciated with infarction (Figs. 12 and 13). A full discussion of this topic is beyond the scope of this article, but it is crucial to appreciate the difference between the causes and outcomes of focal arterial ischemic infarctions versus global cerebral hypoxia and hypoperfusion. In focal arterial ischemic infarc-tions, there is a local injury as a result of arterial occlusion. In hypoxic and ischemic infarctions, there is a global brain insult with maximal injury occurring in regions of maximal vulnerability. These injuries evolve over time and may result in initially negative DWI studies. As in the neonatal population, the out-

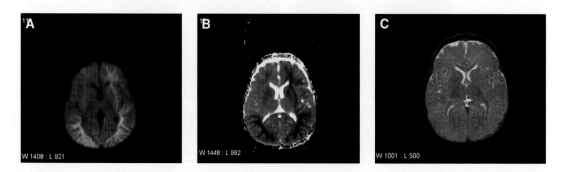

Fig. 13. Anoxic white matter injury: an 8-month-old girl postrespiratory arrest. Unlike arterial ischemic injuries, the anoxic insult is restricted to the white matter and is diffuse; it is not restricted to a standard arterial distribution. DWI (*A*) demonstrates diffusely increased signal intensity in the white matter with corresponding decreased ADC values (*B*). The T2-weighted images (*C*) are more subtle showing diffuse increased T2 signal.

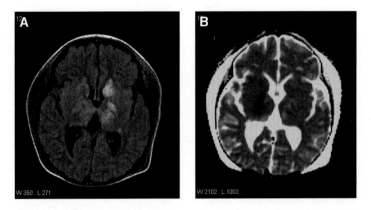

Fig. 14. Pyruvate dehydrogenase deficiency: a 2 -year-old girl was admitted for fever, irritability, and left hypotonia upon awakening. MR imaging demonstrates increased T2 signal on FLAIR (*A*) and mildly decreased diffusion on the ADC map (*B*) in the deep gray nuclei in a nonvascular distribution. The findings are atypical for stroke and are the result of a metabolic disorder that manifested after exacerbation by fever and dehydration.

comes are worse and more difficult to predict in global insults because of the inability of DWI to detect all areas of cellular injury.

Inborn errors of metabolism

When pediatric patients present with an acute neurologic event and a bright DWI lesion, inborn errors of metabolism should be considered, especially if the history is atypical for arterial ischemic stroke, the lesion is not within a vascular territory, or the ADC values are not markedly decreased (Fig. 14). In addition, disorders, such as Leigh syndrome, and urea cycle disorders often present with bilaterally symmetric lesions, unlike arterial ischemic stroke.

However, mitochondrial encephalopathy, lactic acidosis, and strokelike events (MELAS) [95] which may be more difficult to differentiate from arterial ischemic stroke in the acute stages. The clinical presentation varies from migraine-type headaches to seizures to hearing loss—although strokelike symptoms often are present. MELAS is an inherited microdeletion within the mitochondrial DNA. More than 10 different deletions are known. The transmission is maternal, through the ovum, as with other mitochondrial disorders. Strokelike episodes occur in more than 90% of MELAS cases [57]. The exact mechanism of these strokelike episodes is unknown but believed related to either a decrease in oxidative

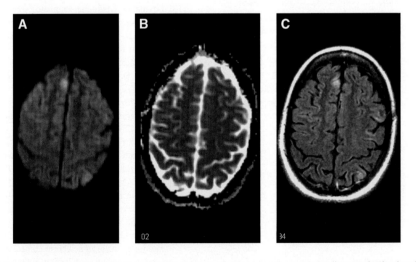

Fig. 15. MELAS: a young girl who had a long-standing history of seizures and a recently diagnosed mitochondrial disorder. MR imaging of the brain demonstrates multiple areas of DWI bright (*A*), ADC isointense (*B*), and FLAIR (*C*) hyperintense cortical lesions on acute presentation.

ATP production or defective mitochondrial functioning within the intravascular smooth muscle leading to impaired autoregulation [96]. MR imaging often demonstrates regional T2 hyperintensity in the white matter, most commonly involving the parietal lobe, temporal lobe, occipital lobe, and basal ganglia, but not in a vascular distribution [97,98]. DWI has increased signal intensity with variable ADC signal (Fig. 15). In many cases, ADC values are isointense to normal brain or even increased (this is believed a result of cellular edema and hyperemia) [99,100].

In addition, enhancement is seen in some of the lesions, likely secondary to breakdown of the blood-brain barrier. This breakdown is supported further by the increased uptake on 99m-Tc-hexamethyl propylene amine oxine single photon emmission CT scans [101] and increased cerebral blood flow on perfusion-weighted MR imaging [102]. Proton spectroscopy often demonstrates increased lactate [103].

Summary

Arterial ischemic stroke and SVT are significant yet under-recognized causes of mortality and morbidity in the pediatric population. With the increased complexity of pediatric stroke etiologies, compared with those of adults, yet a similar urgency for rapid diagnosis and treatment, pediatric stroke teams, like adult stroke teams, likely will become the standard of care. As multidisciplinary teams are developed to diagnose and treat pediatric stroke, however, a common terminology also must be developed to avoid confusing or combining different types of acute cerebral insults—such as focal arterial ischemic stroke and global hypoxia and ischemia—which have different causes and pathophysiologic mechanisms of injury. Increased awareness of these unique pediatric stroke subtypes, their clinical presentation, and their imaging findings will facilitate early identification and development of optimal treatment strategies.

Acknowledgments

We thank the pediatric stroke team at Massachusetts General Hospital.

References

[1] deVeber G. Arterial ischemic strokes in infants and children: an overview of current approaches. Semin Thromb Hemost 2003;29:567–73.

[2] Lynch JK, Hirtz DG, DeVeber G, et al. Report of the National Institute of Neurological Disorders and Stroke workshop on perinatal and childhood stroke. Pediatrics 2002;109:116–23.

[3] Roach Ed G, Riela AR, Wiznitzer M. Recognition and treatment of stroke in children. In: Child Neurology Society Ad Hoc Committee on Stroke in Children. Available at: http://www.stroke-site.org/guidelines/childneuro_stmt.html.

[4] Ozduman K, Pober BR, Barnes P, et al. Fetal stroke. Pediatr Neurol 2004;30:151–62.

[5] deVeber G. Stroke and the child's brain: an overview of epidemiology, syndromes and risk factors. Curr Opin Neurol 2002;15:133–8.

[6] Golomb MR, Dick PT, MacGregor DL, et al. Neonatal arterial ischemic stroke and cerebral sinovenous thrombosis are more commonly diagnosed in boys. J Child Neurol 2004;19:493–7.

[7] Kraus FT, Acheen VI. Fetal thrombotic vasculopathy in the placenta: cerebral thrombi and infarcts, coagulopathies, and cerebral palsy. Hum Pathol 1999; 30:759–69.

[8] Barkovich AJ, Westmark K, Partridge C, et al. Perinatal asphyxia: MR findings in the first 10 days. AJNR Am J Neuroradiol 1995;16:427–38.

[9] Barkovich AJ. MR and CT evaluation of profound neonatal and infantile asphyxia. AJNR Am J Neuroradiol 1992;13:959–72 [discussion: 973–5].

[10] Mercuri E. Early diagnostic and prognostic indicators in full term infants with neonatal cerebral infarction: an integrated clinical, neuroradiological and EEG approach. Minerva Pediatr 2001;53:305–11.

[11] Scher M, Wiznitzer M, BAngert BA. Cerebral infarctions in the fetus and neonate: maternal-placental-fetal considerations. Clin Perinatol 2002;29:693–724.

[12] Ferriero DM. Toward the recognition and treatment of perinatal stroke. Curr Opin Pediatr 2001;13:497–8.

[13] Levine D. Magnetic resonance imaging in prenatal diagnosis. Curr Opin Pediatr 2001;13:572–8.

[14] Levine D. Ultrasound versus magnetic resonance imaging in fetal evaluation. Top Magn Reson Imaging 2001;12:25–38.

[15] Levine D. Fetal magnetic resonance imaging. Top Magn Reson Imaging 2001;12:1–2.

[16] Kim MS, Elyaderani MK. Sonographic diagnosis of cerebroventricular hemorrhage in utero. Radiology 1982;142:479–80.

[17] Lee J, Croen LA, Backstrand KH, et al. Maternal and infant characteristics associated with perinatal arterial stroke in the infant. JAMA 2005;293:723–9.

[18] Howke AM, Oakes DJ, Woodman PD, et al. Prothrombin and PIVKA-II levels in cord blood from newborn exposed to anticonvulsants during pregnancy. Epilepsia 1999;40:980–4.

[19] Sreenan C, Bhargava R, Robertson CM. Cerebral infarction in the term newborn: clinical presentation and long-term outcome. J Pediatr 2000;137:351–5.

[20] Boardman JP, Ganesan V, Rutherford MA, et al. Magnetic resonance image correlates of hemiparesis after

neonatal and childhood middle cerebral artery stroke. Pediatrics 2005;115:321–6.

[21] Kurnik K, Kosch A, Strater R, et al. Recurrent thromboembolism in infants and children suffering from symptomatic neonatal arterial stroke: a prospective follow-up study. Stroke 2003;34:2887–92.

[22] Wu YW, Miller SP, Chin K, et al. Multiple risk factors in neonatal sinovenous thrombosis. Neurology 2002; 59:438–40.

[23] deVeber G, Andrew M, Adams C, et al. Cerebral sinovenous thrombosis in children. N Engl J Med 2001; 345:417–23.

[24] Shapiro SA, Campbell RL, Scully T. Hemorrhagic dilation of the fourth ventricle: an ominous predictor. J Neurosurg 1994;80:805–9.

[25] Roland EH, Flodmark O, Hill A. Thalamic hemorrhage with intraventricular hemorrhage in the full-term newborn. Pediatrics 1990;85:737–42.

[26] Grant PE, Yu D. Acute injury to the immature brain with ypoxia +/− hypperfusion. MRI Clin North Am, in press.

[27] DeVeber G. In pursuit of evidence-based treatments for paediatric stroke: the UK and Chest guidelines. Lancet Neurol 2005;4:432–6.

[28] Roach ES. Etiology of stroke in children. Semin Pediatr Neurol 2000;7:244–60.

[29] Steinlin M, Pfister I, Pavlovic J, et al. The first three years of the Swiss Neuropaediatric Stroke Registry (SNPSR): a population-based study of incidence, symptoms and risk factors. Neuropediatrics 2005;36: 90–7.

[30] Kirkham F, Sebire G, Steinlin M, et al. Arterial ischaemic stroke in children. Review of the literature and strategies for future stroke studies. Thromb Haemost 2004;92:697–706.

[31] Dodds N, Shahidi H, et al. Pediatrics, sickle cell disease. Available at: http://www.emedicine.com/emerg/topic406.htm.

[32] Steen RG, Emudianughe T, Hankins GM, et al. Brain imaging findings in pediatric patients with sickle cell disease. Radiology 2003;228:216–25.

[33] Ohene-Frempong K, Weiner SJ, Sleeper LA, et al. Cerebrovascular accidents in sickle cell disease: rates and risk factors. Blood 1998;91:288–94.

[34] Pegelow CH, Macklin EA, Moser FG, et al. Longitudinal changes in brain magnetic resonance imaging findings in children with sickle cell disease. Blood 2002;99:3014–8.

[35] Miller ST, Macklin EA, Pegelow CH, et al. Silent infarction as a risk factor for overt stroke in children with sickle cell anemia: a report from the Cooperative Study of Sickle Cell Disease. J Pediatr 2001;139: 385–90.

[36] Armstrong FD, Thompson Jr RJ, Wang W, et al. Cognitive functioning and brain magnetic resonance imaging in children with sickle cell disease. Neuropsychology Committee of the Cooperative Study of Sickle Cell Disease. Pediatrics 1996;97:864–70.

[37] Dobson SR, Holden KR, Nietert PJ, et al. Moyamoya syndrome in childhood sickle cell disease: a predictive factor for recurrent cerebrovascular events. Blood 2002;99:3144–50.

[38] Hillery CA, Panepinto JA. Pathophysiology of stroke in sickle cell disease. Microcirculation 2004;11: 195–208.

[39] Adams RJ, McKie VC, Hsu L, et al. Prevention of a first stroke by transfusions in children with sickle cell anemia and abnormal results on transcranial Doppler ultrasonography. N Engl J Med 1998;339:5–11.

[40] Bulas D. Screening children for sickle cell vasculopathy: guidelines for transcranial Doppler evaluation. Pediatr Radiol 2005;35:235–41.

[41] Zimmerman RA. MRI/MRA evaluation of sickle cell disease of the brain. Pediatr Radiol 2005;35:249–57.

[42] Bernaudin F, Verlhac S, Coic L, Lesprit E, Brugieres P, Reinert P. Long-term follow-up of pediatric sickle cell disease patients with abnormal high velocities on transcranial Doppler. Pediatr Radiol 2005;35:242–8.

[43] Hillary CA, Panepinto JA. Pathophysiology of stroke in sickle cell disease. Microcirculation 2004; 11(2):195–208.

[44] Zimmerman RA. MRI/MRA evaluation of sickle cell disease of the brain. Pediatr Radiol 2005;35(3): 249–57.

[45] Lanthier S, Carmant L, David M, et al. Stroke in children: the coexistence of multiple risk factors predicts poor outcome. Neurology 2000;54:371–8.

[46] Tyler HR, Clark DB. Cerebrovascular accidents in patients with congenital heart disease. AMA Arch Neurol Psychiatry 1957;77:483–9.

[47] Knepper LE, Biller J, Adams Jr HP, Bruno A. Neurologic manifestations of atrial myxoma. A 12-year experience and review. Stroke 1988;19:1435–40.

[48] Tanigawara T, Yamada H, Sakai N, et al. Studies on cytomegalovirus and Epstein-Barr virus infection in moyamoya disease. Clin Neurol Neurosurg 1997; 99(Suppl 2):S225–8.

[49] Ogawa K, Nagahiro S, Arakaki R, et al. Anti-alphafodrin autoantibodies in Moyamoya disease. Stroke 2003;34:e244–6.

[50] Yamamoto M, Aoyagi M, Tajima S, et al. Increase in elastin gene expression and protein synthesis in arterial smooth muscle cells derived from patients with Moyamoya disease. Stroke 1997;28:1733–8.

[51] Amano T, Inoha S, Wu CM, et al. Serum alpha1-antitrypsin level and phenotype associated with familial moyamoya disease. Childs Nerv Syst 2003;19: 655–8.

[52] Takanashi J, Sugita K, Honda A, et al. Moyamoya syndrome in a patient with Down syndrome presenting with chorea. Pediatr Neurol 1993;9:396–8.

[53] Schrager GO, Cohen SJ, Vigman MP. Acute hemiplegia and cortical blindness due to moya moya disease: report of a case in a child with Down's syndrome. Pediatrics 1977;60:33–7.

[54] Mito T, Becker LE. Vascular dysplasia in Down syndrome: a possible relationship to moyamoya disease. Brain Dev 1992;14:248–51.

[55] Erickson RP, Woolliscroft J, Allen RJ. Familial occurrence of intracranial arterial occlusive disease (Moyamoya) in neurofibromatosis. Clin Genet 1980; 18:191–6.

[56] Yamada I, Himeno Y, Suzuki S, et al. Posterior circulation in moyamoya disease: angiographic study. Radiology 1995;197:239–46.

[57] Goto Y, Horai S, Matsuoka T, et al. Mitochondrial myopathy, encephalopathy, lactic acidosis, and stroke-like episodes (MELAS): a correlative study of the clinical features and mitochondrial DNA mutation. Neurology 1992;42:545–50.

[58] Numaguchi Y, Gonzalez CF, Davis PC, et al. Moyamoya disease in the United States. Clin Neurol Neurosurg 1997;99(Suppl 2):S26–30.

[59] Ikeda H, Sasaki T, Yoshimoto T, et al. Mapping of a familial moyamoya disease gene to chromosome 3p24.2-p26. Am J Hum Genet 1999;64:533–7.

[60] Suzuki J, Kodama N. Moyamoya disease—a review. Stroke 1983;14:104–9.

[61] Fukui M. Guidelines for the diagnosis and treatment of spontaneous occlusion of the circle of Willis ('moyamoya' disease). Research Committee on Spontaneous Occlusion of the Circle of Willis (Moyamoya Disease) of the Ministry of Health and Welfare, Japan. Clin Neurol Neurosurg 1997;99(Suppl 2): S238–40.

[62] Yamada I, Himeno Y, Nagaoka T, et al. Moyamoya disease: evaluation with diffusion-weighted and perfusion echo-planar MR imaging. Radiology 1999; 212:340–7.

[63] Kassner A, Zhu XP, Li KL, et al. Neoangiogenesis in association with moyamoya syndrome shown by estimation of relative recirculation based on dynamic contrast-enhanced MR images. AJNR Am J Neuroradiol 2003;24:810–8.

[64] Saeki N, Silva MN, Kubota M, et al. Comparative performance of magnetic resonance angiography and conventional angiography in moyamoya disease. J Clin Neurosci 2000;7:112–5.

[65] Fullerton HJ, Johnston SC, Smith WS. Arterial dissection and stroke in children. Neurology 2001;57: 1155–60.

[66] Schievink WI, Mokri B, O'Fallon WM. Recurrent spontaneous cervical-artery dissection. N Engl J Med 1994;330:393–7.

[67] Hofmann LV, Liddell RP, Arepally A, et al. In vivo intravascular MR imaging: transvenous technique for arterial wall imaging. J Vasc Interv Radiol 2003; 14:1317–27.

[68] Lee WL, Dooling EC. Acute Kingella kingae endocarditis with recurrent cerebral emboli in a child with mitral prolapse. Ann Neurol 1984;16:88–9.

[69] Noonan JA, Wilson CB, Spencer FC, et al. Cerebral and cardiac complications from bacterial endocarditis. A successfully managed case with unusual complications. Am J Dis Child 1968;116: 666–74.

[70] Snyder RD, Stovring J, Cushing AH, et al. Cerebral infarction in childhood bacterial meningitis. J Neurol Neurosurg Psychiatry 1981;44:581–5.

[71] Taft TA, Chusid MJ, Sty JR. Cerebral infarction in Hemophilus influenzae type B meningitis. Clin Pediatr (Phila) 1986;25:177–80.

[72] Griesemer D, Barton LL, Reese CM, et al. Amebic meningoencephalitis caused by Balamuthia mandrillaris. Pediatr Neurol 1995;10:249–54.

[73] Askalan R, Laughlin S, Mayank S, et al. Chickenpox and stroke in childhood: a study of frequency and causation. Stroke 2001;32:1257–62.

[74] Ganesan V, Prengler M, McShane MA, et al. Investigation of risk factors in children with arterial ischemic stroke. Ann Neurol 2003;53:167–73.

[75] Sebire G, Meyer L, Chabrier S. Varicella as a risk factor for cerebral infarction in childhood: a case-control study. Ann Neurol 1999;45:679–80.

[76] Lanthier S, Armstrong D, Domi T, et al. Post-varicella arteriopathy of childhood: natural history of vascular stenosis. Neurology 2005;64:660–3.

[77] National Committee on Immunization. Statement on recommended use of varicella virus vaccine. Can Commun Dis Rep 1999. Available at: http://phac-aspc.gc.ca/im/vpd-mev/varicella_e.html.

[78] Frank Y, Lim W, Kahn E, et al. Multiple ischemic infarcts in a child with AIDS, varicella zoster infection, and cerebral vasculitis. Pediatr Neurol 1989; 5:64–7.

[79] Ichiyama T, Houdou S, Kisa T, et al. Varicella with delayed hemiplegia. Pediatr Neurol 1990;6:279–81.

[80] Berger TM, Caduff JH, Gebbers JO. Fatal varicella-zoster virus antigen-positive giant cell arteritis of the central nervous system. Pediatr Infect Dis J 2000; 19:653–6.

[81] Gilden DH, Kleinschmidt-DeMasters BK, LaGuardia JJ, et al. Neurologic complications of the reactivation of varicella-zoster virus. N Engl J Med 2000;342:635–45.

[82] Shuper A, Vining EP, Freeman JM. Central nervous system vasculitis after chickenpox—cause or coincidence? Arch Dis Child 1990;65:1245–8.

[83] Kamholz J, Tremblay G. Chickenpox with delayed contralateral hemiparesis caused by cerebral angiitis. Ann Neurol 1985;18:358–60.

[84] Vilchez-Padilla JJ, Redon J, Ruiz A, et al. CNS varicella-zoster vasculitis. Arch Neurol 1982;39:785.

[85] Bodensteiner JB, Hille MR, Riggs JE. Clinical features of vascular thrombosis following varicella. Am J Dis Child 1992;146:100–2.

[86] Levin M, Eley BS, Louis J, et al. Postinfectious purpura fulminans caused by an autoantibody directed against protein S. J Pediatr 1995;127:355–63.

[87] Fujiwara S, Yamano T, Hattori M, et al. Asymptomatic cerebral infarction in Kawasaki disease. Pediatr Neurol 1992;8:235–6.

[88] Lapointe JS, Nugent RA, Graeb DA, et al. Cerebral infarction and regression of widespread aneurysms in Kawasaki's disease: case report. Pediatr Radiol 1984; 14:1–5.

[89] Nestoridi E, Buonanno FS, Jones RM, et al. Arterial ischemic stroke in childhood: the role of plasma-phase risk factors. Curr Opin Neurol 2002;15:139–44.

[90] Heller C, Heinecke A, Junker R, et al. Cerebral venous thrombosis in children: a multifactorial origin. Circulation 2003;108:1362–7.

[91] Stam J. Thrombosis of the cerebral veins and sinuses. N Engl J Med 2005;352:1791–8.

[92] Barron TF, Gusnard DA, Zimmerman RA, et al. Cerebral venous thrombosis in neonates and children. Pediatr Neurol 1992;8:112–6.

[93] Sebire G, Tabarki B, Saunders DE, et al. Cerebral venous sinus thrombosis in children: risk factors, presentation, diagnosis and outcome. Brain 2005;128: 477–89.

[94] Carvalho KS, Garg BP. Cerebral venous thrombosis and venous malformations in children. Neurol Clin 2002;20:1061–77.

[95] Pavlakis SG, Phillips PC, DiMauro S, et al. Mitochondrial myopathy, encephalopathy, lactic acidosis, and strokelike episodes: a distinctive clinical syndrome. Ann Neurol 1984;16:481–8.

[96] Ohama E, Ohara S, Ikuta F, et al. Mitochondrial angiopathy in cerebral blood vessels of mitochondrial encephalomyopathy. Acta Neuropathol (Berl) 1987;74:226–33.

[97] Allard JC, Tilak S, Carter AP. CT and MR of MELAS syndrome. AJNR Am J Neuroradiol 1988;9: 1234–8.

[98] Barkovich AJ, Good WV, Koch TK, et al. Mitochondrial disorders: analysis of their clinical and imaging characteristics. AJNR Am J Neuroradiol 1993;14: 1119–37.

[99] Yonemura K, Hasegawa Y, Kimura K, et al. Diffusion-weighted MR imaging in a case of mitochondrial myopathy, encephalopathy, lactic acidosis, and strokelike episodes. AJNR Am J Neuroradiol 2001; 22:269–72.

[100] Kolb SJ, Costello F, Lee AG, et al. Distinguishing ischemic stroke from the stroke-like lesions of MELAS using apparent diffusion coefficient mapping. J Neurol Sci 2003;216:11–5.

[101] Ooiwa Y, Uematsu Y, Terada T, et al. Cerebral blood flow in mitochondrial myopathy, encephalopathy, lactic acidosis, and strokelike episodes. Stroke 1993;24: 304–9.

[102] Gropen TI, Prohovnik I, Tatemichi TK, et al. Cerebral hyperemia in MELAS. Stroke 1994;25:1873–6.

[103] Castillo M, Kwock L, Green C. MELAS syndrome: imaging and proton MR spectroscopic findings. AJNR Am J Neuroradiol 1995;16:233–9.

ELSEVIER
SAUNDERS

Neuroimag Clin N Am 15 (2005) 609 – 621

NEUROIMAGING
CLINICS OF
NORTH AMERICA

Vulnerable Plaque Imaging

John W. Chen, MD, PhD[a],*, Bruce A. Wasserman, MD[b]

[a]*Division of Neuroradiology, Department of Radiology, Massachusetts General Hospital, Boston, MA, USA*
[b]*Neuroradiology Division, Russell H. Morgan Department of Radiology and Radiological Science,*
Johns Hopkins Medical Institutions, Baltimore, MD, USA

More than 16 million people die worldwide from cardiovascular diseases (CVD) each year, despite recent advances treatment [1]. Coronary heart disease and stroke are the two leading subsets of CVD that cause significant morbidity and mortality. The common pathway leading to these diseases is atherosclerosis.

Atherosclerosis is the process in which deposits of fatty substances, cholesterol, cellular waste products, calcium, and other substances accumulate in the wall of an artery to form plaque, typically affecting medium- and large-sized arteries. In postmortem, histopathologic studies, patients who have fatal coronary events have severely stenotic coronary artery lesions, with more than 90% cross-sectional diameter narrowing [2–5]. Similarly, the North American Symptomatic Carotid Endarterectomy Trial [6] and the European Carotid Surgery Trial [7] show that patients who have symptomatic carotid stenosis above 70% benefit more from surgical than medical treatment with regard to stroke risk. These studies form the basis for reliance on measurements of vascular lumenal narrowing to predict future CVD events.

With regard to coronary arteries specifically, however, some researchers believe that there is compensatory enlargement of the arterial lumen in response to plaque formation, potentially limiting the use of the angiographic stenosis as a criterion to assess CVD risk [8,9]. Moreover, retrospective studies in patients who have acute myocardial infarction or unstable angina show that 78% to 97% of the culprit lesions

are less than 50% stenotic on the initial arteriogram before an acute event [10–12]—although the culprit lesions causing fatal coronary events have greater than 90% stenosis. This implies that—at least in the cardiac model—there is a sudden change in the degree of stenosis before a fatal event and that the narrowing caused by plaque does not portend the risk for ischemic events fully. Rather, the risk or vulnerability of a plaque suddenly to become critically stenotic (ie, become a culprit lesion) is the most important factor.

Contributing to a plaque's stroke risk are its composition and structure, independent of its hemodynamic effect on the lumen. The features that create a plaque's instability and its potential to disrupt are the basis for the concept of plaque vulnerability [13]. Various terms are used in the literature and by clinicians to refer to vulnerable plaques, including high-risk plaques, hot plaques, unstable plaques, soft plaques, and noncalcified plaques.

Plaque vulnerability

Falk [13] divides plaques into two types, a hard collagen-rich plaque, with barely detectable lipid, and a soft plaque, with a prominent pool of extracellular lipid separated by a fibrous cap, and reports that soft plaque is more vulnerable, because the thin fibrous cap may rupture to expose underlying thrombogenic material to the flowing blood.

Davies and colleagues [14] show that plaques that have undergone ulceration and thrombosis (ie, vulnerable plaques) contain a large lipid core (>40% of the cross-sectional area) and a fibrous cap that con-

---

* Corresponding author.
E-mail address: chenjo@helix.mgh.harvard.edu
(J.W. Chen).

1052-5149/05/$ – see front matter © 2005 Elsevier Inc. All rights reserved.
doi:10.1016/j.nic.2005.08.005

tains a larger volume of monocytes/macrophages than plaques that do not undergo rupture and thrombosis.

Burke and colleagues [15] define a vulnerable coronary plaque further as a plaque with a fibrous cap less than 65 μm thick and an infiltrate of macrophages, with or without plaque rupture; plaques that ruptured had an average thickness of 23 ± 19 μm, with 95% of the caps measuring less than 64 μm. Symptomatic carotid plaques are shown to behave similarly by Carr and coworkers [16], who report fibrous cap thinning in 95% of symptomatic plaques compared with 48% of asymptomatic plaques, with symptomatic plaques more prone to rupture. In addition, they found that foam cell infiltration of the fibrous cap was significantly more common in symptomatic plaques (84% versus 44%), but no significant differences were found between plaque hemorrhage, necrotic core, luminal thrombus, shape, plaque type, and smooth muscle cell infiltration [16].

Inflammatory cells (activated macrophages and T lymphocytes) also play an important role in atherosclerosis [17,18], and adhesion molecules (such as vascular cell adhesion molecule [VCAM]-1 that recruit these cells are elevated in plaques [19]. These inflammatory cells secrete cytokines that can oxidize low-density lipoprotein (LDL) [17] and high-density lipoprotein (HDL) [20] and cause thinning and disruption of the fibrous cap through activation of matrix metalloproteinases that remodel the extracellular matrix [18,21–24]. In addition, serum inflammatory markers, such as C-reactive protein (CRP) [25,26] and myeloperoxidase (MPO) [27,28], are elevated in patients at higher risk for CVD events. Therefore, it is evident that plaque disruption occurs most often where the fibrous cap is the thinnest and most heavily infiltrated by inflammatory/foam cells [29].

Although it is understood that rupture-prone vulnerable plaques often have a large lipid pool, a thin cap, and macrophage-dense inflammation on or beneath its surface [29], the actual site of rupture typically is in an area of increased mechanical stress. Lee and colleagues took in vitro plaque specimens and measured stress at different points in the plaque, and found that the stress is highest at the shoulder region of the plaque, regardless of size [30–32]. When Lee and colleagues replaced the lipid core with calcium, the plaque became more stable.

In addition, according to Laplace law, if all else is equal, the tension created in fibrous caps of mildly stenotic lesions is greater than that created in caps of severely stenotic lesions, because of the smaller lumen size [29]. This may explain why retrospective angiographic studies of culprit coronary lesions show only moderate narrowing, because plaques that are only mild or moderately stenotic may be more prone to rupture than severely stenotic plaques. Histologic examination of thrombosed atherosclerotic arteries show that in advanced plaques, microscopic fissures in the collagen cap exposes thrombogenic material to blood in the lumen, causing small, probably silent, thrombi to form [33].

Although the thin-cap atheroma is a well-accepted model and the most common type of vulnerable plaque, plaque composition is heterogeneous, and multiple factors predispose to thrombus formation in addition to cap thickness. Virmani and colleagues describe a classification of plaques based on analysis of coronary arteries implicated as the cause for sudden cardiac death [34]. In this classification, plaques with thin caps were most likely to rupture [35].

Besides this type of vulnerable plaque, in 25% to 30%, an erosive plaque was identified, for which serial sectioning of a thrombosed arterial segment fails to reveal fibrous cap rupture [34]. In these erosive plaques, the endothelium is absent at the erosion site, with variable macrophage and T-lymphocyte infiltration. Erosive plaques contain high concentrations of proteoglycans, which—when exposed in denuded endothelium—is extremely thrombogenic [34,36].

The most rare type of vulnerable plaque is a calcified nodule and refers to a lesion with fibrous cap disruption and thrombi associated with an eruptive, dense, calcific nodule. This is different from a fibrocalcific lesion, which contains a thick fibrous cap overlying extensive accumulation of calcium in the intima and which usually is stable and less vulnerable to rupture. Intraplaque hemorrhage, although not a type of vulnerable plaque, may represent plaque fissuring and be a precursor of plaque rupture [37].

Neovascularization is found in ruptured plaque specimens in the human aorta [38]. Neovascularity is believed to be reflective of inflammation within a plaque, associated with increased accumulation of macrophages and T lymphocytes and, hence, contributes to plaque vulnerability [39]. Fleiner and coworkers show that, in patients who suffered a cardiovascular event, the carotid, iliac, and renal arteries had a denser network of vasa vasorum [40]. In carotid artery lesions, plaque rupture and hemorrhage were associated with neovascularity within the plaque and fibrous cap [41].

Naghavi and coworkers devised a consensus statement defining major and minor criteria for vulnerable plaque (Box 1) [42,43]. Fig. 1 shows a schematic representation of a vulnerable plaque using the major criteria. It should be emphasized that these criteria are based on retrospective studies that await validation by

High-resolution MR imaging

There is a large body of experience in using MR imaging to distinguish the components of atherosclerotic plaque [44–51]. T2-weighted imaging was believed to offer the best contrast to discriminate plaque components, as demonstrated by Martin and colleagues [52]. Toussaint and coworkers [44] performed T1- and T2-weighted imaging of dissected human arteries, and found, on T2-weighted images, a higher contrast-to-noise ratio (CNR) for the lipid core compared with the more collagenous fibrous cap. Calcification was identified better on T1-weighted images. They also found that this relationship holds regardless of the magnetic field strength used, from 1.5 T to 9.4 T. This was verified in vivo, demonstrating that in addition to distinguishing between the lipid core, fibrous cap, and calcifications, intraplaque hemorrhage also can be identified [53]. T2-weighted imaging alone, however, was insufficient to characterize and classify plaques fully [54].

Shinnar and colleagues [45] show that, using a multisequence approach with T1-, T2-, proton density-, and diffusion-weighted images, high sensitivity and specificity can be achieved for identifying different plaque components, albeit at 9.4 T. Similarly, Yuan and colleagues [55] show that multisequence MR imaging can be sensitive to different types of lipid composition, including triglycerides, unesterified and esterified cholesterol, and phospholipids. Since these initial studies, many investigators have found that MR imaging can detect the gamut of plaque composition, including the detection of a thin fibrous cap and cap rupture [46,47,51], intraplaque hemorrhage [48,50], and necrotic/lipid core [44,45, 48,51]. The clinical usefulness of these measures is reported by Yuan and coworkers [47], who show that a thin or ruptured fibrous cap detected by in-vivo MR imaging of the carotid artery is associated with an

prospective studies. Imaging will play an important role to facilitate these prospective studies, because it can allow noninvasive characterization of the plaque, with identification of vulnerable features. This is insightful particularly for plaques that otherwise are not amenable to pathologic analysis, such as carotid plaque causing low-grade stenosis. Based on these criteria, anatomic and functional imaging modalities will play significant and complementary roles, with the goals of identifying vulnerable plaques before they become culprit lesions and of improved diagnosis and assessment of a patient's risk for future cardiovascular events, so that early prevention and treatment can be instituted.

Noninvasive imaging modalities

MR imaging

MR imaging has the ability to characterize the soft tissue components of plaques based on inherent differences in signal. The ability of MR imaging to resolve small structures, such as the components of plaque, depends on the signal achievable for that structure. With improved surface coil technology and MR imaging scanners using higher field strengths MR imaging has become a powerful tool for this purpose.

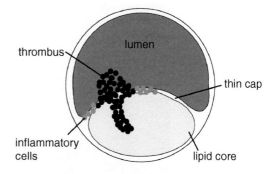

Fig. 1. Schematic representation of a vulnerable plaque. The goal of vulnerable plaque imaging is to identify lesions with these components before significant thrombosis occurs.

odds ratio of 23 for having had a recent transient ischemic attach or stroke.

MR imaging also can be used to image the thrombus associated with plaque rupture. Murphy and coworkers [56] used a T1-weighted fat saturated black blood technique to detect methemoglobin, an intermediate (subacute) breakdown product of blood. They applied this technique to image the carotid arteries of 120 patients who had suspected severe carotid artery stenosis and previous acute cerebral ischemia, and found that high signal, reflecting the presence of methemoglobin, was detected in 60% of the symptomatic patients' ipsilateral carotid arteries versus 36% of their contralateral arteries.

For acute thrombus detection, Viereck and colleagues [57] realized that—unlike hematomas and venous thrombi, which are rich in red blood cells and hemoglobin and, hence, have vastly different MR signal characteristics, depending on the age of the clot—the initial thrombus formed from plaque rupture is more platelet rich. Platelet-rich thrombus may be difficult to distinguish from the vessel wall using standard MR imaging protocols. They demonstrated, in ex-vivo rabbit plaques, that diffusion-weighted images gave the best contrast for distinguishing these platelet-rich thrombi from the vessel wall and can be helpful in identifying the culprit lesion after a vulnerable plaque has caused thrombosis [57]. In this study, however, the field strength used was 11.7 T, which is not clinically practical. At lower field strengths (1.5 T), the investigators were unable to separate the thrombus from the vessel wall [58].

Gadolinium-enhanced MR imaging

Gadolinium is an extracellular contrast agent with uptake mediated by passive diffusion. It is well tolerated and has broad applications because of its ability to detect pathology, including neoplastic processes and inflammation. Its application for plaque characterization is reported by Wasserman and coworkers [49]. In that study, nine subjects who had carotid atherosclerosis were evaluated with double oblique, contrast-enhanced, double inversion-recovery, fast spin-echo MR imaging. Fibrocellular tissue within atheroma selectively enhanced 29% after administration of gadolinium-based contrast. This enhancement helped discriminate fibrous cap from lipid core with a CNR as good as or better than that with T2-weighted MR imaging. In addition, compared with T2-weighted images, there was approximately twice the signal-to-noise ratio, allowing for improved delineation versus the adjacent lipid core. Another study reveals that peak discrimination between the cap and the lipid core is maintained over 30 minutes after gadolinium administration [59]. Fig. 2 demonstrates the enhancing cap after gadolinium administration.

Gadolinium also is known to localize in areas of increased vascularity, a feature that can be exploited when searching for neovascularity within plaque. Kerwin and colleagues show that, in carotid plaque, dynamic imaging with gadolinium correlates well (correlation coefficient 0.80, $P<0.001$) with histologic sections staining for Ulex and CD-31, which reflect angiogenesis [60].

Specific MR imaging contrast agents

There are many ongoing efforts to discover more specific contrast agents, some with well-defined mechanisms of uptake other than diffusion, which can target different components of the vulnerable plaque. This discussion is not meant to be exhaustive, rather, representative of the breadth and promise of contrast agents to increase diagnostic sensitivity in

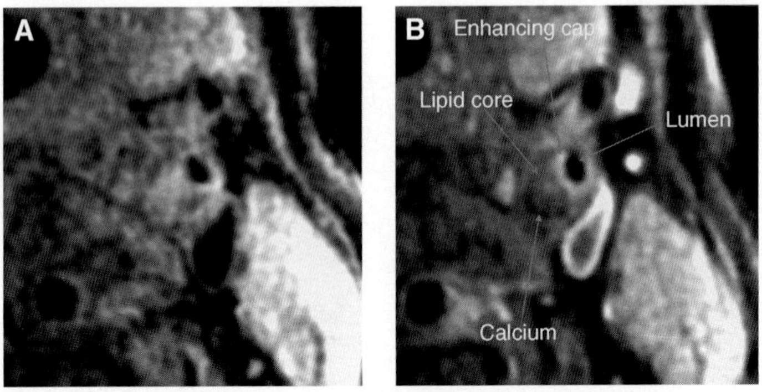

Fig. 2. Postcontrast, high-resolution, T1-weighted, black blood MR imaging demonstrating that there is increased enhancement of the cap after the administration of intravenous gadolinium. (*A*) Precontrast. (*B*) Postcontrast.

identifying vulnerable plaque. Most of these agents are experimental and have limited validation to date in small groups of animals or patients.

Fibrin-binding agents. Fibrin is a predominant component of thrombus, and detection of fibrin can help identify sites of microfissures that may go on to frank disruption, leading to a clinical event. Furthermore, a significant minority of vulnerable plaques do not rupture, rather, are erosive, exposing the underlying matrix proteins and proteoglycans to the blood, causing thrombi to form [34]. Fibrin detection would help to identify these lesions. Yu and coworkers [61] and Flacke and colleagues [62] developed gadolinium-based nanoparticles that accumulate selectively in thrombi. They demonstrate that large CNRs can be achieved in thrombi created in dogs, although a large payload of contrast agent was required. Botnar and colleagues [63] describe the usefulness of a gadolinium-based peptide agent that binds to fibrin, EP-1873. Enhancement with this agent was demonstrated in sites of plaque rupture induced in nine rabbits, with histologic confirmation of uptake of the agent to areas of fibrin. Specificity was not determined, however.

Neovascularization agents. Winter and coworkers report the use of $\alpha_v\beta_3$-integrin–targeted gadolinium nanoparticles to detect sites of neovascularization. They demonstrate enhancement in areas of neovascularity by 47% in a rabbit model injected intravenously with this agent [64]. The tolerance of this agent in humans and its application for identifying vulnerable plaque remain to be tested.

Inflammation agents. The role of inflammation is well established in plaque vulnerability [18,21,25]. Although gadolinium is capable of detecting areas of inflammation, agents that are more specific may provide more useful information regarding the possible role of anti-inflammatory medication for plaque regression [65,66] and more sensitive detection of the inflammatory process that precedes plaque rupture. A variety of potential cellular and molecular targets exists for molecular imaging to detect inflammation.

Ultrasmall paramagnetic iron oxide nanoparticles (USPIO) are taken up by the reticuloendothelial cells, such as macrophages, and can be used to image sites of macrophage accumulation that could reflect significant inflammation within a plaque. Trivedi and coworkers [67] demonstrate USPIO uptake in endarterectomy specimens of seven patients injected with the agent preoperatively, with detectable signal reduction peaking at 24 to 36 hours after injection relative to baseline scans. The USPIO colocalized with activated macrophages on specimen analysis. The source of activated macrophages, however, remains to be determined; these could be derived from migrated blood-borne monocytes, activated macrophages from smooth muscle cells, or foam cells corresponding to macrophages at a later stage [68]. It is a promising agent, although quantification by MR imaging remains to be shown. Fig. 3 demonstrates the use of cross-linked iron oxide nanoparticles in the detection of macrophages in plaques of the aortic root.

Aside from cellular targets of inflammation, another potential molecular target is MPO, an enzyme secreted by activated neutrophils and macrophages in response to inflammation and injury, which has been found in vulnerable plaques [18,69]. MPO usually colocalizes with oxidized LDLs [70]. MPO activity also is linked to the activation of matrix metalloproteinase-7 proenzyme (matrilysin), suggesting that MPO oxidation products may regulate the activity of matrilysin in vivo [23], potentially inducing plaque rupture. MPO also is found to modify

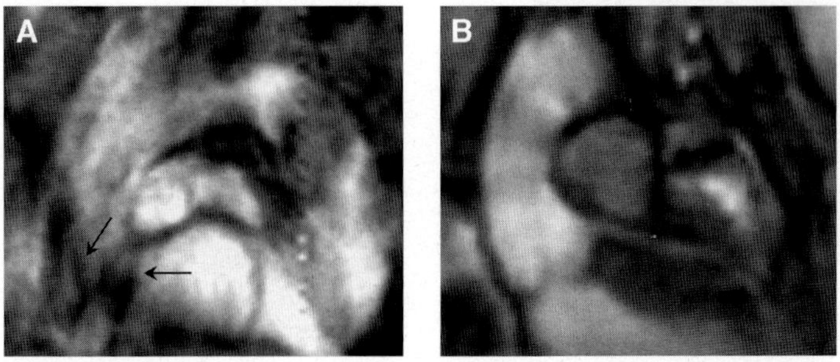

Fig. 3. Cross-linked iron oxide nanoparticles taken up by activated macrophages in plaques cause loss of T2 signal in the atherosclerotic aortic root (*arrows*) in an apoE-knockout mouse, but not in an apoE-knockout mouse injected with saline, at 9.4 T. (*A*) Infected with iron oxide. (*B*) Injected with saline. (Courtesy of Matthias Nahrendorf, MD, and Farouc Jaffer, MD, Charlestown, MA.)

HDL, thereby altering its interaction with scavenger receptors, reversing its protective role [20,71].

A recent study in more than 600 patients established that a single MPO measurement in plasma could predict the risk of major adverse cardiac events within the subsequent 6 months [72]. Another study demonstrates that plasma levels of MPO are elevated in stroke patients [73]. To image MPO activity, Chen and coworkers [74] developed a gadolinium-based agent targeting MPO. In the presence of MPO, the agent is oligomerized. The resulting increased molecular size generates increased T_1 signal by a factor of two relative to nonactivated agents not exposed to MPO (Fig. 4).

Lipophilic agents. As discussed previously, Wasserman and coworkers show that the use of contrast agents can improve the differentiation between the lipid core and fibrous cap by relatively greater enhancement of the cap [49]. Alternative, gadofluorine, originally developed for magnetic resonance lymphography [75,76], seems to target the lipid core [77,78]. Gadofluorine is a macrocyclic gadolinium-based lipophilic agent that forms micelles and may be able bind lipid-rich regions. In one study, Sirol and coworkers [77] demonstrate that there is increased enhancement in the more lipid-rich regions of the plaque.

Frias and coworkers developed a recombinant HDL-like nanoparticle with a gadolinium payload to

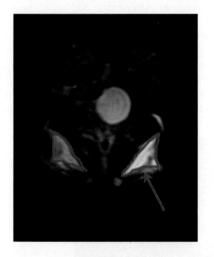

Fig. 4. MPO-sensitive gadolinium-based agent demonstrating nearly twofold increased CNR when activated by MPO. MPO is embedded in a basement membrane extract in the right thigh to simulate a lesion rich in MPO, such as a vulnerable plaque (*arrow*). The contralateral side has no MPO embedded, simulating a lesion such as a stable plaque. (Courtesy of John Chen, MD, PhD, Charlestown, MA.)

target plaques [79]. They show, in an apoE-knockout mouse model, that there is 35% increased enhancement of the wall compared with precontrast images. The nanoparticles seemed to be taken up by macrophages within the plaques.

CT

Electron beam CT and multidetector CT are highly sensitive to calcification and are used as a screening tool for coronary screening asymptomatic individuals [80,81]. The presence and extent of coronary calcium seem to correlate with overall plaque burden [82–85]. The calcium scores generated from CT studies have high negative predictive values, and a high calcium score is associated with increased risk for adverse events.

In 31 patients, calcified plaque of the extracranial carotid artery is 21 times less likely to be symptomatic than is noncalcified plaque [86]. A recent study evaluating the diagnostic accuracy of 16-slice CT scanners in the determination of plaque morphology and composition, using popliteal arteries from amputations, finds 16-slice CT to be reliable in assessing plaque morphology, especially in distinguishing between calcified and noncalcified lesions [87]. CT, however, had low diagnostic accuracy in further classifying plaques as lipid rich or fibrotic. Comparing MR imaging with 16-slice CT, Viles-Gonzalez and coworkers [88] find that CT offers the advantage of very short image acquisition time, which potentially allows it to be more useful for coronary artery imaging. MR imaging, however, provides better tissue characterization.

Ultrasound

For routine clinical evaluation of carotid disease, ultrasound is an important modality to assess the degree of stenosis through B-mode imaging and Doppler velocity measurements. Furthermore, the echogenicity of a plaque is related to its composition. On B-mode imaging, hypoechoic plaques are associated with increased lipid content, macrophage density [89], and intraplaque hemorrhage [90] and are more prone to rupture [91]. A prospective study of 4886 individuals finds that hypoechoic plaques and stenosis greater than 50% are associated with increased risk for future stroke [92], especially in asymptomatic individuals [91]. Although echolucency is associated with increased risk for stroke, because lipid and hemorrhage appear similar and hypoechoic, the major limitations of ultrasound, insofar as vulnerable plaque imaging is concerned, is its insensitivity to characterize vulnerable plaques to stratify risk further. Furthermore, heavy calcification can produce prominent shadowing that can interfere with plaque characterization.

Radionuclide imaging

Like MR imaging, radionuclide imaging relies on innovative radiotracers targeting plaque components to detect vulnerability. Unlike MR imaging, nuclear imaging is highly sensitive, and only a small amount of tracer is needed to detect pathology. Most such agents, however, are in development and remain experimental. Many of these have show initial promise in animal models but have yet to be validated in humans. A few examples are described later.

Single photon emission CT imaging

A variety of radiolabeled substances has been developed to target atherosclerotic lesions. Radiolabeled LDL and oxidized LDL re used to visualize atheroma better, but the presence of LDL does not necessarily indicate a vulnerable plaque [93–98]. Similarly, the apo-B portion of the LDL is radiolabeled and used successfully in rabbits to image atherosclerosis [99]. Antibody-based tracers to proliferating smooth muscle cells also have been developed but with limited success for vulnerable plaque detection [100,101], showing positive uptake in 50% of controls [101].

There also is much effort in designing tracers that can target thrombosis. For example, radiolabeled fibrinogen was developed but did not show much promise because of low sensitivity for arterial thrombus [102]. Fibrin fragments labeled with iodine-123 (^{123}I) and technetium-99m (^{99m}Tc) were used to detect deep venous thrombus in animal models [103], but application to vulnerable plaque detection has yet to be demonstrated. Radiolabeled peptides, mainly targeting GPIIb/IIIa receptors in activated platelets, also have been produced. An example of such an agent is DMP-444-^{99m}Tc, which can identify platelet-rich thrombus in canine coronary arteries and may become useful for detecting culprit lesions and thrombogenic plaques [104]. Annexin V, a small protein that binds to activated platelets and apoptotic vascular smooth muscle cells in the fibrous cap [105–107], is shown to image left atrial thrombus in a porcine model [108]. Blankenberg and coworkers [109] conjected ^{99m}Tc-Annexin V, ^{125}I-MCP-1 (a monomeric polypeptide with high affinity to chemokine receptor expressed on the surface of human monocytes), and fluorodeoxyglucose (FDG) (see discussion later of positron emission tomographic [PET] imaging) into apoE-knockout mice and found that each tracer localized to varying degrees within an atherosclerotic lesion, with distinctly different patterns of plaque localization. These investigators are working on histologic correlation to determine the cellular targets for each tracer to explain the observed differences.

Positron emission tomographic imaging

PET imaging offers improved resolution over single photon emission CT (SPECT), although the short half-lives of these agents make them less practical. Florine-18–FDG is taken up by macrophages [110] and can be used as a measure of inflammation within the plaque [18]. Rudd and coworkers [111] show that FDG is taken up in human carotid atherosclerotic lesions using PET coregistered with CT, with a 27% increased accumulation rate in symptomatic lesions. Ogawa and colleagues [112] show further, in a rabbit model, that the accumulation indeed colocalized to macrophages and not to other cells, such as smooth muscle. Fig. 5 illustrates that FDG/PET imaging can be used in human to localize vascular inflammation.

Although FDG seems a promising agent, challenges include the lack of resolution to localize lesions fully. To this end, the emergence and availability of PET/CT scanners may allow better locali-

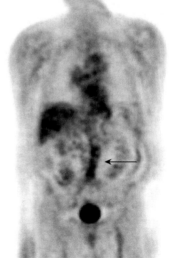

Fig. 5. Increased FDG uptake in an aortic graft infection, demonstrating that PET-FDG can be used to image vascular inflammation. (Courtesy of Alan Fischman, MD, PhD, Boston, MA.)

zation of vulnerable plaques. Comparing FDG uptake with calcium detection in thoracic aorta in 85 consecutive cancer patients, Tatsumi and colleagues [113] find that the site of calcification mostly was distinct from that of FDG uptake and that uptake was increased in women, patients who have hyperlipidemia, and patients who have history of CVD. Despite the potential demonstrated for atherosclerosis imaging by FDG/PET in the aorta and carotid arteries, it may not be possible to image vulnerable plaque in coronary arteries with FDG because of the avid uptake of this agent in myocardium.

Invasive imaging modalities

The inability for conventional angiography to characterize the vulnerable features of plaque has driven the development of invasive modalities to be used to assess the risk of a lesion and, in some cases, provide an opportunity to intervene based on these results.

Intravascular ultrasound

Of the invasive modalities, intravascular ultrasound (IVUS) is the best established. It is a catheter-based technique that can provide high-resolution images of the vessel wall and plaque, because its proximity to the tissue imaged enables the use of high ultrasound frequencies. A miniaturized ultrasound transducer is attached to a catheter and typically operates at 30 to 40 MHz, allowing for a spatial resolution of approximately 150 to 200 μm. IVUS allows the visualization of the full circumference of the vessel wall through tomography. As with conventional ultrasound, IVUS can detect lipid-laden lesions as hypoechoic structures. IVUS is capable of revealing the true plaque size and accounting for vascular remodeling during plaque development [114]. As with conventional ultrasound, however, the echogenicity and texture of different tissue components may exhibit comparable acoustic properties, thus limiting IVUS in the assessment of plaque vulnerability [115].

Optical coherence tomography and angioscopy

Optical coherence tomography uses near-infrared waves and interferometry. It has higher resolution than IVUS, at approximately 10 to 20 μm. Angioscopy uses a camera attached to a catheter, analogous to endoscopy, and can detect fissuring or thrombus. It is able to examine only the luminal surface and cannot penetrate deeper into the plaque to determine composition. In addition, a major drawback of both of these modalities is that they require the inflation of a proximal balloon to obstruct blood flow, which can cause ischemia and vessel injury.

Thermography

Inflammation is an important contributor to plaque disruption, and the goal of thermography is to detect temperature changes associated with this process. Thermography uses a specially designed catheter to measure temperature changes in the wall of the vessel [116]. Ex-vivo studies in human carotid atherosclerotic plaques show that temperature differences within the plaque are related to the cell density of macrophages [117]. In-vivo studies also demonstrate that macrophage mass determines temperature of a plaque [118], and there is a more elevated temperature in patients who have acute coronary syndrome [119]. There is a reduced temperature difference between normal coronary artery walls and plaques treated with statin therapy [120].

Intravascular MR imaging

A potential limitation of noninvasive MR imaging is that of low signal because of the small size of the arteries of interest, for example, the coronary arteries. This may be overcome by placing the coil in near proximity to the plaque (ie, intravascularly via a catheter). Rogers and colleagues [121] show ex-vivo carotid specimens, in which intravascular MR imaging at 0.5 T can be used to detect plaque components, including fibrous cap, lipid core, and calcium. Using hyperlipidemic rabbits, intravascular MR imaging can achieve a resolution of 117×156 μm, compared with 234×468 μm using a surface coil [122].

The vulnerable patient

Recently, a new concept has emerged: the concept of the vulnerable patient. Patients do not have just one vulnerable plaque but often multiple plaques with similar characteristics in different vascular territories [42,43,123–126]. In addition, there is elevation of inflammatory markers in patients who have acute coronary syndrome, such as CRP and MPO [25,27,127]. Imaging combined with serum markers, such as MPO [27] and CRP [26], may be used to identify a vulnerable patient. Any one of the vulnerable plaques in a patient may become the culprit lesion and cause significant morbidity and mortality.

Systemic inflammation, along with significant vulnerable plaque burden, may trigger sudden rupture of vulnerable plaques that cause subsequent catastrophic CVD [124]. The emphasis, therefore, is shifting from the evaluation of an individual plaque to global assessment of the cardiovascular state.

Summary

The concept of vulnerable plaque is well established, owing to increasing evidence from clinical and basic research. With this has come a paradigm shift from focusing on the hemodynamic effect of plaque to its structure and composition. Increasingly, it is evident that methods must be developed to detect and characterize vulnerable plaque. Although MR imaging, CT, and ultrasound provide data regarding the vulnerability of a single lesion, future studies may rely more heavily on nuclear medicine techniques that offer a functional assessment of the entire cardiovascular system.

References

[1] The World Health Report. Geneva (Switzerland): The World Health Organization; 2003.

[2] Horie T, Sekiguchi M, Hirosawa K. Coronary thrombosis in pathogenesis of acute myocardial infarction. Histopathological study of coronary arteries in 108 necropsied cases using serial section. Br Heart J 1978;40:153–61.

[3] Falk E. Plaque rupture with severe pre-existing stenosis precipitating coronary thrombosis. Characteristics of coronary atherosclerotic plaques underlying fatal occlusive thrombi. Br Heart J 1983;50:127–34.

[4] Davies MJ, Thomas A. Thrombosis and acute coronary-artery lesions in sudden cardiac ischemic death. N Engl J Med 1984;310:1137–40.

[5] Qiao JH, Fishbein MC. The severity of coronary atherosclerosis at sites of plaque rupture with occlusive thrombosis. J Am Coll Cardiol 1991;17:1138–42.

[6] North American Symptomatic Carotid Endarterectomy Trial Collaborators. Beneficial effect of carotid endarterectomy in symptomatic patients with high-grade carotid stenosis. N Engl J Med 1991;325: 445–53.

[7] European Carotid Surgery Trialists Collaborative Group. Randomised trial of endarterectomy for recently symptomatic carotid stenosis: final results of the MRC European Carotid Surgery Trial (ECST). Lancet 1998;351:1379–87.

[8] Glagov S, Weisenberg E, Zarins CK, et al. Compensatory enlargement of human atherosclerotic coronary arteries. N Engl J Med 1987;316:1371–5.

[9] Fishbein MC, Siegel RJ. How big are coronary atherosclerotic plaques that rupture? Circulation 1996;94:2662–6.

[10] Ambrose JA. Coronary arteriographic analysis and angiographic morphology. J Am Coll Cardiol 1989; 13:1492–4.

[11] Little WC, Constantinescu M, Applegate RJ, et al. Can coronary angiography predict the site of a subsequent myocardial infarction in patients with mild-to-moderate coronary artery disease? Circulation 1988;78(5 Pt 1):1157–66.

[12] Mulcahy D, Husain S, Zalos G, et al. Ischemia during ambulatory monitoring as a prognostic indicator in patients with stable coronary artery disease. JAMA 1997;277:318–24.

[13] Falk E. Coronary thrombosis: pathogenesis and clinical manifestations. Am J Cardiol 1991;68:28B–35B.

[14] Davies MJ, Richardson PD, Woolf N, et al. Risk of thrombosis in human atherosclerotic plaques: role of extracellular lipid, macrophage, and smooth muscle cell content. Br Heart J 1993;69:377–81.

[15] Burke GL, Evans GW, Riley WA, et al. Arterial wall thickness is associated with prevalent cardiovascular disease in middle-aged adults. The Atherosclerosis Risk in Communities (ARIC) Study. Stroke 1995;26: 386–91.

[16] Carr S, Farb A, Pearce WH, et al. Atherosclerotic plaque rupture in symptomatic carotid artery stenosis. J Vasc Surg 1996;23:755–65.

[17] Berliner JA, Navab M, Fogelman AM, et al. Atherosclerosis: basic mechanisms. Oxidation, inflammation, and genetics. Circulation 1995;91:2488–96.

[18] Libby P. Inflammation in atherosclerosis. Nature 2002;420:868–74.

[19] Davies MJ, Gordon JL, Gearing AJ, et al. The expression of the adhesion molecules ICAM-1, VCAM-1, PECAM, and E-selectin in human atherosclerosis. J Pathol 1993;171:223–9.

[20] Bergt C, Pennathur S, Fu X, et al. The myeloperoxidase product hypochlorous acid oxidizes HDL in the human artery wall and impairs ABCA1-dependent cholesterol transport. Proc Natl Acad Sci USA 2004; 101:13032–7.

[21] Libby P, Ridker PM, Maseri A. Inflammation and atherosclerosis. Circulation 2002;105:1135–43.

[22] Loftus IM, Naylor AR, Goodall S, et al. Increased matrix metalloproteinase-9 activity in unstable carotid plaques. A potential role in acute plaque disruption. Stroke 2000;31:40–7.

[23] Fu X, Kassim SY, Parks WC, et al. Hypochlorous acid oxygenates the cysteine switch domain of promatrilysin (MMP-7). A mechanism for matrix metalloproteinase activation and atherosclerotic plaque rupture by myeloperoxidase. J Biol Chem 2001;276: 41279–87.

[24] Molloy KJ, Thompson MM, Jones JL, et al. Unstable carotid plaques exhibit raised matrix metalloproteinase-8 activity. Circulation 2004;110: 337–43.

[25] Libby P, Ridker PM. Inflammation and atherosclerosis: role of C-reactive protein in risk assessment. Am J Med 2004;116(Suppl 6A):9S–16S.

[26] Danesh J, Wheeler JG, Hirschfield GM, et al. C-reactive protein and other circulating markers of inflammation in the prediction of coronary heart disease. N Engl J Med 2004;350:1387–97.

[27] Brennan ML, Penn MS, Van Lente F, et al. Prognostic value of myeloperoxidase in patients with chest pain. N Engl J Med 2003;349:1595–604.

[28] Baldus S, Heeschen C, Meinertz T, et al. Myeloperoxidase serum levels predict risk in patients with acute coronary syndromes. Circulation 2003;108:1440–5.

[29] Falk E, Shah PK, Fuster V. Coronary plaque disruption. Circulation 1995;92:657–71.

[30] Cheng GC, Loree HM, Kamm RD, et al. Distribution of circumferential stress in ruptured and stable atherosclerotic lesions. A structural analysis with histopathological correlation. Circulation 1993;87:1179–87.

[31] Arroyo LH, Lee RT. Mechanisms of plaque rupture: mechanical and biologic interactions. Cardiovasc Res 1999;41:369–75.

[32] Lee RT. Atherosclerotic lesion mechanics versus biology. Z Kardiol 2000;89(Suppl 2):80–4.

[33] Constantinides P. Cause of thrombosis in human atherosclerotic arteries. Am J Cardiol 1990;66:37G–40G.

[34] Virmani R, Kolodgie FD, Burke AP, et al. Lessons from sudden coronary death: a comprehensive morphological classification scheme for atherosclerotic lesions. Arterioscler Thromb Vasc Biol 2000;20:1262–75.

[35] Burke AP, Farb A, Malcom GT, et al. Coronary risk factors and plaque morphology in men with coronary disease who died suddenly. N Engl J Med 1997;336:1276–82.

[36] Kolodgie FD, Burke AP, Wight TN, et al. The accumulation of specific types of proteoglycans in eroded plaques: a role in coronary thrombosis in the absence of rupture. Curr Opin Lipidol 2004;15:575–82.

[37] Davies MJ, Thomas AC. Plaque fissuring—the cause of acute myocardial infarction, sudden ischaemic death, and crescendo angina. Br Heart J 1985;53:363–73.

[38] Moreno PR, Purushothaman KR, Fuster V, et al. Plaque neovascularization is increased in ruptured atherosclerotic lesions of human aorta: implications for plaque vulnerability. Circulation 2004;110:2032–8.

[39] Jeziorska M, Woolley DE. Local neovascularization and cellular composition within vulnerable regions of atherosclerotic plaques of human carotid arteries. J Pathol 1999;188:189–96.

[40] Fleiner M, Kummer M, Mirlacher M, et al. Arterial neovascularization and inflammation in vulnerable patients: early and late signs of symptomatic atherosclerosis. Circulation 2004;110:2843–50.

[41] McCarthy MJ, Loftus IM, Thompson MM, et al. Angiogenesis and the atherosclerotic carotid plaque: an association between symptomatology and plaque morphology. J Vasc Surg 1999;30:261–8.

[42] Naghavi M, Libby P, Falk E, et al. From vulnerable plaque to vulnerable patient: a call for new definitions and risk assessment strategies: part II. Circulation 2003;108:1772–8.

[43] Naghavi M, Libby P, Falk E, et al. From vulnerable plaque to vulnerable patient: a call for new definitions and risk assessment strategies: part I. Circulation 2003;108:1664–72.

[44] Toussaint JF, Southern JF, Fuster V, Kantor HL. T2-weighted contrast for NMR characterization of human atherosclerosis. Arterioscler Thromb Vasc Biol 1995;15:1533–42.

[45] Shinnar M, Fallon JT, Wehrli S, et al. The diagnostic accuracy of ex vivo MRI for human atherosclerotic plaque characterization. Arterioscler Thromb Vasc Biol 1999;19:2756–61.

[46] Hatsukami TS, Ross R, Polissar NL, Yuan C. Visualization of fibrous cap thickness and rupture in human atherosclerotic carotid plaque in vivo with high-resolution magnetic resonance imaging. Circulation 2000;102:959–64.

[47] Yuan C, Zhang SX, Polissar NL, et al. Identification of fibrous cap rupture with magnetic resonance imaging is highly associated with recent transient ischemic attack or stroke. Circulation 2002;105:181–5.

[48] Yuan C, Mitsumori LM, Ferguson MS, et al. In vivo accuracy of multispectral magnetic resonance imaging for identifying lipid-rich necrotic cores and intraplaque hemorrhage in advanced human carotid plaques. Circulation 2001;104:2051–6.

[49] Wasserman BA, Smith WI, Trout 3rd HH, et al. Carotid artery atherosclerosis: in vivo morphologic characterization with gadolinium-enhanced double-oblique MR imaging initial results. Radiology 2002;223:566–73.

[50] Kampschulte A, Ferguson MS, Kerwin WS, et al. Differentiation of intraplaque versus juxtaluminal hemorrhage/thrombus in advanced human carotid atherosclerotic lesions by in vivo magnetic resonance imaging. Circulation 2004;110:3239–44.

[51] Trivedi RA, U-King-Im JM, Graves MJ, et al. MRI-derived measurements of fibrous-cap and lipid-core thickness: the potential for identifying vulnerable carotid plaques in vivo. Neuroradiology 2004;46:738–43.

[52] Martin AJ, Gotlieb AI, Henkelman RM. High-resolution MR imaging of human arteries. J Magn Reson Imaging 1995;5:93–100.

[53] Toussaint JF, LaMuraglia GM, Southern JF, et al. Magnetic resonance images lipid, fibrous, calcified, hemorrhagic, and thrombotic components of human atherosclerosis in vivo. Circulation 1996;94:932–8.

[54] Serfaty JM, Chaabane L, Tabib A, et al. Atherosclerotic plaques: classification and characterization with T2-weighted high-spatial-resolution MR imaging—an in vitro study. Radiology 2001;219:403–10.

[55] Yuan C, Petty C, O'Brien KD, et al. In vitro and in situ magnetic resonance imaging signal features of atherosclerotic plaque-associated lipids. Arterioscler Thromb Vasc Biol 1997;17:1496–503.

[56] Murphy RE, Moody AR, Morgan PS, et al. Prevalence of complicated carotid atheroma as detected by magnetic resonance direct thrombus imaging in patients with suspected carotid artery stenosis and previous acute cerebral ischemia. Circulation 2003; 107:3053–8.

[57] Viereck J, Ruberg FL, Qiao Y, et al. MRI of atherothrombosis associated with plaque rupture. Arterioscler Thromb Vasc Biol 2005;25:240–5.

[58] Johnstone MT, Botnar RM, Perez AS, et al. In vivo magnetic resonance imaging of experimental thrombosis in a rabbit model. Arterioscler Thromb Vasc Biol 2001;21:1556–60.

[59] Wasserman BA, Casal SG, Astor BC, et al. Wash-in kinetics for gadolinium-enhanced magnetic resonance imaging of carotid atheroma. J Magn Reson Imaging 2005;21:91–5.

[60] Kerwin W, Hooker A, Spilker M, et al. Quantitative magnetic resonance imaging analysis of neovasculature volume in carotid atherosclerotic plaque. Circulation 2003;107:851–6.

[61] Yu X, Song SK, Chen J, et al. High-resolution MRI characterization of human thrombus using a novel fibrin-targeted paramagnetic nanoparticle contrast agent. Magn Reson Med 2000;44:867–72.

[62] Flacke S, Fischer S, Scott MJ, et al. Novel MRI contrast agent for molecular imaging of fibrin: implications for detecting vulnerable plaques. Circulation 2001;104:1280–5.

[63] Botnar RM, Perez AS, Witte S, et al. In vivo molecular imaging of acute and subacute thrombosis using a fibrin-binding magnetic resonance imaging contrast agent. Circulation 2004;109:2023–9.

[64] Winter PM, Morawski AM, Caruthers SD, et al. Molecular imaging of angiogenesis in early-stage atherosclerosis with alpha(v)beta3-integrin-targeted nanoparticles. Circulation 2003;108:2270–4.

[65] Cascieri MA. The potential for novel anti-inflammatory therapies for coronary artery disease. Nat Rev Drug Discov 2002;1:122–30.

[66] Sparrow CP, Burton CA, Hernandez M, et al. Simvastatin has anti-inflammatory and antiatherosclerotic activities independent of plasma cholesterol lowering. Arterioscler Thromb Vasc Biol 2001;21:115–21.

[67] Trivedi RA, U-King-Im JM, Graves MJ, et al. In vivo detection of macrophages in human carotid atheroma: temporal dependence of ultrasmall superparamagnetic particles of iron oxide-enhanced MRI. Stroke 2004; 35:1631–5.

[68] Corot C, Petry KG, Trivedi R, et al. Macrophage imaging in central nervous system and in carotid atherosclerotic plaque using ultrasmall superparamagnetic iron oxide in magnetic resonance imaging. Invest Radiol 2004;39:619–25.

[69] Naruko T, Ueda M, Haze K, et al. Neutrophil in-filtration of culprit lesions in acute coronary syndromes. Circulation 2002;106:2894–900.

[70] Malle E, Waeg G, Schreiber R, et al. Immunohisto-chemical evidence for the myeloperoxidase/H2O2/halide system in human atherosclerotic lesions: colocalization of myeloperoxidase and hypochlorite-modified proteins. Eur J Biochem 2000;267:4495–503.

[71] Marsche G, Hammer A, Oskolkova O, et al. Hypochlorite-modified high density lipoprotein, a high affinity ligand to scavenger receptor class B, type I, impairs high density lipoprotein-dependent selective lipid uptake and reverse cholesterol transport. J Biol Chem 2002;277:32172–9.

[72] Brennan ML, Penn MS, Van Lente F, et al. Prognostic value of myeloperoxidase in patients with chest pain. N Engl J Med 2003;349:1595–604.

[73] Re G, Azzimondi G, Lanzarini C, et al. Plasma lipoperoxidative markers in ischaemic stroke suggest brain embolism. Eur J Emerg Med 1997;4:5–9.

[74] Chen JW, Pham W, Weissleder R, Bogdanov Jr A. Human myeloperoxidase: a potential target for molecular MR imaging in atherosclerosis. Magn Reson Med 2004;52:1021–8.

[75] Misselwitz B, Platzek J, Raduchel B, et al. Gadofluorine 8: initial experience with a new contrast medium for interstitial MR lymphography. MAGMA 1999;8:190–5.

[76] Misselwitz B, Platzek J, Weinmann HJ. Early MR lymphography with gadofluorine M in rabbits. Radiology 2004;231:682–8.

[77] Sirol M, Itskovich VV, Mani V, et al. Lipid-rich atherosclerotic plaques detected by gadofluorine-enhanced in vivo magnetic resonance imaging. Circulation 2004;109:2890–6.

[78] Barkhausen J, Ebert W, Heyer C, et al. Detection of atherosclerotic plaque with Gadofluorine-enhanced magnetic resonance imaging. Circulation 2003;108: 605–9.

[79] Frias JC, Williams KJ, Fisher EA, et al. Recombinant HDL-like nanoparticles: a specific contrast agent for MRI of atherosclerotic plaques. J Am Chem Soc 2004;126:16316–7.

[80] O'Rourke RA, Brundage BH, Froelicher VF, et al. American College of Cardiology/American Heart Association Expert Consensus document on electron-beam computed tomography for the diagnosis and prognosis of coronary artery disease. Circulation 2000;102:126–40.

[81] Stanford W, Thompson BH, Burns TL, et al. Coronary artery calcium quantification at multi-detector row helical CT versus electron-beam CT. Radiology 2004;230:397–402.

[82] Sangiorgi G, Rumberger JA, Severson A, et al. Arterial calcification and not lumen stenosis is highly correlated with atherosclerotic plaque burden in humans: a histologic study of 723 coronary artery segments using nondecalcifying methodology. J Am Coll Cardiol 1998;31:126–33.

[83] Wayhs R, Zelinger A, Raggi P. High coronary artery

calcium scores pose an extremely elevated risk for hard events. J Am Coll Cardiol 2002;39:225–30.

[84] Mohlenkamp S, Lehmann N, Schmermund A, et al. Prognostic value of extensive coronary calcium quantities in symptomatic males—a 5-year follow-up study. Eur Heart J 2003;24:845–54.

[85] Hoff JA, Daviglus ML, Chomka EV, et al. Conventional coronary artery disease risk factors and coronary artery calcium detected by electron beam tomography in 30,908 healthy individuals. Ann Epidemiol 2003;13:163–9.

[86] Nandalur K, Baskurt E, Hagspiel K, et al. Calcified carotid atherosclerotic plaque is associated less with ischemic symptoms than is noncalcified plaque on MDCT. AJR Am J Roentgenol 2004;184:295–8.

[87] Schroeder S, Kuettner A, Wojak T, et al. Noninvasive evaluation of atherosclerosis with contrast enhanced 16 slice spiral computed tomography: results of ex vivo investigations. Heart 2004;90:1471–5.

[88] Viles-Gonzalez JF, Poon M, Sanz J, et al. In vivo 16-slice, multidetector-row computed tomography for the assessment of experimental atherosclerosis: comparison with magnetic resonance imaging and histopathology. Circulation 2004;110:1467–72.

[89] Gronholdt ML, Nordestgaard BG, Bentzon J, et al. Macrophages are associated with lipid-rich carotid artery plaques, echolucency on B-mode imaging, and elevated plasma lipid levels. J Vasc Surg 2002;35: 137–45.

[90] Gronholdt ML, Nordestgaard BG, Schroeder TV, et al. Ultrasonic echolucent carotid plaques predict future strokes. Circulation 2001;104:68–73.

[91] Nordestgaard BG, Gronholdt ML, Sillesen H. Echolucent rupture-prone plaques. Curr Opin Lipidol 2003;14:505–12.

[92] Polak JF, Shemanski L, O'Leary DH, et al. Hypoechoic plaque at US of the carotid artery: an independent risk factor for incident stroke in adults aged 65 years or older. Cardiovascular Health Study. Radiology 1998;208:649–54.

[93] Vallabhajosula S, Paidi M, Badimon JJ, et al. Radiotracers for low density lipoprotein biodistribution studies in vivo: technetium-99m low density lipoprotein versus radioiodinated low density lipoprotein preparations. J Nucl Med 1988;29:1237–45.

[94] Rosen JM, Butler SP, Meinken GE, et al. Indium-111-labeled LDL: a potential agent for imaging atherosclerotic disease and lipoprotein biodistribution. J Nucl Med 1990;31:343–50.

[95] Virgolini I, Rauscha F, Lupattelli G, et al. Autologous low-density lipoprotein labelling allows characterization of human atherosclerotic lesions in vivo as to presence of foam cells and endothelial coverage. Eur J Nucl Med 1991;18:948–51.

[96] Chang MY, Lees AM, Lees RS. Time course of 125I-labeled LDL accumulation in the healing, balloon-deendothelialized rabbit aorta. Arterioscler Thromb 1992;12:1088–98.

[97] Steinberg D, Parthasarathy S, Carew TE, et al. Beyond

cholesterol. Modifications of low-density lipoprotein that increase its atherogenicity. N Engl J Med 1989;320:915–24.

[98] Iuliano L, Signore A, Vallabhajosula S, et al. Preparation and biodistribution of 99m technetium labelled oxidized LDL in man. Atherosclerosis 1996;126: 131–41.

[99] Hardoff R, Braegelmann F, Zanzonico P, et al. External imaging of atherosclerosis in rabbits using an 123I-labeled synthetic peptide fragment. J Clin Pharmacol 1993;33:1039–47.

[100] Narula J, Petrov A, Bianchi C, et al. Noninvasive localization of experimental atherosclerotic lesions with mouse/human chimeric Z2D3 F(ab′)2 specific for the proliferating smooth muscle cells of human atheroma. Imaging with conventional and negative charge-modified antibody fragments. Circulation 1995;92:474–84.

[101] Carrio I, Pieri PL, Narula J, et al. Noninvasive localization of human atherosclerotic lesions with indium 111-labeled monoclonal Z2D3 antibody specific for proliferating smooth muscle cells. J Nucl Cardiol 1998;5:551–7.

[102] Mettinger KL, Larsson S, Ericson K, et al. Detection of atherosclerotic plaques in carotid arteries by the use of 123I-fibrinogen. Lancet 1978;1:242–4.

[103] Knight LC. Scintigraphic methods for detecting vascular thrombus. J Nucl Med 1993;34(3 Suppl): 554–61.

[104] Mitchel J, Waters D, Lai T, et al. Identification of coronary thrombus with a IIb/IIIa platelet inhibitor radiopharmaceutical, technetium-99m DMP-444: a canine model. Circulation 2000;101:1643–6.

[105] Thiagarajan P, Tait JF. Binding of annexin V/placental anticoagulant protein I to platelets. Evidence for phosphatidylserine exposure in the procoagulant response of activated platelets. J Biol Chem 1990; 265:17420–3.

[106] Dachary-Prigent J, Freyssinet JM, Pasquet JM, et al. Annexin V as a probe of aminophospholipid exposure and platelet membrane vesiculation: a flow cytometry study showing a role for free sulfhydryl groups. Blood 1993;81:2554–65.

[107] Flynn PD, Byrne CD, Baglin TP, et al. Thrombin generation by apoptotic vascular smooth muscle cells. Blood 1997;89:4378–84.

[108] Stratton JR, Dewhurst TA, Kasina S, et al. Selective uptake of radiolabeled annexin V on acute porcine left atrial thrombi. Circulation 1995;92:3113–21.

[109] Blankenberg FG, Katsikis PD, Tait JF, et al. In vivo detection and imaging of phosphatidylserine expression during programmed cell death. Proc Natl Acad Sci USA 1998;95:6349–54.

[110] Kubota R, Yamada S, Kubota K, et al. Intratumoral distribution of fluorine-18-fluorodeoxyglucose in vivo: high accumulation in macrophages and granulation tissues studied by microautoradiography. J Nucl Med 1992;33:1972–80.

[111] Rudd JH, Warburton EA, Fryer TD, et al. Imaging

atherosclerotic plaque inflammation with [18F]-fluorodeoxyglucose positron emission tomography. Circulation 2002;105:2708–11.

[112] Ogawa M, Ishino S, Mukai T, et al. (18)F-FDG accumulation in atherosclerotic plaques: immunohistochemical and PET imaging study. J Nucl Med 2004;45:1245–50.

[113] Tatsumi M, Cohade C, Nakamoto Y, et al. Fluorodeoxyglucose uptake in the aortic wall at PET/CT: possible finding for active atherosclerosis. Radiology 2003;229:831–7.

[114] Nissen SE. Application of intravascular ultrasound to characterize coronary artery disease and assess the progression or regression of atherosclerosis. Am J Cardiol 2002;89:24B–31B.

[115] Nissen SE, Yock P. Intravascular ultrasound: novel pathophysiological insights and current clinical applications. Circulation 2001;103:604–16.

[116] Stefanadis C, Diamantopoulos L, Vlachopoulos C, et al. Thermal heterogeneity within human atherosclerotic coronary arteries detected in vivo: a new method of detection by application of a special thermography catheter. Circulation 1999;99:1965–71.

[117] Casscells W, Hathorn B, David M, et al. Thermal detection of cellular infiltrates in living atherosclerotic plaques: possible implications for plaque rupture and thrombosis. Lancet 1996;347:1447–51.

[118] Verheye S, De Meyer GR, Van Langenhove G, et al. In vivo temperature heterogeneity of atherosclerotic plaques is determined by plaque composition. Circulation 2002;105:1596–601.

[119] Stefanadis C, Toutouzas K, Tsiamis E, et al. Increased local temperature in human coronary atherosclerotic plaques: an independent predictor of clinical outcome in patients undergoing a percutaneous coronary intervention. J Am Coll Cardiol 2001;37:1277–83.

[120] Stefanadis C, Toutouzas K, Vavuranakis M, et al. Statin treatment is associated with reduced thermal heterogeneity in human atherosclerotic plaques. Eur Heart J 2002;23:1664–9.

[121] Rogers WJ, Prichard JW, Hu YL, et al. Characterization of signal properties in atherosclerotic plaque components by intravascular MRI. Arterioscler Thromb Vasc Biol 2000;20:1824–30.

[122] Zimmermann-Paul GG, Quick HH, Vogt P, et al. High-resolution intravascular magnetic resonance imaging: monitoring of plaque formation in heritable hyperlipidemic rabbits. Circulation 1999;99: 1054–61.

[123] Rioufol G, Finet G, Ginon I, et al. Multiple atherosclerotic plaque rupture in acute coronary syndrome: a three-vessel intravascular ultrasound study. Circulation 2002;106:804–8.

[124] Tuzcu EM, Schoenhagen P. Acute coronary syndromes, plaque vulnerability, and carotid artery disease: the changing role of atherosclerosis imaging. J Am Coll Cardiol 2003;42:1033–6.

[125] Kato M, Dote K, Habara S, et al. Clinical implications of carotid artery remodeling in acute coronary syndrome: ultrasonographic assessment of positive remodeling. J Am Coll Cardiol 2003;42:1026–32.

[126] Casscells W, Naghavi M, Willerson JT. Vulnerable atherosclerotic plaque: a multifocal disease. Circulation 2003;107:2072–5.

[127] Cusack MR, Marber MS, Lambiase PD, et al. Systemic inflammation in unstable angina is the result of myocardial necrosis. J Am Coll Cardiol 2002; 39:1917–23.

ELSEVIER
SAUNDERS

Neuroimag Clin N Am 15 (2005) 623 – 637

**NEUROIMAGING
CLINICS OF
NORTH AMERICA**

Technical Aspects of Perfusion-Weighted Imaging

Ona Wu, PhD[a,*], Leif Østergaard, MD, PhD[b], A. Gregory Sorensen, MD[a]

[a]*MGH/MIT/HMS Athinoula A. Martinos Center for Biomedical Imaging, Charlestown, MA, USA*
[b]*Center of Functionally Integrative Neuroscience, Department of Neuroradiology, Århus University Hospital, Århus, Denmark*

Perfusion-weighted MR imaging (PWI) is highly sensitive in detecting ischemic tissue at risk of infarction [1–6]. The use of PWI, in conjunction with diffusion-weighted MR imaging, therefore, has gained popularity for the identification of potentially salvageable tissue in acute cerebral ischemia [7–10]. This article explores the technical considerations and potential pitfalls of performing and interpreting PWI. A brief overview of some of the more common techniques used for estimating hemodynamic parameters in PWI also is provided.

MR imaging data acquisition: theoretic considerations

Although there are many ways to perform non-invasive measurement of blood flow, this article is limited to one of the more common clinically performed techniques that estimates cerebral blood flow (CBF) by tracking a bolus of exogenous, non-diffusible, high magnetic susceptibility contrast agent (CA) using MR imaging, followed by tracer kinetic analysis to derive hemodynamic parameters. During the passage of a CA bolus—typically a para-magnetic substance, such as gadolinium-diethylene-triaminepentaacetic acid (Gd-DTPA)—a transient loss of MR signal arises from reduction in the transverse relaxation times (T2 and T2*) as a result of changes in magnetic susceptibility. The relationship between image intensity and change in relaxivity ΔR_2 (or $\Delta R_2{*}$ in gradient-echo [GRE] experiments; Eq. 1) is [11,12]:

$$S(t) = S_0 e^{-TE \cdot \Delta R_2} \tag{1}$$

where S_0 is the baseline MR imaging signal intensity before administration of CA, $R_2 = 1/T_2$ ($R_2{*} = 1/T_2{*}$), and TE is the echo time. Changes in relaxivity, $\Delta R_2{*}$ or ΔR_2, can be measured using either T2-weighted GRE or spin-echo (SE) MR imaging, respectively, although with echo-planar imaging (EPI), SE MR imaging also contains some $R_2{*}$ effects [13].

Studies show a complex interaction between changes in relaxivity and vessel architecture, CA concentration, and MR acquisition parameters [14–18]. For small susceptibility changes, $\Delta\chi$ (dependent on concentration agent type, dosage, and injection rate), a quadratic relationship between CA concentration and $\Delta R_2{*}$ is noted, with linear dependence at large $\Delta\chi$, and transition point dependent on vessel radius and TE [16,17]. For ΔR_2, nonlinear dependencies are noted at all concentrations, with superlinear behavior at low $\Delta\chi$ followed by sublinear relationship at high $\Delta\chi$, with the transition point occurring earlier for larger vessels [17]. This results in SE PWI being less sensitive to vessels of large diameters compared with GRE PWI [17]. Therefore, it is likely no simple relationship exists relating changes in relaxivity with changes in concentration. Using standard clinical

* Corresponding author. MGH Department of Radiology, MGH/MIT/HMS Athinoula A. Martinos Center for Biomedical Imaging, 13th Street, Building 149, Charlestown, MA 02129.

E-mail address: ona@nmr.mgh.harvard.edu (O. Wu).

protocols, however, a linear relationship between CA concentrations and $\Delta R_2/\Delta R_2^*$ can be assumed [19], as often observed for in vivo data. The change in CA concentration over time can then be measured using Eq. 2 [15]:

$$C(t) = -\frac{k}{\mathrm{TE}} \ln \frac{S(t)}{S_0} \qquad (2)$$

where k is a proportionality factor. An example of how this relationship translates clinically is in Fig. 1. After conversion to concentration-time curves, tracer kinetic analysis is used to extract parameters to characterize tissue perfusion status, such as cerebral blood volume (CBV), CBF, and mean transit time (MTT).

In addition to changes in transverse relaxation rates, introduction of Gd-DTPA also shortens longitudinal relaxation time (T_1) leading to enhancement in T_1-weighted images [20]. Assuming an intact blood-brain barrier, however, these effects remain predominantly intravascular since these changes rely on direct access between tissue and CA. Therefore, because these effects scale approximately with the CA distribution space and CBV comprises less than 5% of the total tissue space for typical brain tissue, the observed changes due to T_1 effects are typically smaller than those due to ΔR_2 or ΔR_2^* [11]. When this assumption is violated because of disturbed BBB,

parenchymal enhancement is noted. Measuring dynamic changes in T_1 is sometimes used for characterizing BBB permeability [21]. For now, an intact BBB is assumed and T_1 effects ignored, but T_1 enhancement is covered later when dealing with potential confounds are discussed.

Tracer kinetic analysis

Assuming relaxivity changes are proportional to concentration changes, traditional tracer kinetic models for intravascular agents [22–24] can be extended to dynamic susceptibility contrast MR imaging data for characterizing tissue perfusion status. By integrating the concentration-time curves of CA remaining within the tissue, $C(t)$, with respect to time, CBV can be obtained with Eq. 3 [12,23]:

$$CBV = \frac{\int_0^\infty C(t)dt}{\int_0^\infty C_a(t)dt} \qquad (3)$$

assuming no recirculation or consumption of the CA, and $C_a(t)$ is the concentration at the input artery (the arterial input function [AIF]).

Modeling the vascular bed as a fluid dynamic system consisting of a single inflow and single outflow, with multiple capillary branches in between

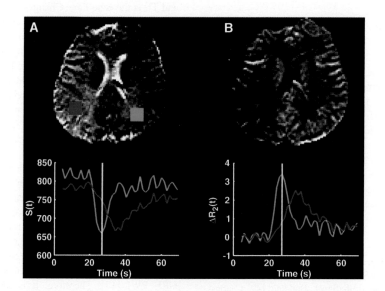

Fig. 1. Examples of (*A*) MR signal changes resulting from injection of a bolus of Gd-DTPA and (*B*) calculated changes in relaxivity in a stroke patient who had occlusion of the right middle cerebral artery, imaged less than 4 hours from symptom onset using SE EPI and TR/TE = 1500/65 ms. The MR signal in the normal hemisphere (*green region of interest*) clearly appears different from the signal measured in the ipsilateral hemisphere (red region of interest). Tracer kinetic analysis can be used to characterize these differences. $\Delta R_2(t)$, change in relaxivity over time in units of s^{-1}; S(t), signal versus time in arbitrary units.

[22], the fraction of CA leaving the bed per unit time can be represented as a transport function (Eq. 4), $h(t)$, where:

$$\int_0^\infty h(t)dt = 1 \tag{4}$$

Furthermore, the fraction of tracer remaining in the system, known as the residue function, $R(t)$, then can be defined as Eq. 5.

$$R(t) = 1 - \int_0^t h(\tau)d\tau \tag{5}$$

$C(t)$ then can be modeled as Eq. 6 [25]:

$$C(t) = F_t C_a(t) \otimes R(t)$$
$$= F_t \int_0^t C_a(\tau)R(t-\tau)d\tau \tag{6}$$

where $\otimes$ represents the convolution operator, and F_t the CBF within the tissue system. CBF then can be measured by deconvolving the signal curve proportional to the concentration remaining in the voxel, $C(t)$, with the AIF, $C_a(t)$ (Eq. 7):

$$F_t R(t) = C(t) \otimes^{-1} C_a(t) \tag{7}$$

where $\otimes^{-1}$ represents the deconvolution operator. Because, by definition, maximum $R(t) = 1$ (ie, the maximum fraction of CA remaining in tissue at any given time is 1), the maximum of the deconvolved signal is assumed to be CBF. This does not necessarily occur at $t = 0$, because of transit delay between the AIF and $C(t)$. The mean of the transit or circulation times then can be calculated using the central volume theorem (Eq. 8) [22,26]:

$$\text{MTT} \equiv \int_0^\infty t\, h(t)dt = \frac{\text{CBV}}{\text{CBF}} \tag{8}$$

Summary statistics of $C(t)$ often are calculated in lieu of measurement of an AIF. For instance, relative CBV or area under $C(t)$ (see Eq. 3), can be determined without knowledge of the AIF, which is assumed common for all voxels in a single acquisition. Therefore, not taking the AIF into consideration results in differences only by a scaling factor [12,17,18]. Other parameters, such as bolus arrival time (BAT), time to peak (TTP), relative TTP (relTTP = TTP-BAT), full-width at half maximum concentration (FWHM), first moment of $C(t)$, and maximum peak concentration (Peak), are indirect measurements of perfusion status that are used as surrogates for MTT and CBF (Fig. 2). Fig. 3 shows examples of these maps calculated either numerically or by fitting the concentration-time curves to a gamma-variate function. Both methods have their benefits and shortcomings. Although easy to calculate, these metrics are not as accurate as techniques that measure the AIF, because of their dependence on

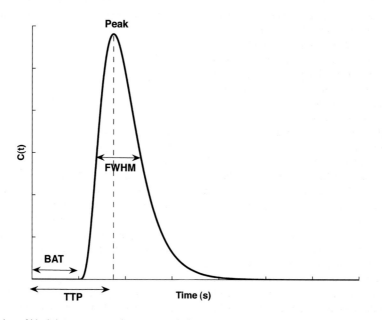

Fig. 2. Representation of ideal tissue concentration curve evolution over time, $C(t)$ (in mm) along with parameters often used to characterize the hemodynamics of tissue voxels.

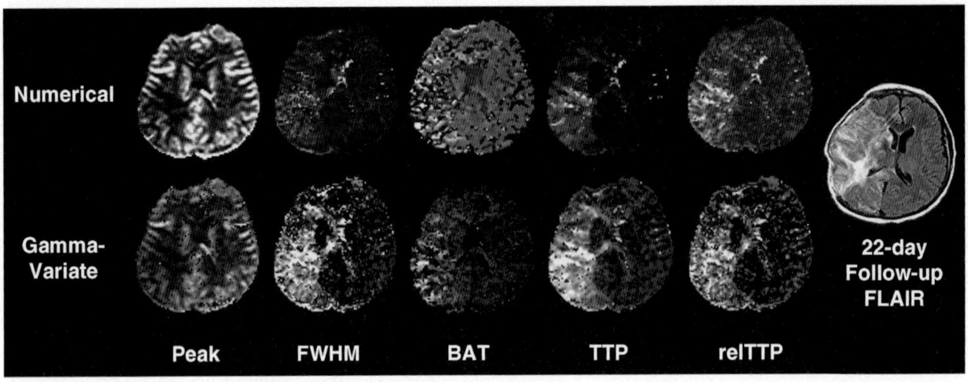

Fig. 3. Example maps of possible summary statistics that can be calculated on a voxel-wise basis from concentration-time curves for the patient shown in Fig. 1. (*Top*) Calculated maps using numeric analysis. (*Bottom*) Calculated maps by fitting concentration-time curves to a gamma-variate function before estimation of summary statistics. The dark spots indicate voxels where the fit failed. Qualitatively, numeric analysis appears to produce superior results with the exception of FWHM and BAT, where noise in the curves leads to artifacts that partly is compensated for by curve fitting. Also shown is the 22-day follow-up for this patient, who developed massive edema and required a hemicraniectomy.

parameters that vary across patients (eg, underlying vascular architecture) [27–29], physiologic factors (eg, cardiac output), and MR acquisitions (eg, injection conditions) [29,30]. As such, interpatient comparisons may be confounded.

Previous studies show that estimating the AIF measured from MR imaging correlates well with values measured directly from arterial blood samples [31]. The AIF is obtained by averaging the signal changes in pixels selected from regions near or in large cerebral vessels in the MR imaging that showed early large increases in ΔR_2 after contrast injection. Various techniques are proposed for the measurement of the AIF, using either manual or automatic approaches [32–34]. It is argued that the AIF can be accurately measured only within a vessel using GRE PWI and in a vessel parallel to the main magnetic field [35]. In other vessels, the change in MR signal as a function of concentration may not be linear as a result of partial volume effects, spatial misregistration, and dependence of induced magnetic field changes on orientation of the large vessel [33,35]. This is true especially for SE PWI, where the degree of signal change also is dependent on vessel size and may be sublinear for large vessels [17]. In practice, the AIF typically is selected in voxels near large vessels using heuristics, such as narrow FWHM, large peak concentration, and early BAT. Without knowledge of the concentration of CA passing through the vessels resulting in the measured AIF, absolute quantitative CBF in terms of mL/100 g/min is not feasible, relegating users to relative flow values that should differ from true CBF by a scale factor. Typically, a single AIF is used for the deconvolution

(see Eq. 6) to calculate relative CBF for all of the voxels in the brain.

Assuming an AIF can be measured accurately from the acquired MR signal, $S_{AIF}(t)$, quantitative CBV and CBF values should be obtainable. There are several studies that attempt to provide quantitative CBV and CBF values by scaling the calculated results with global factors. In one approach for measuring absolute CBV, a correction factor, $k_H = (1 - H_{LV}) / (1 - H_{SV})$ is used to compensate for the differences between the hematocrit in large vessels ($H_{LV} \approx 0.45$) and small vessels ($H_{SV} \approx 0.25$) as shown in Eq. 9:

$$\begin{aligned} CBV &= \frac{k_{tissue}}{k_{AIF}} \frac{k_H}{\rho} \\ &\times \frac{\frac{1}{TE_{tissue}} \int_0^\infty \ln(S_{tissue}(t)/S_{tissue,0}) dt}{\frac{1}{TE_{AIF}} \int_0^\infty \ln(S_{AIF}(t)/S_{AIF,0}) dt} \end{aligned} \quad (9)$$

where $\rho = 1.04$ g/mL is the brain tissue density and k_{tissue} and k_{AIF} are the respective proportionality factors (see Eq. 2) for signals measured from the tissue and AIF and are assumed equal [32,36,37]. For absolute CBF, the calculated CBF values after deconvolution are scaled by the same factors. An alternate approach converts MR-obtained CBF values to correspond to those measured by other techniques, such as positron emission tomography (PET), using a scaling factor that provides equivalent values on an average tissue basis [38,39] or on a reference tissue basis (eg, selecting a scale factor to produce MR-obtained CBF values in white matter equal to 22 mL/100 g/min) [40]. This scaling factor then can be used to obtain absolute CBV values. Scaling results with respect to a reference tissue has the benefit that no assumptions regarding proportionality constants (Eq. 9) are made, but has the downside of assuming normal flow in certain regions [41]. Another approach uses a scaling factor derived from the area of the venous output function measured from the superior sagittal sinus [42]. Methods also are proposed to measure a quantitative AIF (ie, relationship to CA concentration is known) by correcting for partial-volume effects [43] or by using phase changes to measure CA concentration [44].

Underlying many of the techniques for measuring absolute MR-obtained CBF values is an inherent assumption that measured values are relatively correct and that only a scaling factor is needed to obtain absolute values. Relative regional CBF values also may be incorrect, however, as a result of the use of

a single AIF for deconvolution. Errors can arise, because the selected AIF for most tissue is not measured in the actual artery supplying it. There may be delays and dispersion between where the AIF is measured and the true input function, the extent of which varies on an individual voxel basis. This in turn leads to relative CBF values potentially being incorrect. For instance, whether or not the AIF is selected from the ipsilesional or contralesional hemisphere results in large differences in the extent of measured perfusion abnormalities in cerebral vascular diseases [28,45–48]. Recent studies demonstrate that the delay and dispersion between the AIF and concentration-time curves lead to underestimation of CBF values [46,49–51] and may be contributing factors to the sensitivity of CBF and MTT calculation to AIF selection (Fig. 4). The impact of delay on

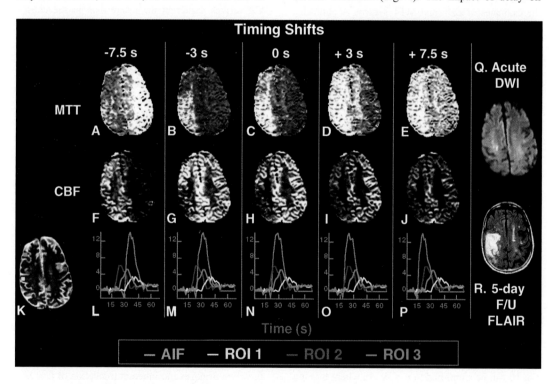

Fig. 4. Artificially shifting an AIF forward and backward in time leads to both over- and underestimation of CBF, demonstrated using acute PWI acquired 5 hours after onset of right middle cerebral artery stroke. Each column represents the calculated (*A–E*) MTT and (*F–J*) CBF for each shift along with (*L–P*) plots of the AIF signal with respect to each region of interest (ROI) signal. (*K*) Three ROIs were selected: one in the ipsilateral hemisphere that is shown to infarct on follow-up imaging (*yellow*; ROI 1), one in the contralateral hemisphere (*magenta,* ROI 2) and one in the ipsilateral hemisphere that does not infarct (*green,* ROI 3). (*L–P*) Bottom row shows the change in relative timing of $\Delta R_2(t)$ in AIF selected ipsilaterally from the right middle cerebral artery and in the three ROIs (*K*). All CBF and MTT maps in a row are scaled using the same dynamic range for better comparison. Also shown are the (*Q*) acute DWI lesion and (*R*) 5-day follow-up FLAIR demonstrating growth of the infarction volume. One sees that shifting the same AIF in time greatly affects the amount of tissue considered abnormal resulting from the heterogeneous distribution of tracer arrival times that can exist even within the same hemisphere. (*From* Wu O, Ostergaard L, Koroshetz WJ, et al. Effects of tracer arrival time on flow estimates in MR perfusion-weighted imaging. Magn Reson Med 2003;50:856–64; with permission.)

CBF values can be compensated for by using tracer-arrival timing-insensitive deconvolution techniques [32,52–54]. To correct for dispersion, there are proposals to use multiple AIFs in local AIF methodologies through use of AIFs that are closer to the tissue of interest [55,56].

Deconvolution methods

Assuming that a $C_a(t)$ can be measured that differs from the true AIF only by a scaling factor but whose shape is the same as the "true" AIF, CBF can be estimated by deconvolving the measured CA concentration time curve with $C_a(t)$ using Eq. 7. Several techniques are available for performing the deconvolution. Choice of deconvolution techniques can affect the estimates of CBF and MTT greatly. A clinically prevalent method, using singular value decomposition (SVD) for the deconvolution, makes no assumptions regarding the residue function $R(t)$ and provides CBF estimates that are independent of the underlying vascular structure and the volume being measured and also performs well in the presence of noise [25]. In the SVD approach, Eq. 6 is reformulated first as a matrix expression in Eq. 10:

$$
\begin{vmatrix} C(t_0) \\ C(t_1) \\ \vdots \\ C(t_{N-1}) \end{vmatrix} = F_t \cdot \Delta t!
$$

$$
\times \begin{vmatrix} C_a(t_0) & 0 & \cdots & 0 \\ C_a(t_1) & C_a(t_0) & \cdots & 0 \\ \vdots & \vdots & \ddots & \vdots \\ C_a(t_{N-1}) & C_a(t_{N-2}) & \cdots & C_a(t_0) \end{vmatrix}
$$

$$
\times \begin{vmatrix} R(t_0) \\ R(t_1) \\ \vdots \\ R(t_{N-1}) \end{vmatrix}
$$

(10)

Eq. 10 can be simplified to $c = A \cdot b$, where b is the elements of $R(t)$ scaled by F_t and A is the matrix scaled by Δt, the temporal resolution which in many cases are equivalent to the TR. Eq. 7 then can be treated as an inverse matrix problem, where $b = A^{-1} \cdot c$. The calculation of A^{-1} is sensitive to noise and can lead to unstable solutions. By decomposing $A = U \cdot S \cdot V^T$, the inverse matrix is simply $A^{-1} = V \cdot W \cdot U^T$, where $W = 1 / S$ along the diagonals. Singular values, which can arise because of noise and lead to unstable solutions, are removed by eliminating diagonal elements in W, corresponding to values where S is less than a preset tolerance threshold, P_{SVD}, usually a percentage of the maximum value of S (typically 15%–20%). Once CBF is calculated, MTT also can be derived in conjunction with the CBV map using Eq. 8, the central volume theorem. In addition to the magnitude, the time point at which the calculated residue function reaches its peak is speculated to represent tracer arrival differences between the AIF and tissue and can be measured from the deconvolved $R(t)$ (Fig. 5) [52].

CBF estimates are highly sensitive to the choice of P_{SVD} [25,52,57], and various methods are proposed for its optimization on a pixel-wise basis [58–60]. Another limitation of the SVD technique is its large sensitivity to delay and dispersion between the AIF and the tissue of interest (described above). In addition, for cases of major vasculopathy where the CA arrives earlier in the tissue than in the chosen AIF, CBF can be either over- or underestimated, depending on the extent of the BAT difference and the underlying hemodynamics of the measured tissue [61]. Approaches modifying the SVD method by using a block-circulant matrix, D, in place of A for deconvolution, produces CBF estimates that are independent of BAT differences but with greater oscillations in the derived residue functions [52]. This can be compensated for, however, through the use of a minimization of oscillation index and local regularization, resulting in a performance comparable to the original SVD technique but without BAT sensitivity (Fig. 6) [52].

Fourier techniques transform the convolution operation (see Eq. 6) in the time domain to multiplication in the frequency domain, such that deconvolution becomes a division problem (Eq. 11):

$$
F_t R(t) = \Im^{-1} \left\{ \frac{\Im\{C(t)\}}{\Im\{C_a(t)\}} \right\}
$$

(11)

where $\Im$ and $\Im^{-1}$ represent the Fourier transform and inverse Fourier transform, respectively. Typically, simple division cannot be performed because of the presence of noise and inherent truncation of $C(t)$ and $C_a(t)$, which can lead to oscillatory results [62]. Therefore, before inverse Fourier transform, $C(t)$ is filtered using a Wiener filter [32], or a modified version of it [25], to reduce noise contamination. This Fourier-based technique is insensitive to delay in tracer arrival; however, it generates flow values whose accuracy is a function of flow rate, resulting in the underestimation of true flow at high flow rates in the presence of noise [25,63].

Methods that assume the residue function follows an a priori assumed form typically produce accurate

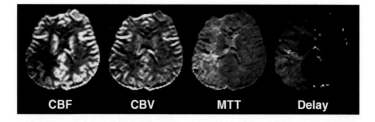

Fig. 5. Example maps of possible parameters that can be calculated on a voxel-wise basis from concentration-time curves using an AIF measured from imaging data for the patient shown in Fig. 1. Note the similarity between CBF and Peak signal change and between Delay and TTP in Fig. 3.

CBF estimates only if the modeled $R(t)$ matched the true residue function [25,64]—which for cases of pathophysiology often does not hold true. Model-dependent approaches that fit for delay and dispersion [65] also show promise in terms of more accurate flow estimates than achieved by SVD; however, their performances have yet to be evaluated in cases of ischemic disease or major vasculopathy, where the assumptions that they are based on may no longer be valid. Studies also show that the shape of $R(t)$ as well as the residue function amplitude (ie, CBF) may be important for characterizing tissue viability in stroke patients [65–68]. As such, techniques that produce smoother $R(t)$ while maintaining accurate CBF estimates are desirable [53,59,69,70]. The performance of these promising methods in terms of identifying tissue at risk of infarction remains to be examined for a large cohort of stroke patients.

MR imaging data acquisition: practical considerations

MR acquisition parameters must be kept in mind when interpreting perfusion maps. Affecting the characteristics of the calculated perfusion metrics are various factors, such as number of baseline points, acquisition duration, TE, TR, peak signal drop, and CA [19,71,72]. These in turn also are affected by which pulse sequence (eg, SE or GRE) is used. For CBV, 50 baseline images are recommended to reduce baseline noise contribution to 10% of the total CBV map [19]. Because of existing scanner hardware constraints, typical PWI acquisitions use approximately 10 baseline images resulting in 34% more noise. As the signal-to-noise ratio (SNR) of the raw images increases, however, baseline noise becomes less important. The total number of points to use for CBV

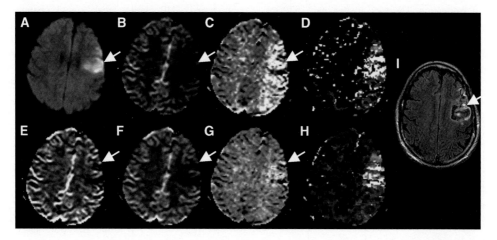

Fig. 6. Example case of a mismatch in DWI and PWI lesion volumes when using standard SVD and no mismatch when using a block-circulant matrix with minimization of oscillation index (oSVD). Acute imaging studies for a patient with a left middle cerebral artery stroke acquired less than 7 hours from symptom onset: (*A*) DWI; (*B*) sCBF; (*C*) sMTT; (*D*) sDelay maps; (*E*) CBV; (*F*) oCBF; (*G*) oMTT; and (*H*) oDelay maps; and (*I*) 4-month follow-up FLAIR shows an infarction that is well matched with the patient's acute DWI, CBV, oCBF, and oMTT studies (*arrows*). (*From* Wu O, Ostergaard L, Weisskoff RM, et al. Tracer arrival timing-insensitive technique for estimating flow in MR perfusion-weighted imaging using singular value decomposition with a block-circulant deconvolution matrix. Magn Reson Med 2003;50:164–74; with permission.)

calculation is recommended to be long enough to encompass the duration of the first-pass bolus of all voxels sufficiently. Too many points, however, may lead to additional noise contamination or to errors resulting from recirculation effects [19], leading to overestimation of CBV [73]. Alternatively, too short an acquisition can lead to signal truncation, which can result in the potentially more problematic underestimation of CBF [74] and CBV [73]. Fitting $C(t)$ to a gamma-variate function to compensate for these potential sources of errors can be done but can result in worse performance for cases of low SNR (see Fig. 3) [19]. On a relative basis, integrating over the entire image range (typically 40–50 volume datasets) produces more accurate CBV and CBF values [73]. In terms of absolute values, however, integrating the deconvolved signal, $R(t)$, generates more accurate estimates [73].

The choice for optimal TE is approximately equal to T2 (or T2*) of the baseline signal [19,72] for moderate peak signal changes (10%–70%) [19,71]. For very large peak signal reductions, long TEs lead to large reductions in SNR in the calculated CBV maps, whereas short TEs produce high-quality maps [19]. For SE sequences, choice of TE also affects the microvascular selectivity (ie, signal change is greater at lower TEs for capillaries than for macrovessels) at the cost of overall SNR [17]. For TR, the optimal value is dependent on the sequence. For SE sequences, the optimal TR is approximately 1.26 T_1 [19]. For GRE, a short as possible TR is optimal. For flow estimation, TR rates greater than 1500 ms underestimate CBF [30,72].

In addition to short TR, as short as possible an input bolus duration is desired to maximize CA concentration and, therefore, maximize signal change [19], which in turn produces higher-quality CBF

images [75]. For SE sequences, greater microvascular selectivity is observed as CA dosage increases [19]. Input bolus width and peak signal drop also are affected by molarity (gadolinium concentration) and dosage [75]. The dosage by bodyweight needed to generate sufficient signal change is dependent on the sequence used and the field strength of the MR scanner [76]. For example, for 1.5 T, dosages of 0.2 mmol/kg typically are used for SE sequences, whereas for 3 T, 0.1 mmol/kg can be used. For GRE sequences, 0.1 mmol/kg typically are used at 1.5 T and 3 T. Injection rates also can affect bolus width. Rates less than 3 mL/s result in the underestimation of CBF [30]. For higher rates, the diameter of the cannula for the intravenous (IV) line needs to be larger than the typical 20 gauge, leading to increased logistic difficulty, including patient discomfort. Furthermore, doubling the injection rate from 5 mL/s to 10 mL/s shows little benefit in terms of improving bolus shape (Fig. 7) and the resulting estimated CBF [30]. There also are practical issues. For example, at injection rates greater than 5 mL/s, actual measured rates are much lower than that set depending on the gauge of the IV line, with smaller diameters resulting in larger errors [76]. CAs typically are administered using a power injector to obtain consistent high injection rates.

Whether to use GRE or SE for PWI data acquisition likely depends on several factors, such as SNR, available CA dosage, and desired vessel-size sensitivity [17]. GRE sequences have the benefit of increased SNR, larger peak signal change as a function of CA concentration, and linear behavior at large concentrations. GRE are sensitive to all vessel sizes, however, with greater sensitivity for macrovessels than for small microvessels with diameters less than approximately 5 μm. GRE-based

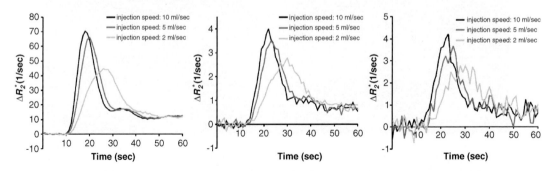

Fig. 7. Influence of injection speed on bolus shapes. Simulated curves are generated for the injection of 30 mL of CA at 10 mL/s, 5 mL/s, or 2 mL/s and a chaser of saline of 20 mL injected with the corresponding speed. (*Left*) Simulated AIF ($SNR_{DSC-MRI} = 30$). (*Middle*) Simulated contrast passage through tissue ($SNR_{DSC-MRI} = 30$). (*Right*) Simulated contrast passage through tissue ($SNR_{DSC-MRI} = 12$). (*From* van Osch MJ, Vonken EJ, Wu O, et al. Model of the human vasculature for studying the influence of contrast injection speed on cerebral perfusion MR imaging. Magn Reson Med 2003;50:614–22; with permission.)

PWI metrics, therefore, may overestimate CBF and CBV as a result of contamination from partial volume effects in tissue near large vessels (Fig. 8) [77]. In contrast, SE sequences exhibit greater signal changes for microvessels than for macrovessels with peak signal change at vessel diameters of approximately 5 μm [17] and may, therefore, provide a more specific estimate of CBF and CBV as long as sufficient SNR is available. This is at the cost of being able to accurately image large vessels, however (see Fig. 8).

There are several studies that compare SE and GRE sequences. For tumor studies, it is suggested that GRE PWI may be better for assessing tumor vascularity than SE PWI [78–80]. For investigating capillary perfusion, however, it is reported that SE PWI is better and produces relative CBF values with ratios of gray-matter to white-matter flow that are consistent with those reported for PET studies, with less intersubject variability in tissue near large vessels

[81]. Other studies find that CBF and CBV increases are detected with GRE PWI but that SE PWI detects increases only in CBV and MTT in response to acetazolamide [82]. Another study finds no difference other than global scaling factors between relative CBF and CBV values acquired with SE or GRE PWI and that both techniques are able to measure increases in CBF and CBV in response to hypercapnia [83]. To address these issues, sequences that acquire simultaneous SE and GRE acquisitions can be used (see Fig. 8) [84]. Such sequences have the additional benefit of allowing for vessel size imaging and, therefore, potential evaluation of angiogenesis [78,85,86].

Pitfalls and artifacts

Even with an optimal PWI acquisition protocol, there are several potentially confounding factors in

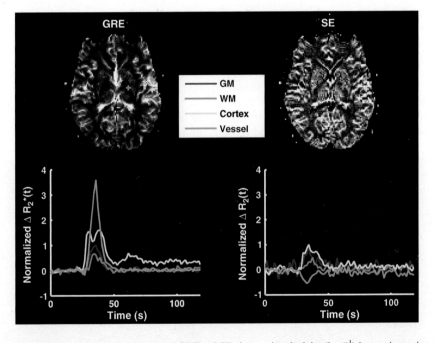

Fig. 8. Differences between simultaneously measured GRE and SE changes in relaxivity (in s^{-1}) in a patient using a dual echo acquisition on a 3 T system with $TR/TE_{GRE}/TE_{SE} = 1500/34/103$ ms. (*Left*) GRE CBV map and concentration-time curves for different tissue of interest—deep gray matter (GM), white matter (WM), cortical gray matter (Cortex) and macrovessel (Vessel). (*Right*) SE CBV map and concentration-time curves for the same tissue voxels shown for GRE CBV. Concentration-time curves were normalized to peak signal change in the gray matter voxel for all graphs. To avoid additional partial volume artifacts from postprocessing, no spatial prefiltering was performed before CBV calculation. As expected, GRE shows equal sensitivity to large vessels, resulting in very large signal changes for large vessels (Vessel). For SE acquisitions, however, almost no signal is apparent for that particular vessel. Note, that SE PWI is not completely insensitive to large vessels, only less sensitive than GRE as apparent by the presence of cortical vessels. Also note that for cortical GM, in the GRE data a dip is evident, indicating likely partial volume effects, whereas for the SE acquisition, the amplitude is on the same order of magnitude as for deep GM. This suggests that SE PWI may be more sensitive for detecting hemodynamic changes in the parenchyma especially for tissue neighboring large vessels.

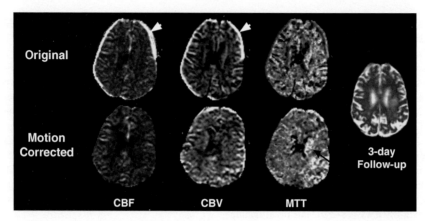

Fig. 9. Example of motion artifacts on calculated perfusion parameters for a stroke patient imaged 6 days from symptom onset. (SE EPI acquisition on 1.5 T scanner TR/TE = 1500/65 ms). (*Top*) Perfusion indices calculated from original data. (*Bottom*) Perfusion indices calculated from same data after motion correction. Hyperintense regions surrounding the cortex on both CBF and CBV maps (*white arrowheads*) are indicative of patient motion. Motion correction can reduce the artifacts, allowing the detection of lesions (*black arrow*) that otherwise may be obscured.

the interpretation of perfusion maps. One source of error is poor cardiac output or low gauge catheter, which could result in insufficient CA concentration to induce change in relaxivity. This easily is recognizable by lack of signal change in the raw data. This phenomenon illustrates that all of these hemodynamic measurement techniques are in some sense flow weighted. For example, in an extreme case, if no CA arrives, no signal change takes place and no CBV measurement can be made, even though the vasculature may be dilated with elevated CBV. Lesser flow abnormalities also can influence hemodynamic measurement, sometimes in a subtle way, particularly if image acquisition is obtained for only a short time window.

Another potential confound in the interpretation of perfusion maps is patient motion (Fig. 9). This manifests itself in the postprocessed CBV maps as

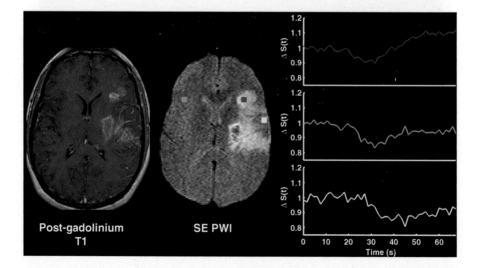

Fig. 10. Example of the effect of BBB damage in acute stroke patient imaged 14 hours from symptom onset of left middle cerebral artery stroke (TR/TE = 1500/75 ms). (*Left*) Postgadolinium T_1-weighted image indicates BBB disturbance. (*Middle*) Raw SE PWI data from a 1.5 T scanner and regions of interest in normal (*green*), BBB damaged (*red*), and hypoperfused (*yellow*) tissue. (*Right*) Change in signal intensities (in arbitrary units and normalized to baseline) for the three regions of interest. T_1 enhancement is evident in the area of disturbed BBB as an increase in signal intensity at later time points as compared with tissue signal in the normal hemisphere and hypoperfused area.

areas of hyperintensity, especially around the cortex. Motion correction can be used to correct this [36]. In cases of severe motion leading to signal loss within a single image, the offending time point should be removed from the calculation of the maps and interpolation performed.

Finally, another potential artifact is the result of disruption of the BBB. As described previously, PWI assumes that the CA stays within the vasculature. Once this assumption is no longer valid, however, the assumed linear relationship between CA and signal attenuation no longer is true. In the case of disturbed BBB with Gd-DTPA tracer, T_1 becomes shortened, which in turn leads to hyperintensity on T_1-weighted images. This change in T_1 relaxation also contaminates the PWI signal. Without any correction, CBV appears artificially low and in extreme circumstances can appear negative (Fig. 10) [78,87]. This in turn may affect not only CBV but also CBF.

Previously, disturbances to BBB have not been considered a major problem in acute stroke imaging.

With the advent of thrombolytic therapy and increased risk of hemorrhagic transformation, however, a method to measure the integrity of the endothelium before therapy might prove clinically useful [88]. Attempts to compensate for leakage have consisted mostly of predosing patients with small amounts of gadolinium (.025 or .05 mmol/kg), 5 to 10 minutes before bolus injection, to allow presaturation of the T_1 enhancement [76]. An alternate approach is to include T_1 effects in the change in signal intensity (see Eq. 2) and correct for it mathematically [78,87]. This approach not only has the benefit of being able to correct for leakage but also provides an assessment of BBB permeability—although the degree of correction possible with these postprocessing approaches is currently limited. These correction schemes perform well in cases of elevated or normal flow (eg, for some tumor cases) and work by first estimating a permeability map and using that to correct the CBV maps. In cases of low flow, however, the correction algorithm may fail and result in overestimation of

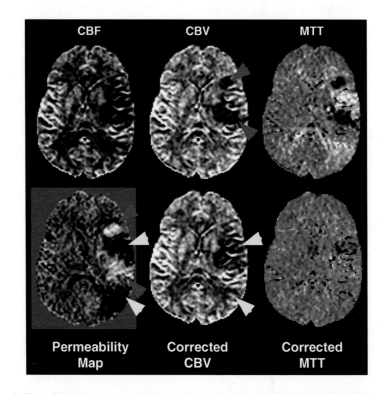

Fig. 11. Example of effects of BBB damage on calculated perfusion maps for same patient as in Fig. 10. Uncorrected CBV maps in regions of high permeability appear hypointense, because signal increases over the baseline become negative relaxivity changes resulting in negative CBV values (*red arrowheads*). In regions of low CBF, however, permeability maps are underestimated resulting in corrections that underestimate CBV, as seen in the corrected CBV maps (*yellow arrowheads*). Visualization of the lesions, therefore, can be obscured as is evident on the corrected MTT maps.

CBV—potentially misleading in stroke patient management (Fig. 11). Research is underway to correct for these errors in low flow conditions [89].

Summary

Appropriate acquisition, reconstruction, and interpretation of MR-based PWIs involve several factors. These include choice of CA type and rate of administration, MR acquisition protocol (ie, TR and TE settings and SE versus GRE acquisition), perfusion parameters (eg, MTT or TTP), and deconvolution techniques. All of these options can influence the accuracy of perfusion assessment. Despite the variety of potential confounding factors presented here and elsewhere [25,46,49,65], MR PWI is an important clinical tool because of its many desirable characteristics, including speed of acquisition, repeatability, and high sensitivity in identifying ischemic tissue at risk of infarction [1,4,5,90–92]. It is important, however, to keep in mind the potential limitations of the technique when interpreting PWI maps. As ongoing research improves perfusion estimates by reducing bias factors such as delay and dispersion, more accurate identification of hypoperfused tissue will be attained, extending the role that PWI plays in guiding stroke therapy.

Acknowledgments

We would like to acknowledge Dr. Christopher Wiggins and Dr. Thomas Benner of the MGH Athinoula A. Martinos Center for Biomedical Imaging for assistance in data acquisition for the dual-echo gradient and spin-echo datasets and Joanie Cacciola and the staffs of the Massachusetts General Hospital Departments of Neurology and Radiology for assistance in the clinical data acquisition. We also would like to thank Dr. Matthias J. P. van Osch of Leiden University Medical Center for manuscript review and feedback.

References

[1] Sorensen AG, Copen WA, Østergaard L, et al. Hyperacute stroke: simultaneous measurement of relative cerebral blood volume, relative cerebral blood flow, and mean tissue transit time. Radiology 1999;210:519–27.

[2] Darby DG, Barber PA, Gerraty RP, et al. Pathophysio-

logical topography of acute ischemia by combined diffusion- weighted and perfusion MRI. Stroke 1999; 30:2043–52.

[3] Neumann-Haefelin T, Wittsack HJ, Wenserski F, et al. Diffusion- and perfusion-weighted MRI. The DWI/ PWI mismatch region in acute stroke. Stroke 1999;30: 1591–7.

[4] Parsons MW, Yang Q, Barber PA, et al. Perfusion magnetic resonance imaging maps in hyperacute stroke: relative cerebral blood flow most accurately identifies tissue destined to infarct. Stroke 2001;32:1581–7.

[5] Sunshine JL, Bambakidis N, Tarr RW, et al. Benefits of perfusion MR imaging relative to diffusion MR imaging in the diagnosis and treatment of hyperacute stroke. AJNR Am J Neuroradiol 2001;22:915–21.

[6] Schaefer PW, Ozsunar Y, He J, et al. Assessing tissue viability with MR diffusion and perfusion imaging. AJNR Am J Neuroradiol 2003;24:436–43.

[7] Parsons MW, Barber PA, Chalk J, et al. Diffusion- and perfusion-weighted MRI response to thrombolysis in stroke. Ann Neurol 2002;51:28–37.

[8] Davis SM, Donnan GA, Butcher KS, et al. Selection of thrombolytic therapy beyond 3 h using magnetic resonance imaging. Curr Opin Neurol 2005;18:47–52.

[9] Hjort N, Butcher K, Davis SM, et al. Magnetic resonance imaging criteria for thrombolysis in acute cerebral infarct. Stroke 2005;36:388–97.

[10] Hacke W, Albers G, Al-Rawi Y, et al. The Desmoteplase in Acute Ischemic Stroke Trial (DIAS): a phase II MRI-based 9-hour window acute stroke thrombolysis trial with intravenous desmoteplase. Stroke 2005;36: 66–73.

[11] Villringer A, Rosen BR, Belliveau JW, et al. Dynamic imaging with lanthanide chelates in normal brain: contrast due to magnetic susceptibility effects. Magn Reson Med 1988;6:164–74.

[12] Rosen BR, Belliveau JW, Chien D. Perfusion imaging by nuclear magnetic resonance. Magn Reson Q 1989; 5:263–81.

[13] Heiland S, Kreibich W, Reith W, et al. Comparison of echo-planar sequences for perfusion-weighted MRI: which is best? Neuroradiology 1998;40:216–21.

[14] Fisel CR, Ackerman JL, Buxton RB, et al. MR contrast due to microscopically heterogeneous magnetic susceptibility: numerical simulations and applications to cerebral physiology. Magn Reson Med 1991;17: 336–47.

[15] Weisskoff RM, Zuo CS, Boxerman JL, et al. Microscopic susceptibility variation and transverse relaxation: theory and experiment. Magn Reson Med 1994; 31:601–10.

[16] Yablonskiy DA, Haacke EM. Theory of NMR signal behavior in magnetically inhomogeneous tissues: the static dephasing regime. Magn Reson Med 1994;32: 749–63.

[17] Boxerman JL, Hamberg LM, Rosen BR, et al. MR contrast due to intravascular magnetic susceptibility perturbations. Magn Reson Med 1995;34:555–66.

[18] Kiselev VG. On the theoretical basis of perfusion

measurements by dynamic susceptibility contrast MRI. Magn Reson Med 2001;46:1113–22.

[19] Boxerman JL, Rosen BR, Weisskoff RM. Signal-to-noise analysis of cerebral blood volume maps from dynamic NMR imaging studies. J Magn Reson Imaging 1997;7:528–37.

[20] Strich G, Hagan PL, Gerber KH, et al. Tissue distribution and magnetic resonance spin lattice relaxation effects of gadolinium-DTPA. Radiology 1985; 154:723–6.

[21] Tofts PS. Modeling tracer kinetics in dynamic Gd-DTPA MR imaging. J Magn Reson Imaging 1997;7: 91–101.

[22] Meier P, Zierler KL. On the theory of the indicator-dilution method for measurement of blood flow and volume. J Appl Physiol 1954;6:731–44.

[23] Lassen NA, Perl W. Tracer kinetic methods in medical physiology. New York: Raven Press; 1979.

[24] Todd-Pokropek A. Estimating blood flow by deconvolution of the injection of radioisotope tracers. In: Rescigno A, Boicelli A, editors. Cerebral blood flow: mathematical models, instrumentation, and imaging techniques, vol. 153. New York: Plenum Press; 1988. p. 107–19.

[25] Østergaard L, Weisskoff RM, Chesler DA, et al. High resolution measurement of cerebral blood flow using intravascular tracer bolus passages. Part I: mathematical approach and statistical analysis. Magn Reson Med 1996;36:715–25.

[26] Stewart GN. Researches on the circulation time in organs and on the influences which affect it. Parts I–III. J Physiol 1994;15:1–30.

[27] Weisskoff RM, Chesler D, Boxerman JL, et al. Pitfalls in MR measurement of tissue blood flow with intravascular tracers: which mean transit time? Magn Reson Med 1993;29:553–8.

[28] Yamada K, Wu O, Gonzalez RG, et al. Magnetic resonance perfusion-weighted imaging of acute cerebral infarction: effect of the calculation methods and underlying vasculopathy. Stroke 2002;33:87–94.

[29] Perthen JE, Calamante F, Gadian DG, et al. Is quantification of bolus tracking MRI reliable without deconvolution? Magn Reson Med 2002;47:61–7.

[30] van Osch MJ, Vonken EJ, Wu O, et al. Model of the human vasculature for studying the influence of contrast injection speed on cerebral perfusion MRI. Magn Reson Med 2003;50:614–22.

[31] Porkka L, Neuder M, Hunter G, et al. Arterial input function measurement with MRI. In: Proceedings of the 10th Annual Meeting of the Society for Magnetic Resonance in Medicine. San Francisco, California, August 10–16, 2001. p. 120.

[32] Rempp KA, Brix G, Wenz F, et al. Quantification of regional cerebral blood flow and volume with dynamic susceptibility contrast-enhanced MR imaging. Radiology 1994;193:637–41.

[33] Rausch M, Scheffler K, Rudin M, et al. Analysis of input functions from different arterial branches with gamma variate functions and cluster analysis for quantitative blood volume measurements. Magn Reson Imaging 2000;18:1235–43.

[34] Carroll TJ, Rowley HA, Haughton VM. Automatic calculation of the arterial input function for cerebral perfusion imaging with MR imaging. Radiology 2003; 227:593–600.

[35] van Osch MJ, Vonken EJ, Viergever MA, et al. Measuring the arterial input function with gradient echo sequences. Magn Reson Med 2003;49:1067–76.

[36] Smith AM, Grandin CB, Duprez T, et al. Whole brain quantitative CBF, CBV, and MTT measurements using MRI bolus tracking: implementation and application to data acquired from hyperacute stroke patients. J Magn Reson Imaging 2000;12:400–10.

[37] Vonken EJ, van Osch MJ, Bakker CJ, et al. Measurement of cerebral perfusion with dual-echo multi-slice quantitative dynamic susceptibility contrast MRI. J Magn Reson Imaging 1999;10:109–17.

[38] Østergaard L, Smith DF, Vestergaard-Poulsen P, et al. Absolute cerebral blood flow and blood volume measured by magnetic resonance imaging bolus tracking: comparison with positron emission tomography values. J Cereb Blood Flow Metab 1998;18:425–32.

[39] Østergaard L, Johannsen P, Host-Poulsen P, et al. Cerebral blood flow measurements by magnetic resonance imaging bolus tracking: comparison with [(15)O]H2O positron emission tomography in humans. J Cereb Blood Flow Metab 1998;18:935–40.

[40] Mukherjee P, Kang HC, Videen TO, et al. Measurement of cerebral blood flow in chronic carotid occlusive disease: comparison of dynamic susceptibility contrast perfusion MR imaging with positron emission tomography. AJNR Am J Neuroradiol 2003;24: 862–71.

[41] Grandin CB. Assessment of brain perfusion with MRI: methodology and application to acute stroke. Neuroradiology 2003;45:755–66.

[42] Lin W, Celik A, Derdeyn C, et al. Quantitative measurements of cerebral blood flow in patients with unilateral carotid artery occlusion: a PET and MR study. J Magn Reson Imaging 2001;14:659–67.

[43] van Osch MJ, Vonken EJ, Bakker CJ, et al. Correcting partial volume artifacts of the arterial input function in quantitative cerebral perfusion MRI. Magn Reson Med 2001;45:477–85.

[44] Akbudak E, Conturo TE. Arterial input functions from MR phase imaging. Magn Reson Med 1996;36: 809–15.

[45] Calamante F, Ganesan V, Kirkham FJ, et al. MR perfusion imaging in Moyamoya Syndrome: potential implications for clinical evaluation of occlusive cerebrovascular disease. Stroke 2001;32:2810–6.

[46] Calamante F, Gadian DG, Connelly A. Quantification of perfusion using bolus tracking magnetic resonance imaging in stroke: assumptions, limitations, and potential implications for clinical use. Stroke 2002;33: 1146–51.

[47] Thijs VN, Somford DM, Bammer R, et al. Influence of arterial input function on hypoperfusion volumes

measured with perfusion-weighted imaging. Stroke 2004;35:94–8.

[48] Neumann-Haefelin T, Wittsack HJ, Fink GR, et al. Diffusion- and perfusion-weighted MRI: influence of severe carotid artery stenosis on the DWI/PWI mismatch in acute stroke. Stroke 2000;31:1311–7.

[49] Calamante F, Gadian DG, Connelly A. Delay dispersion effects in dynamic susceptibility contrast MRI: simulations using singular value decomposition. Magn Reson Med 2000;44:466–73.

[50] Wu O, Ostergaard L, Koroshetz WJ, et al. Effects of tracer arrival time on flow estimates in MR perfusion-weighted imaging. Magn Reson Med 2003;50:856–64.

[51] Calamante F, Yim PJ, Cebral JR. Estimation of bolus dispersion effects in perfusion MRI using image-based computational fluid dynamics. Neuroimage 2003;19(2 Pt 1):341–53.

[52] Wu O, Ostergaard L, Weisskoff RM, et al. Tracer arrival timing-insensitive technique for estimating flow in MR perfusion-weighted imaging using singular value decomposition with a block-circulant deconvolution matrix. Magn Reson Med 2003;50:164–74.

[53] Vonken EP, Beekman FJ, Bakker CJ, et al. Maximum likelihood estimation of cerebral blood flow in dynamic susceptibility contrast MRI. Magn Reson Med 1999;41:343–50.

[54] Smith MR, Lu H, Trochet S, et al. Removing the effect of SVD algorithmic artifacts present in quantitative MR perfusion studies. Magn Reson Med 2004;51:631–4.

[55] Alsop D, Wedmid A, Schlaug G. Defining a local input function for perfusion quantification with bolus contrast MRI [abstract]. In: Proceedings of the 10th Annual Meeting of the International Society of Magnetic Resonance in Medicine. Honolulu, Hawaii, May 18–22, 2002. p. 659.

[56] Calamante F, Morup M, Hansen LK. Defining a local arterial input function for perfusion MRI using independent component analysis. Magn Reson Med 2004;52:789–97.

[57] Murase K, Shinohara M, Yamazaki Y. Accuracy of deconvolution analysis based on singular value decomposition for quantification of cerebral blood flow using dynamic susceptibility contrast-enhanced magnetic resonance imaging. Phys Med Biol 2001;46:3147–59.

[58] Liu HL, Pu Y, Liu Y, et al. Cerebral blood flow measurement by dynamic contrast MRI using singular value decomposition with an adaptive threshold. Magn Reson Med 1999;42:167–72.

[59] Sourbron S, Luypaert R, Van Schuerbeek P, et al. Deconvolution of dynamic contrast-enhanced MRI data by linear inversion: choice of the regularization parameter. Magn Reson Med 2004;52:209–13.

[60] Koh TS, Wu XY, Cheong LH, et al. Assessment of perfusion by dynamic contrast-enhanced imaging using a deconvolution approach based on regression and singular value decomposition. IEEE Trans Med Imaging 2004;23:1532–42.

[61] Wu O, Østergaard L, Benner T, et al. Perfusion calcu-

lations using singular value decomposition are biased by tracer arrival timing [abstract]. In: Proceedings of the 10th Annual Meeting of the International Society of Magnetic Resonance in Medicine. Honolulu, Hawaii, May 18–24, 2002. p. 660.

[62] Gobbel GT, Fike JR. A deconvolution method for evaluating indicator-dilution curves. Phys Med Biol 1994;39:1833–54.

[63] Wirestam R, Andersson L, Østergaard L, et al. Assessment of regional cerebral blood flow by dynamic susceptibility contrast MRI using different deconvolution techniques. Magn Reson Med 2000;43:691–700.

[64] Chen JJ, Smith MR, Frayne R. Advantages of frequency-domain modeling in dynamic-susceptibility contrast magnetic resonance cerebral blood flow quantification. Magn Reson Med 2005;53:700–7.

[65] Østergaard L, Chesler DA, Weisskoff RM, et al. Modeling cerebral blood flow and flow heterogeneity from magnetic resonance residue data. J Cereb Blood Flow Metab 1999;19:690–9.

[66] Østergaard L, Sorensen AG, Chesler DA, et al. Combined diffusion-weighted and perfusion-weighted flow heterogeneity magnetic resonance imaging in acute stroke. Stroke 2000;31:1097–103.

[67] Simonsen CZ, Rohl L, Vestergaard-Poulsen P, et al. Final infarct size after acute stroke: prediction with flow heterogeneity. Radiology 2002;225:269–75.

[68] Perkio J, Soinne L, Ostergaard L, et al. Abnormal intravoxel cerebral blood flow heterogeneity in human ischemic stroke determined by dynamic susceptibility contrast magnetic resonance imaging. Stroke 2005;36:44–9.

[69] Calamante F, Gadian DG, Connelly A. Quantification of bolus-tracking MRI: Improved characterization of the tissue residue function using Tikhonov regularization. Magn Reson Med 2003;50:1237–47.

[70] Andersen IK, Szymkowiak A, Rasmussen CE, et al. Perfusion quantification using Gaussian process deconvolution. Magn Reson Med 2002;48:351–61.

[71] Smith MR, Lu H, Frayne R. Signal-to-noise ratio effects in quantitative cerebral perfusion using dynamic susceptibility contrast agents. Magn Reson Med 2003;49:122–8.

[72] Knutsson L, Stahlberg F, Wirestam R. Aspects on the accuracy of cerebral perfusion parameters obtained by dynamic susceptibility contrast MRI: a simulation study. Magn Reson Imaging 2004;22:789–98.

[73] Perkiö J, Aronen HJ, Kangasmaki A, et al. Evaluation of four postprocessing methods for determination of cerebral blood volume and mean transit time by dynamic susceptibility contrast imaging. Magn Reson Med 2002;47:973–81.

[74] Smith AM, Grandin CB, Duprez T, et al. Whole brain quantitative CBF and CBV measurements using MRI bolus tracking: comparison of methodologies. Magn Reson Med 2000;43:559–64.

[75] Tombach B, Benner T, Reimer P, et al. Do highly concentrated gadolinium chelates improve MR brain perfusion imaging? Intraindividually controlled ran-

domized crossover concentration comparison study of 0.5 versus 1.0 mol/L gadobutrol. Radiology 2003;226: 880–8.

[76] Sorensen AG, Reimer P. Cerebral MR perfusion imaging: principles and current applications. New York: Georg Thieme Verlag; 2000.

[77] Carroll TJ, Haughton VM, Rowley HA, et al. Confounding effect of large vessels on MR perfusion images analyzed with independent component analysis. AJNR Am J Neuroradiol 2002;23:1007–12.

[78] Donahue KM, Krouwer HG, Rand SD, et al. Utility of simultaneously acquired gradient-echo and spin-echo cerebral blood volume and morphology maps in brain tumor patients. Magn Reson Med 2000;43: 845–53.

[79] Uematsu H, Matsuda T, Takahashi M, et al. Susceptibility-induced changes in signal intensity from spin-echo versus gradient-echo sequences. Clin Imaging 2002; 26:367–70.

[80] Sugahara T, Korogi Y, Kochi M, et al. Perfusion-sensitive MR imaging of gliomas: comparison between gradient-echo and spin-echo echo-planar imaging techniques. AJNR Am J Neuroradiol 2001;22:1306–15.

[81] Speck O, Chang L, DeSilva NM, et al. Perfusion MRI of the human brain with dynamic susceptibility contrast: gradient-echo versus spin-echo techniques. J Magn Reson Imaging 2000;12:381–7.

[82] Marstrand JR, Rostrup E, Rosenbaum S, et al. Cerebral hemodynamic changes measured by gradient-echo or spin-echo bolus tracking and its correlation to changes in ICA blood flow measured by phase-mapping MRI. J Magn Reson Imaging 2001;14:391–400.

[83] Simonsen CZ, Ostergaard L, Smith DF, et al. Comparison of gradient- and spin-echo imaging: CBF, CBV, and MTT measurements by bolus tracking. J Magn Reson Imaging 2000;12:411–6.

[84] Bandettini PA, Wong EC, Jesmanowicz A, et al. Spin-echo and gradient-echo EPI of human brain activation using BOLD contrast: a comparative study at 1.5 T. NMR Biomed 1994;7:12–20.

[85] Dennie J, Mandeville JB, Boxerman JL, et al. NMR imaging of changes in vascular morphology due to tumor angiogenesis. Magn Reson Med 1998;40:793–9.

[86] Jensen JH, Chandra R. MR imaging of microvasculature. Magn Reson Med 2000;44:224–30.

[87] Weisskoff RM, Boxerman JL, Sorensen AG, et al. Simultaneous blood volume and permeability mapping using a singleGd-based contrast injection [abstract]. In: Proceedings of the 2nd Annual Meeting of the Society for Magnetic Resonance in Medicine. San Francisco, California, August 6–12, 1994. p. 279.

[88] Latour LL, Kang DW, Ezzeddine MA, et al. Early blood-brain barrier disruption in human focal brain ischemia. Ann Neurol 2004;56:468–77.

[89] Wu O, Schwamm LH, Weisskoff RM, et al. Measuring changes in blood-brain barrier permeability with perfusion-weighted MRI in human cerebral ischemia [abstract]. Stroke 2003;34:263.

[90] Baird AE, Warach S. Magnetic resonance imaging of acute stroke. J Cereb Blood Flow Metab 1998;18: 583–609.

[91] Grandin CB, Duprez TP, Smith AM, et al. Which MR-derived perfusion parameters are the best predictors of infarct growth in hyperacute stroke? Comparative study between relative and quantitative measurements. Radiology 2002;223:361–70.

[92] Sorensen AG. What is the meaning of quantitative CBF? AJNR Am J Neuroradiol 2001;22:235–6.

**ELSEVIER
SAUNDERS**

Neuroimag Clin N Am 15 (2005) 639 – 653

**NEUROIMAGING
CLINICS OF
NORTH AMERICA**

Sodium MR Imaging of Acute and Subacute Stroke for Assessment of Tissue Viability

Keith R. Thulborn, MD, PhD[a],*, Denise Davis, BS[b], James Snyder, MD[c],
Howard Yonas, MD[d], Amin Kassam, MD[e]

[a]Center for Magnetic Resonance Research, University of Illinois at Chicago Medical Center, Chicago, IL, USA
[b]Department of Radiology, University of Pittsburgh Medical Center, Pittsburgh, PA, USA
[c]Department of Anesthesiology/Critical Care Medicine, University of Pittsburgh Medical Center, Pittsburgh, PA, USA
[d]Department of Neurosurgery, University of New Mexico, Albuquerque, NM, USA
[e]Department of Neurological Surgery, University of Pittsburgh Medical Center, Pittsburgh, PA, USA

The design of treatments to minimize the impact of stroke on clinical recovery has been a goal for stroke researchers for many years [1]. Early intervention is accepted as an important step in minimizing tissue loss, thereby improving recovery. The time from symptom onset has been used as an important criterion in clinical trials across a range of intervention strategies. The only thrombolysis strategy approved by the US Food and Drug Administration (FDA) remains intravenous recombinant tissue plasminogen activator (rt-PA) with a 3-hour window [2], whereas intra-arterial thrombolytic agents have been used at longer times [3]. Such times have been based on goals for improved clinical outcomes as well as avoidance of the complication of hemorrhagic transformation of the stroke. The use of the 3-hour window criterion is based on improved outcome measures determined from a large clinical trial [2]. Methods that may better characterize the pathophysiology of the stroke in individual patients have also been suggested

as aids in management decisions [4]. These methods include measurements of tissue x-ray attenuation with CT [5] diffusion- and perfusion-weighted MR imaging [6–8], ligand binding measurements with positron emission tomography (PET) [9], and, more recently, measurement of tissue sodium concentration (TSC) with sodium MR imaging [4]. It is important to distinguish these methods from those used for diagnosis of stroke, such as diffusion-weighted MR imaging, which is now replacing or complementing conventional CT in this role [10,11].

A therapeutic question arises after the diagnosis of nonhemorrhagic stroke has been made and a perfusion study has demonstrated that a thrombus is present. Is the tissue involved in the stroke viable or nonviable? This fundamental question in stroke has been difficult to address directly. Statements have been made that apparent diffusion coefficient (ADC) measures the core of a stroke (ie, the infarction volume), whereas the volume of abnormal perfusion measures the area at risk [6–8]. This approach may be an oversimplification, because cases of reversible ADC maps have been reported [12,13]. Although a method to establish the volume of tissue at risk for infarction remains important, consideration should also be given to the volume of tissue already infarcted. The extent of tissue infarction may relate to the likelihood of complications of hemorrhagic transformation in the presence of thrombolytic therapy.

This work was supported by Public Health Service grants PO1 NS35949 and R01 NS386760, with technical support from General Electric Healthcare.

* Corresponding author. Center for Magnetic Resonance Research, University of Illinois at Chicago Medical Center, 1801 West Taylor Street, OCC (MC707), Room 1307, Chicago, IL 60612.

 E-mail address: kthulbor@uic.edu (K.R. Thulborn).

Tissue viability requires an operational definition. Perfusion has been used as a surrogate marker of viability, but perfusion is not a switch. Loss of viability is a complex function of the degree of reduction of perfusion and its duration. The unpredictable collateral circulation plays an important role in maintaining flow, albeit at reduced levels, to provide a variable therapeutic window. It is the unpredictable nature of this collateral flow for individual patients, except in the setting of extremely low or no flow, that is problematic for clinical decision-making. In the latter case, the aerobic tissue of the brain is rapidly irreversibly damaged. Even dead tissue has some degree of perfusion, however.

A more direct measure of tissue viability is to use one of the many biochemical parameters that depict cellular function. To be useful in the clinical setting of stroke, the parameter must be measurable as an image at a spatial resolution (ie, a few mL) that is useful for assessment across the distribution of the stroke and in an acquisition time that is acceptable for patients and does not delay treatment (ie, less than 10 minutes). Although this parametric map allows the risks and benefits of therapy to be weighed, the acquisition time should be minimized.

The single most effective and accessible biochemical imaging parameter that reflects tissue viability is the TSC [4]. Tissue sodium homeostasis is a fundamental property of viable cells, as depicted in Fig. 1. Loss of cellular energy production in the form of ATP results in loss of function of the sodium-potassium transporter, with concomitant rapid loss of ion balance across the cell membrane. The integrity of cell membranes is rapidly lost. The interstitial space with high sodium concentration (140 mmol/L) and low potassium (4 mmol/L) is buffered by the sodium and potassium homeostatic mechanisms of the entire body. The loss of cell membrane integrity effectively increases the interstitial space and TSC. The rate of increase in TSC reflects the loss of cells and subsequent decline in cell density.

The measurement of TSC has been demonstrated in the acute care setting of stroke in human beings [4]. An elevation of approximately 50% above the value in the homologous region of the contralateral hemisphere was consistent with completed infarction. For human cortex, this value corresponded to approximately 70 mmol/L as compared with less than 45 mmol/L in normal tissue. In a nonhuman primate model of embolic stroke, a TSC value greater than approximately 70 mmol/L was found at 6 hours, corresponding to histologically verified infarction. This same animal model suggested that values of TSC less than 55 mmol/L indicated potential rever-

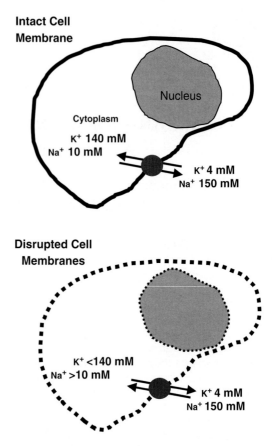

Fig. 1. Two-compartment model of sodium ion homeostasis in the brain. The small interstitial space (<20% of brain tissue volume) in the tightly packed brain tissue is buffered systemically at a high sodium concentration (~150 mmol/L) and low potassium concentration (~4 mmol/L). The large intracellular volume has concentrations for low sodium (~10 mmol/L) and high potassium (~140 mmol/L), which are maintained by hydrolysis of ATP by ion pumps on the cell membrane. Loss of blood flow and oxygen prevents oxidative phosphorylation to produce ATP, ultimately causing loss of cellular integrity and ion homeostasis.

sibility of stroke [4]. Such data are provocative, because such a parameter may link decisions about stroke management to the metabolic status of the tissue of individual patients rather than to a sometimes ambiguous time parameter based on an empirically established risk/benefit ratio from large population studies.

The parameter of TSC derived from sodium MR imaging has been proposed from animal models [4,14] and human studies [4]. Not only may TSC be important in the assessment of acute stroke but in the subacute setting of malignant middle cerebral artery syndrome [15–17]. Malignant middle cerebral artery syndrome is a not infrequent occurrence in which a patient with a large stroke involving one or more vascular territories, usually that of the large middle cerebral artery, survives for the initial few days; however, subsequent brain swelling from edema compresses the brain stem, with onset of cranial nerve palsies, respiratory depression, and death [15–17]. The resection of infarcted tissue (ie, strokectomy) would provide a means of reducing the mass effect that leads to brain stem compression and subsequent death. The surgical question is to define the region of nonviable tissue that can be resected. Although perfusion studies can establish regions of absent perfusion, and infarcted tissue by implication, even dead tissue can be perfused, albeit at a reduced level. Thus, the sodium imaging method, which is based on a biologic parameter that can be used as an operational definition of tissue viability—the ability of tissue to maintain sodium ion homeostasis—may provide a more direct means for answering this clinical question.

Sodium imaging

Conventional MR imaging uses the signal derived from the protons in water and fat. The proton is a spin 1/2 nucleus with a signal that decays exponentially with relatively long (many tens to thousands of milliseconds) transverse and longitudinal relaxation times. The slow relaxation times allow imaging to be achieved by a straightforward two-dimensional or three-dimensional Fourier transform of the time domain data (k-space), distributed on a Cartesian grid by rectilinear frequency and phase encoding. In contrast, the sodium MR signal has a 3/2 spin with bi-exponential behavior and extremely short relaxation times. Most of the sodium signal decays with a transverse relaxation time of less than 1.5 ms, whereas the longer component decays with a relaxation time of less than 15 ms. Conventional pulse sequences do not yield acceptable quality.

The standard approach for imaging of MR signals with short relaxation times is to use projection imaging, in which the time domain data are acquired on radial lines originating from the center of k-space and uniformly distributed in three dimensions. This type of acquisition oversamples the center of k-space but increasingly undersamples the k-space data further away from the center unless many projections are acquired. Thus, the acquisition times become excessively long. This problem was overcome by using a customized pulse sequence, termed *twisted projection imaging* (TPI), in which the k-space trajectory was designed to fill k-space uniformly on the surface of a sphere located away from the center by using twisted rather than simple radial projections [18].

This three-dimensional acquisition allows extremely short echo time (TE) values (<0.3 ms) to be achieved, because a short rectangular radiofrequency (RF) pulse can be used for excitation and frequency encoding can begin immediately after the pulse is turned off. Because it is a three-dimensional acquisition, no time is wasted with slice selection gradients. Because the center of k-space is acquired on every projection, signal to noise is improved and the strategy is self-correcting for motion artifacts. The use of projections does require correction for regridding the k-space data onto a Cartesian grid before the three-dimensional Fourier transform. The quality of the sodium images that can be achieved at 3.0 T is illustrated with the clinical examples later in this article.

Cell death

Another important point to be considered in understanding stroke is the nature of cell death. It is clear that stroke is a catastrophic event for the tissue in which the blood flow is severely and abruptly interrupted. Aerobic brain tissue rapidly spirals into a low-energy state from which the tissue cannot recover. Energy metabolism through oxidative phosphorylation ceases without oxygen, and the limited capacity of substrate level phosphorylation fails to maintain cell functions, including adequate ion homeostasis. As the cellular metabolic machinery ceases to function, the cell membranes fall apart, releasing toxic excitatory amino acids and destructive enzymes. The cascade of reactions associated with this catastrophic core endangers neighboring tissue (ie, penumbra), propagating destruction and thereby enlarging the core. Such cell death is termed *necrosis*.

Another type of cell death triggered by the prolonged stress of reduced blood flow and oxygen deprivation is that of apoptosis. This energy-requiring and tightly regulated cascade of events in the self-destruction process is less dramatic than necrosis. It occurs over a longer interval of time, and once initiated, it may not be reversed by a simple reperfusion intervention. The longer temporal evolution of stroke is seldom considered from an imaging perspective. Having no approved interventions beyond reperfusion in the acute setting, serial imaging of stroke seems redundant outside unexplained changes in clinical status. With biochemical imaging, such as sodium MR imaging, however, the pathophysiology of evolving stroke can be documented in human beings. Such information can be expected to be important for designing and monitoring new interventions aimed at later stages of evolving stroke. As a quantitative measure of stroke progression, TSC maps allow the therapeutic window to be tailored to the individual patient rather than to a population-derived average time before which some therapeutic benefit is derived from thrombolysis.

This report presents the current accumulated data from the relevant nonhuman primate models of human stroke, normal volunteers, and patient studies to support the role of TSC as a parameter relevant to stroke management. The animal model allows detailed assessment of the time course of TSC evolution in acute stroke out to 10 hours, in parallel to current imaging parameters (diffusion and anatomy) and histopathologic findings. These normal values of TSC, reported from normal human volunteers, allow the dynamic biochemical picture of evolving stroke to be derived in patient studies from serial sodium MR imaging.

Nonhuman primate studies

Although much has been learned about the pathophysiology of stroke using small animal models, the lack of success in extrapolating results from such models to stroke interventions in human patients suggests that such models are unreliable predictors of successful strategies in human beings. The nonhuman primate brain has a size, metabolic rate, and vascular physiology that are closely matched to those of the human brain. These animals also allow a more realistic model of human embolic stroke by providing arteries large enough for placement of catheters, through which autologous clot can be embolized. This avoids surgically altering normal cerebral physiology with surgically induced stroke.

Animal model

This nonhuman primate model has been previously reported [4] and has now been used to follow stroke out to longer than 10 hours after induction. Briefly, a monkey (Macaca mulatta, 15 kg, male, 12 years of age) was induced (ketamine, 22 mg/kg,

administered intramuscularly and acepromazine, 0.2 mg/kg, administered intramuscularly) and anesthetized (phenobarbital, 5 mg/kg, administered intravenously every 45 minutes as titrated based on the absence of a blink reflex). Vascular volume was maintained by balancing urine output, monitored via a bladder catheter, with intravenous fluids (normal saline). The trachea was intubated to maintain the airway during the extended period of anesthesia in the supine position, although the animal was allowed to breathe spontaneously. Venous catheters were placed in the femoral and brachial vessels for fluid replacement therapy and drug administration. The animal was placed in a supine position in a temperature-controlled animal cradle during fluoroscopy and MR imaging. Catheter sheaths were also placed in the femoral arteries for blood pressure monitoring and for transfemoral catheterization of the right internal carotid artery. This procedure was guided by iodinated contrast fluoroscopic angiography. Once in place in the right internal carotid artery, the catheter (5 French) was used for embolization of autologous clot to induce the stroke. After anatomic, diffusion, and sodium images were acquired in the MR imaging scanner, the animal was returned to the angiography suite. The stroke was induced by embolization with autologous clot (1 mL) through the catheter placed in the right internal carotid artery and followed by a physiologic saline flush (5 mL). The obstruction of the right middle artery was confirmed by an immediate conventional contrast arteriogram of the right and left common carotid arteries. A thermoplastic mask was placed over the head of the animal and secured to the cradle to ensure that no head motion would occur after the monkey was returned to the MR imaging scanner over the next 10 hours of imaging. The results of TSC followed in a representative monkey surviving more than 10 hours after stroke induction are shown in Fig. 2.

The physiologic status of the animal was closely monitored and maintained over the duration of the experiment. The vital signs (heart rate and blood pressure), monitored via the indwelling catheters, were stable. Respiratory rate, rectal temperature, blood gases, and electrolytes, monitored periodically, were in the normal range.

Histopathologic findings

After 10 hours, the animal was killed by exsanguination under general anesthesia. After the top of the calvarium was removed, the brain was removed carefully but rapidly by transecting the brain stem, cranial nerves, and vascular structures.

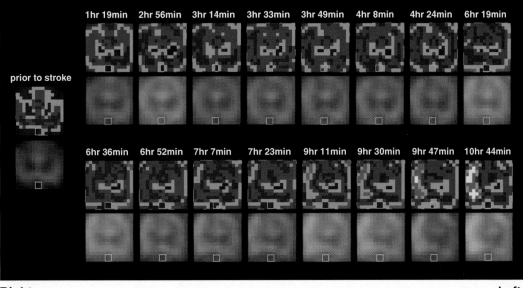

Right **Left**

Fig. 2. Time samples (as labeled) of the colorized tissue sodium concentration maps (*colored rows*) and the corresponding partition from the three-dimensional sodium imaging (*gray-scale rows*) before and over the first 10 hours after stroke induction by embolization in the animal model. The color scale (range: 31–83 mmol/L) is the same as in Fig. 1F. The stroke progressed from normal to encompass much of the right cerebral hemisphere. There was also a small stroke in the superior portion of the left cerebral hemisphere. The yellow square was placed in a common location in the field of view on all images to demonstrate alignment.

The brain was processed immediately for gross sections and histologic examination. The fresh brain was sliced into 6-mm-thick slabs along the plane of the imaging study. One central slice was selected for preservation in formalin (4%) for histologic examination. The other slices were placed in 2,3,5-triphenyl tetrazolium chloride (2% TTC) solution (10 g per 500 mL of saline) for 45 minutes without exposure to light. The TTC-stained specimens were then photographed digitally and compared directly with the MR images and maps, as shown in Fig. 3. The TTC-stained tissue was then compared visually with the corresponding MR images and maps. Conventional histopathologic examinations (hematoxylin and eosin stain) and apoptotic stain (terminal deoxynucleotidyl transferase–mediated deoxyuridine triphosphate nick end-labeling [TUNEL]) were performed (results not shown).

MR imaging protocol

Imaging was performed on a 3.0-T whole-body MR imaging scanner (Signa; General Electric Medical Systems, Milwaukee, Wisconsin) equipped with resonant gradient, echo-planar, and broadband capabilities as described elsewhere [19–21]. The manufacturer's proton RF birdcage head coil was used for proton imaging, whereas a custom-designed sodium quadrature RF birdcage coil was used for sodium imaging [22].

Sodium imaging was performed at 3.0 T with TPI as described previously [4,18,23], with an effective TE of 0.3 ms, repetition time (TR) of 100 ms, and 984 projections, achieving an isotropic spatial resolution of $5 \times 5 \times 5$ mm^3. Two concentration calibration phantoms (31 and 92 mmol/L) were placed within the RF coil beside the head to use for a two-point concentration calibration of sodium signal intensity within the brain [4]. Sodium images were reconstructed from the k-space data using a modification of a regridding and three-dimensional Fourier transform algorithm described previously [18,23]. Homogeneity of the B_1 field was performed as reported elsewhere [24].

Anatomic proton MR imaging was performed and analyzed as described previously [4,20,25]. Images were acquired with dual-echo spin-echo imaging (TR = 2000 ms, TE = 30/80 ms, 9 slices at 4-mm

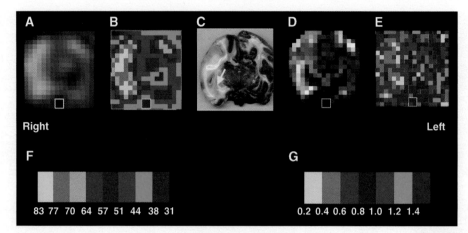

Fig. 3. Representative images, quantitatively colorized maps, and gross pathologic findings of a selected slice through the nonhuman primate brain 10 hours after induction of stroke by embolization of autologous clot through a catheter placed in the right internal carotid artery. (*A*) Sodium twisted projection image. (*B*) Map of TSC colorized according to the concentration scale (*F*, range: 83–31 mmol/L) derived from *A*. (*C*) 2,3,5-Triphenyl tetrazolium chloride–stained gross anatomy with yellow arrow showing region sampled for histologic examination. Diffusion-weighted echo-planar image (*D*) and map of ADC trace (ADC_{trace}) (*E*) colorized according to the ADC scale (*G*, range: $0.2–1.4 \times 10^{-3}$ mm²/s) derived from *D*. Radiologic convention is followed, with the right side of the subject on the left side of the page.

thickness, 1-mm gap, 16×12 cm² field of view, and 256×192 acquisition matrix) and axial three-dimensional, gradient-echo, T1-weighted images (TR = 25 ms, TE = 5 ms, 40° flip angle, 24×18 cm² field of view, 256×192 acquisition matrix, and 124 contiguous slices at 1.5-mm thickness).

In brief, diffusion-weighted imaging was performed with b-values of 0 and 687 s/mm² with spin-echo echo-planar imaging (TR=6000 ms, TE=140 ms, 9 slices at 4-mm thickness, 1-mm gap, 40×20 field of view, and 128×64 acquisition matrix). Three diffusion gradient directions (687 s/cm² in the x, y, and z directions) were used. The trace of the ADC matrix was calculated on a voxel-by-voxel basis to produce an ADC map [25].

Image data analysis

All images and maps were displayed using custom-designed software called CliniViewer [26].

Sodium images were converted to TSC maps by color-coding the ranges of TSC values (<30, 31–38, 39–44, 45–51, 52–57, 58–64, 65–70, 71–77, and 78–83 mmol/L) for ease of quantitative viewing. These maps were generated for each time point as well as across the entire brain before stroke and before the animals were killed. The maps were analyzed for rate of change in TSC (mmol/L/h) at the center and periphery of the cortical and basal ganglia portions of the lesion.

The diffusion-weighted images were used to calculate ADC maps. These ADC maps were color-coded (0.2–0.4, 0.4–0.6, 0.6–0.8, 0.8–1.0, 1.0–1.2, 1.2–1.4, and $>1.4 \times 10^{-3}$ mm²/s) for ease of quantitative viewing. These maps were generated across the entire brain for each time point.

The time courses of TSC and ADC from selected regions across the stroke from the core to the periphery and from homologous contralateral areas were plotted and characterized as the rates of change in both parameters as the first derivative of the time courses.

The volume (mL) of the lesion enclosed by specific values of TSC (> 70 mmol/L) and ADC (0.5×10^{-3} mm²/s) was determined using customized segmentation software called Morph [27] and the known voxel volume of each type of image. A value of 70 mmol/L for the boundary condition for the TSC map was selected assuming that this and higher values implied loss of tissue viability [4]. Similarly, a value of ADC of 0.5×10^{-3} mm²/s was used as a measure of nonviable tissue.

Results from the nonhuman primate model

The time course of the change in the distribution of the TSC in the stroke regions over 10 hours is shown on the TSC maps in Fig. 2. The digital photograph of the TTC-stained brain slice at 10 hours after stroke induction matches the changes present in the corresponding sodium and diffusion images and TSC and ADC maps just before the animals were killed, as shown in Fig. 3. The right hemisphere has a large region that is unstained by the vital TTC stain, consistent with nonviable mitochondria and infarction. The smaller area of reduced TTC staining in the superior aspect of the left hemisphere also indicated infarction. Both areas were confirmed as being involved in the stroke based on restricted diffusion (reduced ADC) and by conventional histologic staining. In both areas, mean regional TSC values were elevated to greater than 70 mmol/L.

The time course of TSC maps from Fig. 2 is reduced to numeric time courses for selected cortical and basal ganglia regions in Figs. 4 and 5, respectively. The cortical areas of the stroke lesion (see Fig. 4) showed linearly increasing TSC values to greater than 75 mmol/L within the core centrally and peripheral TSC values of greater than 65 mmol/L in the first 10 hours. In contrast, the involved areas of the basal ganglia (see Fig. 5) showed an initially slowly increasing phase up to approximately 400 minutes in which the core TSC values reached 45 mmol/L (normal=34 mmol/L) and then an increasing rate of change reaching core TSC values of 65 mmol/L after 10 hours. The distribution of elevated TSC visually matched that of the nonstained area of the corresponding TTC-stained brain slice (see Fig. 2). The area of abnormal ADC values also matched this

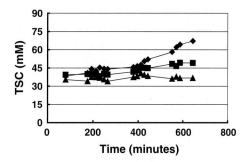

Fig. 5. Time courses for the change in TSC in the basal ganglia over the first 10 hours after stroke induction by embolization in the animal model. Tissue sodium concentration values refer to regions of interest sampled in the contralateral normal left cerebral hemisphere (▲) and at the periphery (■) and core (◆) of the stroke in the right basal ganglia. The greater rates of change in TSC in the core of the stroke as compared with the periphery (1.4 mmol/L/h) seem to be nonlinear (1.8 mmol/L/h, increasing to 5.0 mmol/L/h after 400 minutes).

same region, although no significant central or peripheral changes occurred over the entire 10-hour period.

Two observations are important. The first is that two different temporal patterns of increasing TSC values are present, being near linear in the cortex but biphasic in the basal ganglia. The second observation is that rates of change in TSC are regionally variable across the cortex and basal ganglia. The rate of change of TSC in the cortex was as high as 2.9 mmol/L/h in the center of the cortical lesion but only 1.2 mmol/L/h in the periphery of the cortical lesion. In contrast, the rate of change in TSC value in the early phase (<400 minutes) in the center of the lesion in the basal ganglia was only 1.8 mmol/L/h but rose to 5.0 mmol/L/h in the later phase. In the periphery of the basal ganglia, the rate of change in TSC was approximately 1.4 mmol/L/h.

The ADC map in Fig. 6 demonstrated an initial rapid decrease in ADC and then little further temporal change. There were regional variations, with the center of the lesion showing more depressed ADC values than the periphery, however, as has been reported elsewhere [10,11].

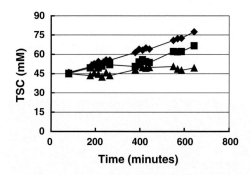

Fig. 4. Time courses for the change in TSC in the brain cortex over the first 10 hours after stroke induction by embolization in the animal model. Tissue sodium concentration values refer to regions of interest sampled in the contralateral normal left cerebral hemisphere (▲) and at the periphery (■) and core (◆) of the stroke in the right cerebral hemisphere. The greater rates of change in TSC in the core (2.9 mmol/L/h) compared with the periphery (1.2 mmol/L/h) of the stroke seem to be linear.

Implications of animal studies to patient studies

The detailed documentation of the evolution of TSC and ADC in this nonhuman primate model provides the essential information for the interpretation of these parameters in patient studies. These

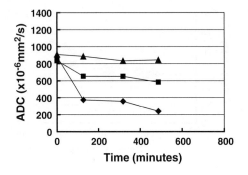

Fig. 6. Time courses for the change in ADC trace (ADC$_{trace}$) in the brain cortex over the first 10 hours after stroke induction by embolization in the animal model. Apparent diffusion coefficient values refer to regions of interest sampled in the contralateral normal left cerebral hemisphere (▲) and at the periphery (■) and core (◆) of the stroke in the right cerebral cortex. The greater change in ADC in the core (300×10^{-6} mm^2/s) of the stroke as compared with the periphery (650×10^{-6} mm^2/s) does not change significantly over the first 10 hours after the initial rapid decrease.

parameters are quantitative and, unlike conventional anatomic proton imaging, have a direct biologic interpretation. The imaging studies in human beings have been performed on the same clinical 3.0-T scanner with an identical RF coil, imaging sequences, and parameters. The extrapolation of the observations in the animal model to the patient setting is a reasonable step, given that the human studies do not permit many imaging sessions or histologic verification, except in rare cases. The 3-hour window approved for thrombolytic therapy can be given a biologic interpretation as the time before which TSC has reached 70 mmol/L, the concentration at which stroke has become irreversible infarction. The figure of 70 mmol/L comes from TSC measured in

completed strokes of animals and human beings. There may well be a lower value of TSC at which a stroke has progressed to irreversible infarction. Because normal TSC is less than 45 mmol/L, the rate of change in TSC must be less than 8.5 mmol/L/h over 3 hours for the clinical window to apply. The animal model had a maximal rate of only 5 mmol/L/h in the basal ganglia, suggesting that the window may be wider in cases in which the collateral circulation may be sufficient to slow the rate of change in TSC. The model does suggest that TSC acts as a physiologic timer of stroke progress by which therapeutic decisions may be made objectively and efficiently in individual patients.

Human studies

Healthy adult volunteers (n = 5) as well as the patients or their families (n = 4) gave written informed consent for serial MR imaging at 1.5 or 3.0 T as approved by the Institutional Review Board. All MR imaging studies were performed within FDA guidelines. These representative patient cases of serial MR imaging were recruited from the neurologic intensive care unit. The results of single imaging studies from a much larger number of subjects (n=68) have been published elsewhere [4]. Imaging protocols matched those described for the animal model. The functional imaging study with blood oxygenation level–dependent (BOLD) contrast in case 4 was performed with four separate block design paradigms. Each paradigm was with unilateral movement of the wrist or ankle (1 Hz, 30-second block) alternated with rest (30-second block) across 4.5 cycles, starting and ending on rest [19–21,28]. Head motion was less than 0.5 voxel [29]. The activation maps were

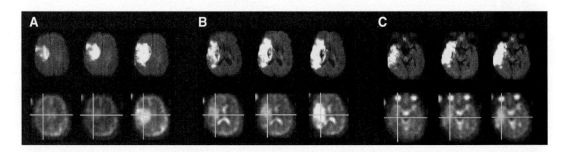

Fig. 7. Case 1. Temporal evolution of a human stroke in the right middle cerebral artery territory shown by diffusion weighted imaging (*upper row*) and sodium images (*lower row*) at 19 hours (*first column*), 34 hours (*second column*), and 87 hours (*third column*) at each of three levels: centrum semiovale (*A*), lateral ventricles (*B*), and temporal lobes (*C*). The yellow horizontal and vertical lines depict the regional profiles of TSC over time, as shown in Fig. 8.

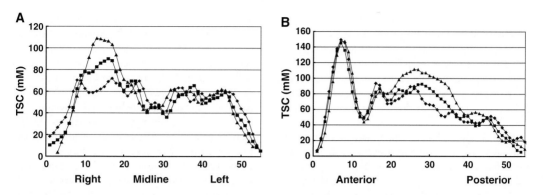

Fig. 8. Medial-lateral (*A*) and anterior-posterior (*B*) profiles of TSC values (millimoles) through the right middle cerebral artery stroke, shown as the horizontal and vertical yellow lines, respectively, in Fig. 7A through C (*bottom row*) demonstrating regional temporal changes in TSC values at 19 hours (◆), 34 hours (■) and 87 hours (▲). The level is through the temporal lobes. The profiles show the increase in volume of the stroke in both dimensions. The large TSC in B is the globe of the eye at close to 150 mmol/L, which represents a useful internal calibration. These are representative profiles, but all the levels and directions indicated in Fig. 7 were analyzed with similar results.

calculated with a two-tailed *t* test ($P < .05$) without filtering and were presented as a color scale superimposed over high-resolution anatomic images using AFNI software [29].

Case 1 is a representative patient illustrating the evolution of stroke as observed by serial MR imaging. This was a 78-year-old right-handed woman with a history of rheumatic heart disease who found that she was unable to get out of bed on the evening of day 1 because of left-sided weakness. Medical evaluation at a local hospital with CT showed no evidence of cerebral hemorrhage and a questionable right middle cerebral artery stroke. After transfer to our hospital, further evaluation at 4 hours after the first observation of symptoms revealed a left gaze preference and left hemiparesis.

A xenon-enhanced CT brain perfusion examination showed reduced perfusion in the right middle cerebral artery territory. Conventional angiography confirmed the occlusion of the right middle cerebral artery. Treatment with intra-arterial urokinase thrombolysis was unsuccessful. Comprehensive MR imaging examinations, including anatomic, diffusion-weighted, and sodium imaging, were performed at 19 hours, 35 hours, and 87 hours after onset of symptoms (Fig. 7). The diffusion-weighted imaging maps (see Fig. 7, top row) and TSC maps (see Fig. 7, bottom row) of this case are presented for three slices through the brain (at the level of the centrum semiovale, lateral ventricles, and temporal lobes in Fig. 7A–C, respectively) at three time points (19, 34, and 87 hours in the first column, second column, and third column, respectively). Horizontal and vertical

lines across the TSC maps were used to produce the profile patterns through the stroke of the changes in TSC and ADC over time (Fig. 8A and B, respectively) to demonstrate the quantitative temporal progression of the stroke. The progressive enlargement of infarction as a volume fraction of cerebral hemispheric volume, defined operationally as the volume in which TSC is greater than 70 mmol/L and ADC is less than 50% of normal, is shown in Fig. 9.

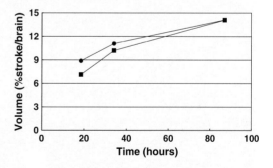

Fig. 9. The percentage brain volume of the stroke as a function of time for the lesion shown in Fig. 7. The volume was assessed by TSC greater than 70 mmol/L (■) and by 50% reduction in ADC (●) compared with the contralateral side. Both parameters converge on a 14% lesion volume by 87 hours. The lesion volume is calculated as a percentage of the hemispheric volume to ensure consistency over time. The brain volume was 1400 ± 28 mL, and the final lesion volume was 198 mL. (*From* Imaging of the nervous system. In: Latchaw RE, Kucharczzyk J, Moseley ME, editors. Philadelphia: Elsevier Mosby; 2005.)

Three other patients were also imaged serially and are discussed in comparison with the first case.

Case 2 was an 80-year-old right-handed woman found with left-sided weakness and slurred speech. Imaging showed a stroke in the territory of the right middle cerebral artery. MR imaging was performed at 31, 77, and 97 hours as the patient improved clinically (Fig. 10).

Case 3 was a 71-year-old right-handed woman who presented with slurred speech, headache, and confusion with progressive left-sided weakness and, ultimately, loss of responsiveness. A right middle cerebral artery hemorrhagic stroke was diagnosed. MR imaging was performed at 29, 47, and 71 hours as the patient improved clinically. These results are not shown because they emulate those of case 2.

Case 4 was a 34-year-old right-handed man who presented with left-sided weakness but was otherwise alert and cooperative. Imaging showed a stroke spanning the territories of the right middle and anterior cerebral arteries. MR imaging was performed

at 9 and 42 hours as the patient became increasingly somnolent (Fig. 11). Although there was concern for the development of malignant middle cerebral artery syndrome, cranial nerve findings did not occur until 56 hours; at that time, a strokectomy of the infarcted tissue was performed involving removal of the right motor and somatosensory cortices. The strokectomy was guided by the TSC map in which the regions of elevated TSC greater than 70 mmol/L were resected. The patient recovered from surgery with resolution of the cranial nerve findings and was discharged from hospital within 10 days of surgery. At 67 days after his initial hospital admission, he returned for follow-up. At that time, he was able to use the left side of his body and to ambulate with a cane and left knee brace. To understand this functional recovery, despite resection of the right motor cortex, functional MR imaging was performed. Functional MR imaging used BOLD contrast and four separate block design paradigms (Fig. 12).

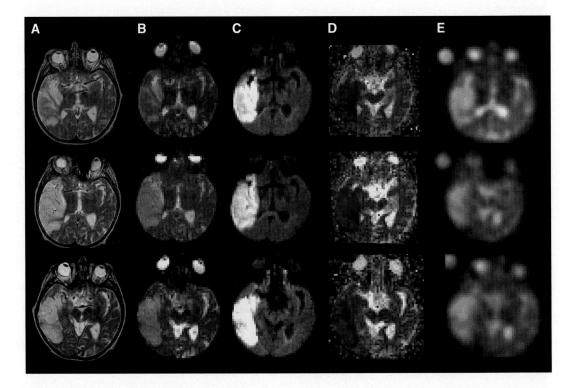

Fig. 10. Case 2. This patient showed no changes in the volume or distribution of changes at 31 (*top row*), 77 (*middle row*), or 97 (*bottom row*) hours after onset of symptoms in any of the images acquired, including T2-weighted fast spin-echo images (*A*); T2-weighted, spin-echo, echo-planar images (*B*); diffusion-weighted echo-planar images (*C*); ADC maps calculated from B and C (*D*); and sodium images (*E*). No change is discernible by visual inspection or by volume measurements. Case 3 is a similar pattern and not shown. (*From* Imaging of the nervous system. In: Latchaw RE, Kucharczzyk J, Moseley ME, editors. Philadelphia: Elsevier Mosby; 2005.)

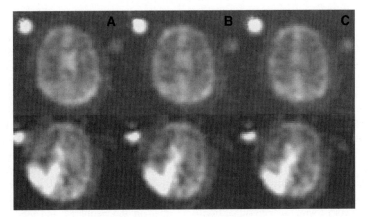

Fig. 11. Case 4. Selected sodium images at lateral ventricles (*A*), centrum semiovale (*B*), and vertex (*C*) at 9 hours (*upper row*) and 42 hours (*lower row*) after onset of left hemiplegia in this initially cognitive alert and cooperative patient. By 42 hours, the patient was somnolent, not readily following instructions, and moving as shown by the head rotation and degraded image quality. The bright circular signal above and to the right side of the brain is the higher concentration of the two calibration phantoms. The similar fainter intensity to the left is the lower concentration phantom. The TSC map shows only slightly elevated TSC values at 9 hours but a large increase by 42 hours to greater than 70 mmol/L, suggesting that viable tissue at the time of 9 hours was nonviable by 42 hours.

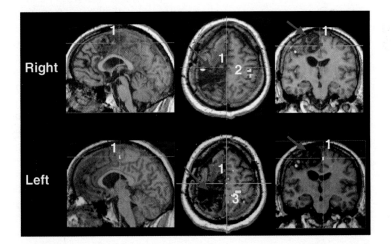

Fig. 12. Activation maps in the sagittal, axial, and coronal planes (*green lines*) for right (*upper row*) and left (*lower row*) wrist flexion/extension generated by functional MR imaging with BOLD contrast in a 4.5-minute block-designed paradigm of the patient at 67 days after strokectomy. The surgery removed the right motor and somatosensory cortices (*red arrow*). The patient was able to walk with a cane and knee brace. The normal activation pattern, shown as colored statistically significant activation, for the right upper extremity (*upper row*) shows the supplementary motor area (1) and motor and somatosensory areas (2). (3) Left upper extremity (*lower row*) mapped onto the primary motor cortex into the left hemisphere but to a slightly different area. The activation map was calculated using a Student's *t* test to compare the rest condition (30 seconds) with the active condition of wrist flexion and extension (30 seconds) in a block-designed paradigm with 4.5 cycles. The activation map was superimposed over high-resolution T1-weighted images for improved visualization in three planes. The tissue loss from resection of the right posterior frontoparietal region is seen on the axial and coronal images (*red arrow*). (*From* Imaging of the nervous system. In: Latchaw RE, Kucharczzyk J, Moseley ME, editors. Philadelphia: Elsevier Mosby; 2005.)

Results from human studies

The calibration of TSC measurements at 3.0 T in the structures of normal human brain (voxel dimensions of $5 \times 5 \times 5$ mm^3) using the same acquisition and reconstruction strategies employed in the animal model is presented in Table 1. These numbers represent averages of TSC values sampled from each region averaged over healthy normal volunteers (n = 5). The corresponding TSC numbers at 1.5 T (voxel dimension of $6 \times 6 \times 6$ mm^3) obtained from the same volunteers with the same total acquisition time revealed higher values, presumably because of partial volume averaging of cortex with the high signal from cerebrospinal fluid (results not shown). The TSC values for cortical gray matter (40.4 ± 0.7 mmol/L) are significantly (two-tailed t test, $P < .005$) higher than the TSC values of the white matter (33.1 ± 0.5 mmol/L). The relatively higher value of TSC for the hippocampus (46.9 ± 0.3 mmol/L) most likely represents contamination from the much higher surrounding cerebrospinal fluid, even at the higher resolution at 3.0 T available in much the same way as for the overly high TSC values of superficial cortex for the lower spatial resolution results at 1.5 T.

Table 1

Tissue sodium concentration values for regions of the brain measured at 3.0 Tesla and sampled with voxel resolution of $5 \times 5 \times 5$ mm^3

Brain region	TSC (mean ± SD) in mmol/L	
	Right	Left
Hemisphere		
Frontal cortex	37.5 ± 2.8	37.9 ± 2.6
Parietal lobe	38.1 ± 3.1	42.2 ± 2.5
Temporal lobe	42.1 ± 3.0	41.4 ± 2.8
Occipital lobe	41.7 ± 1.6	41.8 ± 1.1
Gray matter average	**39.9 ± 2.4**	**40.8 ± 2.0**
Forceps major	35.5 ± 2.1	37.0 ± 1.3
Forceps minor	34.2 ± 3.0	35.9 ± 2.5
Corona radiata	33.2 ± 3.1	33.2 ± 3.1
Centrum semiovale	28.1 ± 3.4	27.8 ± 3.5
White matter average	**32.8 ± 3.2**	**33.5 ± 4.1**
Thalamus	32.8 ± 3.2	32.1 ± 2.6
Putamen	37.3 ± 4.1	39.1 ± 3.2
Dentate nucleus	35.5 ± 2.6	33.6 ± 2.1
Hippocampus	47.1 ± 2.5	46.7 ± 2.1
Midbrain	36.7 ± 1.6	37.0 ± 1.9
Brainstem	31.3 ± 1.5	30.9 ± 2.9

Values were averaged from 5 healthy adults using a 2-point concentration calibration corrected for B_1 inhomogeneities. Boldface represents mean of values listed above.

Adapted from Imaging of the nervous system. In: Latchaw RE, Kucharczyk J, Moseley ME, editors. Philadelphia: Elsevier Mosby; 2005.

Case 1 was selected from the studies of clinical stroke patients as a representative example of the temporal evolution of a hemorrhagic stroke (see Fig. 7). This case shows a pattern of stroke evolution from 19 to 87 hours after initial onset of symptoms in the right middle artery territory. The volume of the lesion, as defined by decreased ADC and elevated TSC, extended superiorly (see Fig. 7A, columns 1–3), posteriorly (see Fig. 7B, columns 1–3), and inferiorly (see Fig. 7C, columns 1–3). These regional results are more easily appreciated quantitatively on the profiles (see Fig. 8) showing that TSC increased faster in the central regions of the stroke than in the periphery and that considerable lesion expansion occurred after 34 hours. The right globe in the profile of Fig. 8B acts as an internal standard of approximately 150 mmol/L to show that the quantification of TSC maps over time is reproducible, unlike the MR imaging signal intensity of an image that is dependent on instrument settings. The volume of stroke based on the ADC and the TSC maps increased with time and converged on approximately 14% hemispheric volume at the last time point (87 hours), as shown in Fig. 9.

In comparison to this case, cases 2 and 3 were patients who showed completed strokes without change in the volume of distribution of TSC or ADC after approximately 25 hours from onset of symptoms up to almost 100 hours (case 2, see Fig. 10). In these cases, the stroke core contained TSC values in excess of 70 mmol/L that did not change over the observation period. In comparison, the contralateral normal side showed TSC values in the normal range as defined in Table 1.

Case 4 provided an example of the use of TSC maps after tissue infarction and the development of malignant middle cerebral artery syndrome. At the first time point at 9 hours after symptom onset (see Fig. 11), the TSC values were less than 55 mmol/L, indicating viable tissue with intact sodium ion homeostasis. By 42 hours (see Fig. 11), however, a large volume of the stroke had TSC values greater than 70 mmol/L, indicating that the stroke had progressed to infarction over an increasing volume. The rising TSC values seemed to coincide with the development of somnolence yet preceded by many hours the development of the cranial nerve palsies that characterize malignant middle cerebral artery syndrome. This information formed the basis for deciding on the strokectomy intervention that saved the patient's life, with subsequent rapid recovery of cranial nerve palsies and discharge from acute care within 10 days. The resection of motor cortex would normally not be contemplated, because residual surviving tissue within the stroke zone has been thought to be the basis of functional recovery. Given that TSC indicated the stroke had progressed to completed infarction and the prognosis for middle cerebral artery syndrome was grim, resection was performed to save the life of this patient. The right motor cortex was resected with the expectation of a permanent left hemiplegia, but this was not observed. Such excellent recovery of the left upper and lower extremities in this case could not be attributed to surviving neurons within the stroke region. Functional imaging (see Fig. 12) performed at 67 days provided the explanation in that the control of the left extremities had been transferred to the left hemisphere, as has been reported elsewhere [30–32]. The activations in the left cerebral hemisphere during movement of the left extremities were not attributable to mirroring of movements from the right extremities, because the activation regions are not in exactly the same areas as those induced by movement of the right extremities.

Implications of serial sodium MR imaging in stroke management

The natural evolution of TSC (see Figs. 2–5) and ADC (see Figs. 3 and 6) over the first 10 hours in the animal model of embolic stroke shows considerable regional variation, albeit monotonically increasing change across the superficial gray matter and structures within the basal ganglia. Higher rates of change in the basal ganglia may reflect the lack of any collateral supportive circulation for the end arteries supplying this region. Superficial cortex has a collateral blood supply that may allow sodium homeostasis to be maintained for longer times, thereby causing TSC to increase more slowly. This is reflected in a gradual but variable rate of increase in TSC values. The ADC parameter shows less change after the initial rapid decrease, making it useful in the diagnosis of stroke but less sensitive for monitoring changes over time. The monotonically increasing TSC serves as a means to monitor the progressive loss of tissue viability. If a threshold of TSC reversibility can be determined, as has been suggested previously from the same primate animal model [4], this parameter may become useful as a physiologic measure by which to decide whether to proceed with a therapeutic intervention.

A TSC value of 70 mmol/L, previously proposed as an indicator of irreversible tissue loss [4], might be useful for deciding when not to intervene, at least

with thrombolytic agents. The most direct evidence that a TSC value of 70 mmol/L indicates irreversible tissue loss is the close correlation with the TCC stain (see Fig. 3), as previously reported over a shorter period [4]. Although at 3 hours, lack of TTC staining may understate infarct size and histologic signs of infarction continue to evolve over a longer period, the TTC method establishes final infarction size by 6 hours, when occlusion is permanent, as it was in this case [33]. Although our understanding of the complex pattern of cell death in stroke remains incomplete [34], the importance of an in vivo parameter, such as TSC, that can be used across animal and human investigations is emphasized. The different rates of loss of tissue viability, as reflected in the different rates of change in TSC values between cortex and basal ganglia, suggest that clinical decisions to use thrombolytic agents may use different time windows depending on the location of the stroke. Cortical stroke may have a wider time window than basal ganglia involvement.

Sodium imaging is clearly of a quality and duration that is practical for clinical applications. The representative human studies show two patterns of evolution over the first few days after stroke onset. Case 1, in which the stroke volume expanded, is indicative of the incorporation of the stroke penumbra into the core. Although the penumbra has been reported as being the difference between the ADC and perfusion parameters, termed the *diffusion-perfusion mismatch*, the current work suggests a refinement of this description. The ADC overestimates the core in the first few days, although TSC and ADC converge to the same volume when no intervention is made successfully (see Fig. 9). The expansion of the core with recruitment of the penumbra was not uniform. In case 1 (see Figs. 7 and 8), extension occurred superiorly and posteriorly, probably reflecting collateral circulation and changes in perfusion patterns concomitant with mass effect from the edema. Although ADC showed small changes, the accurate measurement of these small changes, after the initial large change in ADC used for diagnosis of stroke and probably reflecting similar processes being monitored by TSC, proved more difficult to quantify accurately than TSC.

Not all patients demonstrate delayed evolution of stroke, as was shown in cases 2 and 3 (see Fig. 10), in which all imaging parameters remained unchanged after approximately 30 hours up to approximately 100 hours.

The TSC maps are not limited to the loss of tissue viability for the triaging of acute patients to therapy. This information can also be used in patient management during the subacute stages of malignant middle cerebral artery syndrome, which occurs in 3% to 10% of stroke patients [15–17]. Although case 4 is a single case, its documentation is important to show how this TSC measure of tissue viability can be used to manage such patients by defining the scope of tissue resection, despite the traditional view of the expected outcome of permanent hemiplegia (see Figs. 11 and 12). The rapid recovery of function on clinical follow-up examination is a testimony to the plasticity of the brain in the face of even severe insults. The biologic basis of such rapid recovery may be attributable to the known small fraction of ipsilaterally connected neurons in the corticospinal tracts [30–32].

Summary

Sodium imaging of acute and subacute stroke patients can be performed efficiently and repeatedly on a clinical imaging service, yielding useful information for tailored clinical management of individual patients. Maps of TSC and ADC yield complementary information. The monotonically increasing function of TSC evolution is useful for monitoring the progressive loss of viable tissue and may provide a useful parameter to guide therapeutic decision making for individual patients rather than using the empirically based 3-hour time window currently employed for deciding on the use of thrombolysis.

Although some may argue that serial MR imaging is expensive and unnecessary, clinical experience indicates that the initial CT examination is usually followed by several MR imaging examinations performed to confirm the initial diagnosis and then to explain the evolution of symptoms as the disease progresses. A more efficient algorithm may be actively planned serial imaging with quantitative parameters that can be predictive of disease progression. This would be preferable to imaging in response to new clinical findings, resulting in emergent reactive, and therefore delayed, decisions in medical or neurosurgical management. Such serial imaging in the acute care setting may provide advanced warning of lesion progression, often accompanied by brain swelling and the development of malignant middle cerebral artery syndrome [15–17]. The use of a comprehensive imaging approach, including sodium imaging when appropriate, may provide considerable insight into stroke pathophysiology in individual patients, allowing efficient yet tailored management.

References

[1] Kalafut MA, Saver JL. The acute stroke patient: the first 6 hours. In: Cohen SN, editor. Management of ischemic stroke. New York: McGraw-Hill; 2000. p. 17–52.

[2] National Institutes of Neurological Disorders and Stroke rt-PA Stroke Study Group. Tissue plasminogen activator for acute ischemic stroke. N Engl J Med 1995;333:1581–7.

[3] Ernst R, Pancioli A, Tomsick T, et al. Combined intravenous and intra-arterial recombinant tissue plasminogen activator in acute ischemic stroke. Stroke 2000;31:2552–7.

[4] Thulborn KR, Gindin TS, Davis D, et al. Comprehensive MRI protocol for stroke management: tissue sodium concentration as a measure of tissue viability in a non-human primate model and clinical studies. Radiology 1999;139:26–34.

[5] Grond M, von Kummer R, Sobesky J, et al. Early x-ray hypoattenuation of brain parenchyma indicates extended critical hypoperfusion in acute stroke. Stroke 2001;31:133–9.

[6] Parsons MW, Yang Q, Barber PA, et al. Perfusion magnetic resonance imaging maps in hyperacute stroke relative cerebral blood flow most accurately identifies tissue destined to infarct. Stroke 2001;32:1581–7.

[7] Wu O, Koroshetz WJ, Ostergaard L, et al. Predicting tissue outcome in acute human cerebral ischemia using combined diffusion and perfusion-weighted MR imaging. Stroke 2001;32:933–42.

[8] Chalela JA, Alsop DC, Gonzalez-Atavales JB, et al. Magnetic resonance perfusion imaging in acute ischemic stroke using continuous arterial spin labeling. Stroke 2000;31:680–7.

[9] Heiss W-D, Kracht L, Grond M, et al. Early [11C] flumazenil/H2O positron emission tomography predicts irreversible ischemic cortical damage in stroke patients receiving acute thrombolytic therapy. Stroke 2000;31:366–9.

[10] Desmond PM, Lovell AC, Rawlinson AA, et al. The value of apparent diffusion coefficient maps in early cerebral ischemia. AJNR Am J Neuroradiol 2001;22: 1260–7.

[11] Helpern JA. The missing element [editorial]. AJNR Am J Neuroradiol 2001;22:1235–6.

[12] Kidwell CS, Alger JR, Di Salle F, et al. Diffusion MRI in patients with transient ischemic attacks. Stroke 1999;30:1174–80.

[13] Grant PE, He J, Halpern EF, et al. Frequency and clinical context of decreased apparent diffusion coefficient reversal in the human brain. Radiology 2001;221: 43–50.

[14] Lin S-P, Song S-K, Miller JP, et al. Direct longitudinal comparison of 1H and 23Na MRI after transient focal cerebral ischemia. Stroke 2001;32:925–32.

[15] Rieke K, Schwab S, Krieger D, et al. Decompressive surgery in space occupying hemispheric infarction:

results of an open, prospective study. Crit Care Med 1995;23:1576–87.

[16] Schwab S, Steiner T, Aschoff A, et al. Early hemicraniectomy in patients with complete middle cerebral artery infarction. Stroke 1998;29:1888–93.

[17] Hacke W, Schwab S, Horn M, et al. Malignant middle cerebral artery territory infarction: clinical course and prognostic signs. Arch Neurol 1996;53:309–15.

[18] Boada FB, Gillen JS, Shen GX, et al. Fast three dimensional sodium imaging. Magn Reson Med 1997; 37:706–15.

[19] Thulborn KR, Davis D. Clinical fMRI. In: Haacke EM, editor. Current protocols in magnetic resonance imaging. New York: Wiley and Sons; 2001. p. A6.0.1–.6.

[20] Thulborn KR, Davis D, Erb P, et al. Clinical fMRI: implementation and experience. Neuroimage 1996; 4(Suppl):S101–7.

[21] Thulborn KR, Martin C, Voyvodic J. fMRI using a visually guided saccade paradigm in Alzheimer's disease. AJNR Am J Neuroradiol 2000;21:524–31.

[22] Shen GX, Wu J, Boada FE, Thulborn KR. An experimentally verified theoretical design of dual-tuned, low-pass birdcage RF resonators for MRI and MRS of human brain at 3.0 Tesla. Magn Reson Med 1999;41:268–75.

[23] Chesler D, Vevea JM, Boada FE, et al. Rapid 3-D reconstruction from 1-D projections for metabolic MR imaging of short T2 species. In: Proceedings of 11th Annual Meeting Society Magnetic Resonance in Medicine Berlin, Germany. Berkeley (CA): Society of Magnetic Medicine; 1992. p. 665.

[24] Thulborn KR, Boada FE, Shen GX, et al. Correction of B1 inhomogeneities using echo-planar imaging of water. Magn Reson Med 1998;39:369–75.

[25] Thulborn KR, Uttecht S, Betancourt C, et al.

A functional, physiological and metabolic toolbox for clinical magnetic resonance imaging: integration of acquisition and analysis strategies. Int J Imaging Syst Technol 1997;8:572–81.

[26] Uttecht S, Thulborn KR. Software for efficient visualization and analysis of multiple, large, multi-dimensional data sets from magnetic resonance imaging. Comput Med Imaging Graph 2001;16:73–89.

[27] Thulborn KR, Uttecht S. Volumetry and topography of the human brain by MRI. Int J Imaging Syst Technol 2000;11:198–208.

[28] Thulborn KR. Clinical fMRI. In: Atlas SW, editor. Magnetic resonance imaging of the brain and spine. Philadelphia: Lippincott Williams & Wilkins; 2001. p. 1973–92.

[29] Cox RW. AFNI, software for analysis and visualization of functional magnetic resonance neuroimages. Comput Biomed Res 1996;29:162–73.

[30] Naidich TP, Hof PR, Yousry TA, et al. The motor cortex. Anatomic substrates of function. Neuroimaging Clin N Am 2001;11:171–93.

[31] Tanji J, Okano K, Sato KC. Neuronal activity in cortical motor areas related to ipsilateral, contralateral and bilateral digit movements of the monkey. J Neurophysiol 1988;60:325–43.

[32] Tanji J, Okano K, Sato KC. Relation of neurons in the nonprimary motor cortex to bilateral hand movement. Nature 1987;327:618–20.

[33] Aronowski J, Cho KH, Strong R, et al. Neurofilament proteolysis after focal ischemia; when do cells die after experimental stroke? J Cereb Blood Flow Metab 1999;19:652–60.

[34] Lipton P. Ischemic cell death in brain neurons. Physiol Rev 1999;79:1431–568.

ELSEVIER
SAUNDERS

Neuroimag Clin N Am 15 (2005) 655–665

Diffusion Tensor Imaging and Fiber Tractography in Acute Stroke

Pratik Mukherjee, MD, PhD*

Neuroradiology Section, Department of Radiology, University of California at San Francisco, San Francisco, CA, USA

Diffusion tensor imaging (DTI) is an area of burgeoning research in technical refinements and clinical applications. Diffusion MR imaging reflects information on a microscopic spatial scale, allowing researchers and clinicians an unprecedented ability to probe tissue microarchitecture noninvasively. Fiber tractography based on DTI can reveal the three-dimensional (3-D) white matter connectivity of the human brain. In this article, current methods for performing DTI and tractography are examined, followed by a brief review of the normal anatomy of the human brain studied with DTI. Finally, areas of ongoing clinical research and developing clinical applications of DTI and tractography for stroke are presented.

Diffusion tensor imaging methods

Acquisition

The most widely used techniques for acquiring DTI are the same as for routine clinical diffusion-weighted imaging (DWI): single-shot, spin-echo echo-planar imaging (EPI), a method for rapid imaging that freezes bulk macroscopic motion, thereby permitting imaging of water diffusion at microscopic spatial scales. DTI requires higher signal-to-noise

ratio (SNR), however, for accurate assessment of diffusion anisotropy, preferably greatly exceeding a SNR of 20 [1]. DTI fiber tractography also requires better spatial resolution than DWI for detailed visualization of small white matter tracts, preferably cubic voxels 2.5 mm on a side or smaller. The use of cubic voxels, which have the same length in all three orthogonal dimensions, is recommended for tractography to avoid biasing the 3-D tracking algorithm toward the direction of poorer spatial resolution. EPI can provide sufficient spatial resolution with adequate SNR for DTI tractography at 1.5 T in a clinically feasible acquisition time [2]. Higher field magnets (3 T and above) enable DTI at higher spatial resolution or shorter acquisition times. Geometric warping artifacts common to EPI may limit anatomic fidelity, however, especially in areas of high magnetic field susceptibility resulting from brain-air-bone interfaces, such as the skull base and the posterior fossa. These susceptibility artifacts can be problematic even at 1.5 T and increase markedly at higher field strengths. Pulsation artifacts from cerebrospinal fluid also create artifacts, especially in the posterior fossa and in regions of the supratentorial brain bordering the lateral ventricles [3–5]. To optimize DTI of the brainstem and cerebellum, where susceptibility and pulsation artifacts are greatest, segmented EPI with phase navigation and cardiac gating is used [6], although these strategies lengthen the examination time for patient preparation and image acquisition. New advances in gradient strength and speed, multichannel radio-frequency (RF) coils, and parallel imaging can address these problems.

The new multichannel, phased-array head RF coils with better SNR characteristics than the standard birdcage head RF coils have enhanced DTI, which is

This article is adapted from Edelman RR, Hesselink JR, Zlatkin MB, et al. Clinical magnetic resonance imaging. 3rd edition. Philadelphia: Elsevier; 2005; with permission.

* Neuroradiology Section, Department of Radiology, University of California at San Francisco, 505 Parnassus Avenue, Box 0628, San Francisco, CA 94143-0628.

E-mail address: pratik@radiology.ucsf.edu

an SNR-limited imaging modality. The multichannel RF coils also enable parallel imaging, a technical advance that can improve the image quality of DTI [7]. Parallel imaging techniques, such as SMASH (simultaneous acquisition of spatial harmonics), SENSE (sensitivity encoding), ASSET (array spatial sensitivity encoding technique), and iPAT (integrated parallel acquisition techniques), all can be used to shorten the echo train length of EPI, thereby mitigating geometric warping artifacts and reducing the blurring of image contrast that occurs with extended EPI echo trains. These gains increase with the acceleration factor used in parallel imaging, but must be balanced against the greater loss of SNR. With current 8-channel head RF coils, acceleration factors of 2 to 3 are optimal [7]. Parallel imaging is instrumental for ameliorating the greater EPI susceptibility artifacts that occur at 3 T and above, thereby permitting high-field DTI with superior image quality.

Another important hardware consideration for performing DTI is the gradient performance of the MR scanner for the diffusion gradients and the EPI readout gradients. Stronger and faster gradients enable stronger diffusion weighting in a shorter period of time and reduce the time required to form an EPI image. This permits DTI to be acquired at a shorter echo time (TE), which improves SNR and reduces geometric warping artifacts. Hence, the latest generation of MR images, with 4 G/cm gradient strength, allows DTI with high spatial resolution and anatomic fidelity.

Other variables that may affect the quality of DTI and tractography include the b value (diffusion weighting factor) and the number of directions in 3-D space in which diffusion gradients are applied. A b value of 1000 s/mm^2 has become the standard for clinical DWI and also is used for DTI in many studies. The brains of newborns and infants have much longer T2 relaxation times and much higher apparent diffusion coefficients (ADC) than adults [8]; therefore, it is standard to use lower b values (eg, 600 s/mm^2) for DWI and DTI. The superior gradient performance of the latest generation of MR scanners permits the acquisition of DTI at diffusion-weighting factors much greater than 1000 s/mm^2, and applications for ultrahigh b factor DTI are an area of active investigation [9]. The minimum number of diffusion-sensitizing directions needed to solve for the diffusion tensor is six, although each six-direction whole brain acquisition needs to be repeated several times and averaged to provide sufficient SNR at high enough spatial resolution on a 1.5 T scanner for DTI tractography. DTI performance improves, however, with greater numbers of diffusion-encoding directions isotropically distributed in 3-D space [10,11].

DTI can be performed with other types of fast imaging sequences besides EPI to avoid the artifacts inherent in single-shot EPI. Examples include line scan [12], single-shot, fast spin-echo [13], and PROPELLER (periodically rotated overlapping parallel lines with enhanced reconstruction) [14]. All of these other sequences suffer from less SNR per unit time compared with EPI and, thus, longer acquisition times. They may be of benefit for evaluating ischemia near the skull base, however, in the posterior fossa or in the spinal cord.

Postprocessing and visualization

DTI postprocessing and visualization require the generation of parametric maps, the most popular of which are spatially-averaged ADC (also called D_{av}, and mean diffusivity), diffusion anisotropy, directionally encoded color anisotropy, and the eigenvalues of the diffusion tensor. Calculation of DTI parametric maps and 3-D tractography may require postprocessing on a dedicated image workstation, although vendors increasingly incorporate on-line DTI visualization tools in their latest MR scanner software releases.

There are many different measures of diffusion anisotropy described in the literature, the most popular of which are: (1) fractional anisotropy (FA), which is the most sensitive to low anisotropy values; (2) volume ratio (VR), which is the most sensitive to high anisotropy values; and (3) relative anisotropy (RA), which is more linear across the entire range of anisotropy values than the other two metrics. The three eigenvalues of the diffusion tensor represent the magnitude of diffusion along the three principal directions in 3-D space, which are mutually orthogonal. The eigenvalue with the maximum value (the major eigenvalue) is the magnitude of diffusion along the orientation in which water diffuses most freely, whereas the two other eigenvalues (the minor eigenvalues) represent the magnitude of diffusion along the directions orthogonal to this preferred orientation. The mean of the three eigenvalues is equivalent to the ADC, and the variance of the three eigenvalues is related to the diffusion anisotropy.

White matter anatomy of the human brain

Anisotropy of white matter tracts

DTI excels at depicting the white matter architecture of the human brain. In conventional T1- and T2-weighted MR imaging, white matter appears homogeneous throughout the normal adult brain. DTI can differentiate among different white matter tracts via two distinct contrast mechanisms: (1) the magnitude of anisotropy within the white matter tract and (2) the orientation of the fibers within the white matter tract. White matter tracts of the cerebral hemispheres may be classified into three distinct types: (1) association—those that connect two different regions of the cerebral cortex within the same hemisphere; (2) projection—those that connect the cerebral cortex to subcortical structures, such as the thalamus and spinal cord; and (3) commissural—those that connect cortical regions of the left hemisphere with those of the right hemisphere. In general, the anisotropy values of association tracts are less than those of projection tracts, which in turn are lower than those of commissural tracts [15]. Within the association category, the anisotropy of short association fibers connecting adjacent regions of cortex, also known as subcortical U-fibers, is less than those of long association fibers running in large bundles, such as the superior longitudinal fasciculus (SLF) and the inferior longitudinal fasciculus (ILF). Gray matter of the cerebral cortex is believed to have zero anisotropy in adults, to within the limits of measurement noise [15,16].

Although water diffuses more freely parallel to highly collimated axonal bundles than in the plane perpendicular to the fiber bundles, the biologic basis for this diffusion anisotropy is not elucidated completely. It is likely that structural elements, such as the plasma membrane of axons (the axolemma) and their myelin sheaths, hinder water diffusion across fiber bundles. Biophysical processes, such as ion fluxes across the axolemma and fast axonal transport, also are implicated. Measurements of diffusion anisotropy in vivo and in formalin-fixed myelinated white matter show similar values, although the ADC is much lower in fixed tissue, indicating that the determinants of anisotropy in mature myelinated white matter likely are microstructural and not physiologic [17,18].

Fiber orientation of white matter tracts

The three major types of white matter tracts also can be distinguished by the direction of the axons within their fiber bundles on directionally encoded color anisotropy maps. Water diffuses more freely parallel to white matter fibers than orthogonal to them, which is the basis for white matter diffusion anisotropy. The fiber orientation of white matter pathways can be determined from the direction of maximal diffusivity. This direction corresponds to the primary eigenvector of the diffusion tensor, which is

associated with the major eigenvalue (defined previously). The projection of the primary eigenvector on each of three orthogonal axes (left-right, anteroposterior, and craniocaudal) can be encoded by different colors. In the most widely accepted directional encoding scheme, the left-right direction is assigned to red, the anteroposterior dimension is assigned to green, and the craniocaudal direction is assigned to blue [19]. This works well for differentiating large association tracts, which usually are green because they connect anterior and posterior cortical regions within a single cerebral hemisphere, from projection pathways, which often are blue because they connect superior cortical areas to inferior subcortical regions, and also from commissural fibers, which appear red because of their left-right orientation across the two hemispheres. DTI cannot distinguish between anterograde and retrograde axonal directions along a single orientation, for example, the corticospinal tract cannot be separated from the somatosensory radiation on the basis that, in the former, the axons project from the cortex down to a subcortical structure, whereas, in the latter, the axons project from a subcortical structure up to the cortex. Both projection pathways appear blue on directionally encoded color FA maps because both have a predominantly craniocaudal orientation.

The normal white matter anatomy of the adult human brain is illustrated in Fig. 1 with DTI parametric maps. The optimized DTI technique used to acquire these images at 1.5 T includes 4 G/cm gradients, a high-sensitivity eight-channel head RF coil, and parallel imaging. This optimized technique permits high-quality imaging even in regions of high susceptibility and cerebrospinal fluid pulsatility, such as the brainstem, without the need for segmented EPI, cardiac gating, or phase navigation [20].

Three-dimensional fiber tractography of white matter

Because white matter pathways in the brain exist in 3-D, even sophisticated 2-D representations, such as directionally encoded color anisotropy maps, intrinsically are limited. Moreover, these color anisotropy maps cannot differentiate adjacent white matter tracts that have the same fiber orientation. These obstacles can be overcome with 3-D fiber tractography. There are many techniques for performing fiber tractography described in the literature, but most of them are variations on the same underlying idea of tracking bidirectionally along the orientation of the primary eigenvector of the diffusion tensor from voxel to voxel in 3-D [21–23]. DTI tractography cannot distinguish forward from backward along a fiber tra-

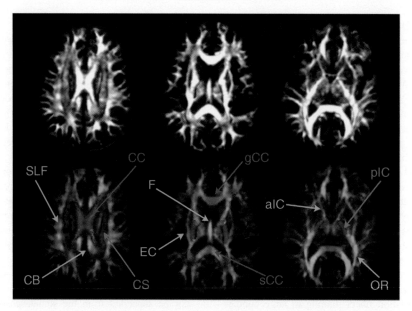

Fig. 1. DTI of the supratentorial brain in a normal adult. Axial FA images (*top row*) and the corresponding directionally-encoded color FA images (*bottom row*) are shown at the level of the roof of the lateral ventricles (*left*), the genu and splenium of the corpus callosum (*middle*), and the basal ganglia and thalami (*right*). The top row of FA images show that the commissural and projectional white matter tracts of the corpus callosum and internal capsule, respectively, have higher FA than the long association tracts of the SLF or the short association pathways in the subcortical U-fibers. The color FA images display fiber orientation within white matter as red for left-right, green for anteroposterior, and blue for craniocaudal. Fibers oriented oblique to these three canonical axes display mixtures of these three colors. aIC, anterior limb of the internal capsule; CB, cingulum bundle; CC, body of the corpus callosum; CS, centrum semiovale; EC, external capsule; F, body of the fornix; gCC, genu of the corpus callosum; OR, optic radiation; pIC, posterior limb of the internal capsule, sCC; splenium of the corpus callosum.

jectory. Tractography can be used to separate functionally distinct white matter pathways using the multiple region-of-interest (ROI) method [21], in which a priori knowledge concerning the origin and termination of a white matter tract is used to delineate its entire 3-D trajectory. The fiber tracking is initiated at an ROI defined at one end of the pathway, and only those fiber tracks that pass through the ROI defined at the other end of the pathway are retained. Any other tracks that do not connect to both ROIs are filtered out. In Fig. 2, the two-ROI tractography method is used to "dissect" out the commissural, projection, and association white matter connections of the left visual cortex. Additional ROIs positioned at intermediate points along the expected course of the white matter tract can be used to further guide and refine the 3-D fiber tracking. In this fashion, functionally distinct axonal pathways that are located adjacent to each other within a white matter structure, such as the pyramidal tract and the somatosensory radiation within the internal capsule, can be differentiated from each other. DTI tractography also can delineate the topographic relation-

ship of fibers within a single white matter pathway, such as the somatotopy of the somatosensory cortex. The 3-D trajectory information from tractography also can be used to measure tract-based ADC, anisotropy, or other DTI parameters. The advantages of this tract-based quantitation over traditional ROI measurements within white matter structures are that it is more specific to the functionally distinct axonal pathway of interest and that it reflects the entire 3-D course of the pathway rather than just one location within the pathway.

Currently, there are several limitations to DTI fiber tracking that must be considered when applying this technology. Insufficient spatial resolution to resolve adjacent axonal pathways may cause fiber tracks to artifactually "jump" from one tract to another, invalidating the calculated fiber trajectories. White matter fibers that make hairpin turns, such as the optic radiations at Meyer's loop, may be difficult to track. Currently, DTI tractography cannot reliably track through white matter regions where fibers from distinct axonal pathways cross each other at a microscopic scale, such as the laterally projecting fibers of

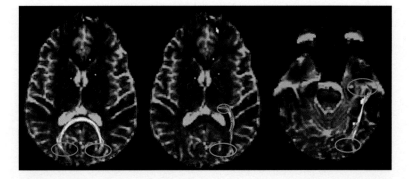

Fig. 2. DTI with 3-D fiber tractography of the white matter connectivity of the left visual cortex in a normal adult. 2-D axial projections of the 3-D tractography show the commissural visual pathways in the splenium of the corpus callosum (*left*), projection tracts of the optic radiation (*center*), and association tracts of the ILF (*right*). 3-D fiber tractography was performed with the two-ROI method for defining white matter pathways based on their origin and termination. 2-D slices of the 3-D ROI used for initiating fiber tracking in the left occipital lobe are displayed as green ellipses, and 2-D slices of the 3-D ROIs used for filtering the resulting fiber tracks in the right occipital lobe (*left*), lateral geniculate nucleus of the thalamus (*center*), and anterior temporal lobe (*right*) are shown as blue ellipses. The color within the fiber tracts indicates the magnitude of anisotropy, varying continuously from bright white (high anisotropy) to dark orange (low anisotropy). The commissural, projection, and association tracts all show higher anisotropy at the center of their 3-D trajectory and lower anisotropy toward both termini. This generally is true of most long white matter pathways, because their fibers tend to be more highly collimated and tightly bundled in the middle of their course than at their origins and terminations.

the pyramidal tract at the corona radiata, representing the motor homunculus of the upper part of the body, which pass through the anteroposteriorly oriented fibers of the SLF. Additionally, DTI tractography may not be able to distinguish between "crossing" fiber tracts and "kissing" fiber tracts, which abut each other but do not pass through each other. Further advances to DTI tractography are being developed to address the problem of crossing fibers [24].

Normal development and normal aging cause alterations in brain water diffusion; therefore, DTI can characterize age-related changes in white matter and in gray matter noninvasively [5,25]. During infancy and childhood, the ADC decreases throughout the brain and anisotropy increases in developing white matter tracts. Conversely, during aging, FA of white matter declines and ADC values rise. These changes of normal development and aging must be taken into account when interpreting DTI results in pediatric stroke and in cerebrovascular disease of the elderly, respectively.

Applications to stroke

Acute cerebral ischemia in the adult brain

Apparent diffusion coefficients

The most well established clinical application of diffusion imaging is for the early detection of acute ischemic stroke. ADC decreases within minutes of the onset of cerebral ischemia and is reduced by 50% or more in the acute stage of infarction [26,27]. Therefore, DWI has revolutionized the diagnosis of hyperacute stroke, allowing delineation of the region of ischemia/infarction within the first 3 to 6 hours after symptom onset, when interventions, such as intravenous or intra-arterial thrombolysis, may be effective. Furthermore, DWI has found clinical usefulness in distinguishing acute infarctions from more chronic lesions in patients who have suffered multiple episodes of cerebral ischemia. The ADC of large territorial infarctions pseudonormalizes within the first week after onset of ischemia and continues to increase to supranormal values thereafter [28]. The time evolution of ADC in watershed infarctions may be more prolonged, remaining reduced for a month or longer before pseudonormalization [29].

Quantitative diffusion imaging also can distinguish the cytotoxic edema of acute ischemia from vasogenic edema in disorders where both processes may coexist [30,31]. ADC is reduced strongly in cytotoxic edema, whereas ADC is increased in vasogenic edema, which is characterized by accumulation of interstitial water. The diffusion anisotropy is reduced strongly in vasogenic edema, whereas changes in anisotropy in cytotoxic edema are smaller and less consistent [32]. This is illustrated in Fig. 3 for a case of impaired cerebrovascular autoregulation leading to the reversible posterior leukoencephalopathy syndrome complicated by acute cerebral ischemia.

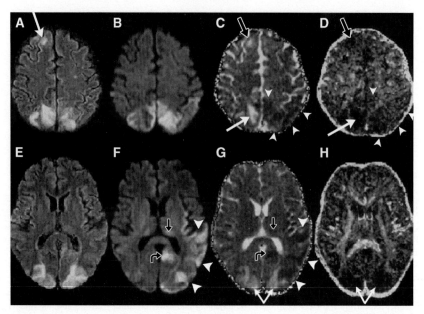

Fig. 3. DTI can distinguish vasogenic edema from cytotoxic edema in a case of posterior leukoencephalopathy complicated by acute cerebral ischemia. The patient had a history of lupus nephritis and presented with hypertension and seizures. The top row (*A−D*) of axial images illustrates findings in the posterior parietal lobes and the bottom row (*E−H*) illustrates findings more caudally in the occipital lobes. (*A*) The FLAIR (fluid attenuated inversion recovery) image demonstrates asymmetrically increased T2-weighted signal intensity in the gray matter and subcortical white matter of the parietal lobes, right greater than left. There also is a smaller focus of increased T2-weighted signal intensity in the right frontal lobe (*arrow*). (*B*) DWI also shows asymmetrically increased signal intensity in both parietal lobes, but left greater than right. (*C*) ADC image reveals increased diffusion in the right parietal lobe (*closed arrow*) and right frontal lobe (*open arrow*), consistent with vasogenic edema, whereas the reduced diffusion in the left parietal lobe (*arrowheads*) reflects cytotoxic edema. (*D*) There is markedly reduced anisotropy within the regions of vasogenic edema (*open and closed arrows*) with relatively preserved anisotropy within the area of cytotoxic edema (*arrowheads*). (*E*) FLAIR image shows T2-weighted hyperintensity in a cortical/subcortical distribution in both occipital lobes. (*F*) DWI shows the greatest hyperintensity in the left temporal lobe (*arrowheads*), left thalamus (*straight open arrow*), and isthmus of the left cingulate gyrus (*curved open arrow*). (*G*) ADC image confirms that the areas of DWI hyperintensity show the reduced diffusion characteristic of cytotoxic edema, whereas the occipital poles show the increased diffusion characteristic of vasogenic edema (*closed arrows*). (*H*) Again markedly reduced anisotropy is seen within the areas of vasogenic edema (*closed arrows*) with relatively preserved anisotropy within the regions of acute ischemia. (*Reproduced from* Mukherjee P, McKinstry RC. Reversible posterior leukoencephalopathy syndrome: evaluation with diffusion-tensor MR imaging. Radiology 2001;219:756−65; with permission.)

Although DWI has found a role in the evaluation of acute cerebral ischemia, the added value for performing DTI in this clinical setting is not yet established. Moreover, DTI requires longer acquisition and postprocessing times than DWI, which is undesirable for the assessment of hyperacute stroke. Hence, to date there are few studies of DTI in acute cerebral ischemia. Unlike DWI alone, DTI can distinguish white matter from gray matter based on differences in anisotropy and thereby separately quantify changes of ADC in ischemic gray matter and ischemic white matter (Fig. 4). In patients who have acute to early subacute territorial infarctions, differences in the time evolution of ADC between white matter and gray matter are documented with DTI [32–34].

In the first few days after infarction, the ADC remains reduced in white matter for longer than in gray matter, where pseudonormalization requires less time. A difference in ADC values between white matter and gray matter in response to ischemia, however, has not been observed in the hyperacute phase of stroke [35].

Diffusion anisotropy and tensor eigenvalues

In addition to the well-known decrease of ADC in acutely infarcted gray and white matter, alterations in diffusion anisotropy also are observed in acute white matter ischemia. The data on anisotropy changes in acute stroke are conflicting, with some studies show-

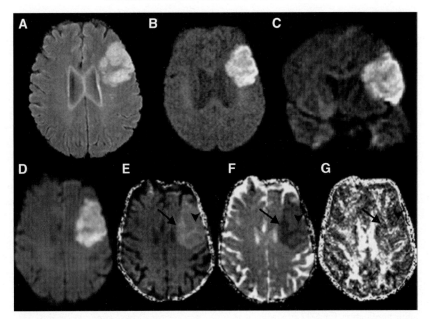

Fig. 4. DTI shows greater reductions in white matter ADC than in gray matter ADC in a 71-year-old woman imaged 46 hours after onset of left middle cerebral artery ischemia. Axial FLAIR (*A*) and DWI (*B–D*) images show hyperintensity within the left middle cerebral artery branch infarction. Exponential DWI (*E*) and the ADC image (*F*) confirm that there is reduced diffusion within the infarction. Comparison with the anisotropy image (*G*) shows that ADC is more reduced within white matter (*arrows, arrowhead*) than gray matter. There also is reduced white matter anisotropy in this early subacute stage of infarction, although the anisotropy loss is not as severe as typically seen with pure vasogenic edema (see Fig. 3). (*Reproduced from* Mukherjee P, Bahn MM, McKinstry RC, et al. Differences between gray matter and white matter water diffusion in stroke: diffusion-tensor MR imaging in 12 patients. Radiology 2000;215:211–20; with permission.)

ing an increase in anisotropy [32,36] and others showing a decrease in anisotropy [34,35,37]. Ozsunar and colleagues have attempted to resolve this issue with results showing that FA and T2 signal intensity are correlated negatively in patients who have acute stroke, whereas FA and ADC are not correlated at all [38]. Therefore, FA tends to be elevated above normal values in ischemic regions with normal T2 signal intensity and is reduced in regions of T2 prolongation. The individual diffusion tensor eigenvalues also have been measured in acute ischemic white matter lesions; the greatest change is a marked decrease in the major eigenvalue, which corresponds to the diffusivity parallel to the axonal bundles [35]. This reduction in the major eigenvalue leads to a decrease in ADC, as is universally observed in acute stroke, and a decrease in anisotropy, as is usually, although not invariably, found in acute stroke.

Despite the intense research interest over the past several years, no compelling evidence has been found for the clinical usefulness of anisotropy or eigenvalue measures in acute cerebral ischemia; hence, DTI is not yet applied widely to acute stroke diagnosis,

given the additional acquisition time needed to perform DTI, especially if sufficient SNR and spatial resolution for fiber tractography are desired. A comparison between DWI and DTI in hyperacute stroke shows that DTI anisotropy measures, such as RA, FA, and VR, are not sensitive to cerebral ischemia during the first 6 hours, although the investigators suggest a potential role for anisotropy in differentiating hyperacute stroke from acute or subacute stroke [39]. Other potential applications for DTI in early stroke include using directionally encoded color anisotropy images and 3-D fiber tractography to localize acute stroke lesions in relation to functionally-specific pathways, which also may allow more accurate prognosis of long-term recovery or disability [40–43]. Not only can the location of an acute ischemic lesion relative to white matter tracts be identified with DTI, but also disruption or distortion of white matter tracts can be inferred in patients who have subacute stroke [44]. Delayed involvement of functionally important white matter pathways by interval enlargement of the infarction between the acute and subacute stages of ischemia is documented by

DTI fiber tractography, accounting for the worsening symptoms in a subgroup of patients who have stroke [43].

Chronic cerebral ischemia in the adult brain

Compared with hyperacute and acute stroke, diffusion anisotropy changes in subacute to chronic cerebral ischemia are well characterized. As illustrated in Fig. 5, diffusion anisotropy in involved white matter becomes progressively more reduced during the subacute to chronic stages of infarction [32,37,45]. A longitudinal DTI study of 32 patients who had ischemic stroke finds varying degrees of residual FA in white matter tracts within the infarction zone at 3 months' follow-up, indicating that some microstructural integrity may persist in a subgroup of patients [34]. This suggests that residual white matter FA may have usefulness for predicting patient outcome.

Another major application for DTI in stroke is to quantitatively characterize wallerian degeneration of long white matter tracts remote from the infarction zone secondary to subacute or chronic ischemia, even those tracts that appear normal on conventional MR imaging [45–48]. Anisotropy metrics, such as FA,

are more sensitive than ADC for wallerian degeneration [47,48]. The decrease in FA, which results from a decrease in the major eigenvalue and increase in the minor eigenvalues, can be detected as soon as 2 weeks after infarction and correlates with the motor deficit when the pyramidal tract is involved [48]. Therefore, DTI may provide useful prognostic information for recovery of motor function after stroke. DTI with fiber tracking also is used to demonstrate selective reduction in somatosensory fibers in a case of central poststroke pain syndrome [49], providing structure-function correlation for yet another dimension of patient outcome after cerebral ischemia.

Cerebral autosomal dominant arteriopathy with subcortical infarctions and leukoencephalopathy (CADASIL) is a small-vessel vasculopathy that leads to recurrent ischemia predominantly affecting subcortical white matter. Increasing ADC and decreasing anisotropy of white matter, including normal-appearing white matter on conventional MR imaging, provides a marker for disease progression in CADASIL [50,51]. Elevated ADC in the thalamus of CADASIL patients correlate directly with white matter ADC and the ischemic burden and correlate inversely with Mini–Mental State Examination score, suggesting wallerian degeneration of thalamocortical axonal pathways [52].

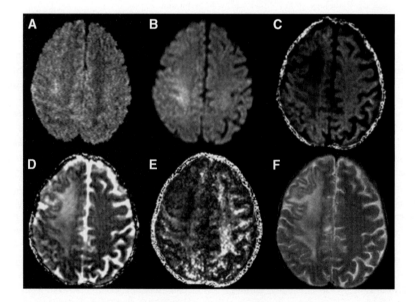

Fig. 5. DTI shows elevated ADC and strongly reduced anisotropy in the subacute stage of infarction. MR imaging was performed 16 days after onset of postoperative right middle cerebral ischemia due to right carotid endarterectomy. DWI (*A and B*) shows only faint ill-defined hyperintensity in the right frontoparietal region, consistent with pseudonormalization. The exponential DWI (*C*) and ADC (*D*) images, however, reveal elevated diffusion throughout the right middle cerebral artery territory, which is typical 2 weeks after territorial infarction. There is severe loss of anisotropy throughout the involved white matter (*E*). The subacute infarction also is seen as hyperintensity on T2-weighted imaging (*F*).

Hypoxic-ischemic injury in the developing brain

There are several DTI studies of hypoxic-ischemic injury in the developing human brain. Diffusion imaging may be more sensitive than conventional MR imaging for detecting perinatal brain injury. One study finds that abnormal decreases in ADC may demonstrate and define the extent of perinatal brain injury better than conventional MR imaging, especially when obtained between the second and fourth days of life [53]. The investigators also demonstrate, however, that DTI might underestimate the extent of injury if obtained during the first 24 hours of life or after a week has elapsed. In a study of preterm infants imaged shortly after birth and again near term-equivalent age, infants who had moderate to severe white matter injury of prematurity, also known as periventricular leukomalacia, did not demonstrate the expected decrease in ADC and increase in anisotropy observed during preterm maturation in infants without white matter injury [54]. Those neonates who had only minimal white matter injury of prematurity showed the normal decrease in ADC but did not show the expected increase in frontal white matter anisotropy. Abnormally decreased anisotropy at the site of the central white matter injury and in the ipsilateral internal capsule has been identified in premature newborns, suggesting impaired development

of the corresponding fiber tracts [55]. A DTI tractography study of four infants and children who had unilateral congenital hemiparesis, ranging in age from 10 to 44 months, showed increased ADC and reduced anisotropy of the pyramidal tract controlling motor function to the hemiparetic side compared with the contralateral pyramidal tract (Fig. 6) [56]. In a complementary study of two 6-year-old boys who had spastic quadriplegia secondary to white matter injury of prematurity, DTI tractography demonstrated attenuation of the posterior thalamic radiation projecting to and from occipital and parietal lobes, rather than the corticospinal tracts, suggesting that the pathophysiology of motor disability in white matter injury of prematurity may be at least in part the result of abnormal somatosensory connectivity [57]. In the future, DTI and fiber tractography may prove useful in elucidating alterations in brain connectivity resulting from neuroplasticity after stroke.

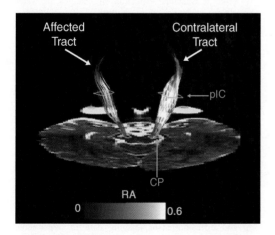

Fig. 6. Coronal projection of 3-D fiber tractography shows asymmetrically reduced volume and reduced RA of the pyramidal tract governing motor function to the affected side of the body in a child with unilateral congenital hemiparesis. 3-D DTI tractography of the pyramidal tracts was performed bilaterally using the two-ROI approach with ROIs defined at the posterior limb of the internal capsule (pIC) (*green ellipses*) and at the cerebral peduncles (CP) (*green ellipses*). (Courtesy of Roland Henry, PhD, San Francisco, CA.)

References

[1] Bastin ME, Armitage PA, Marshall I. A theoretical study of the effect of experimental noise on the measurement of anisotropy in diffusion imaging. Magn Reson Imaging 1998;16:773–85.

[2] Jones DK, Williams SC, Gasston D, et al. Isotropic resolution diffusion tensor imaging with whole brain acquisition in a clinically acceptable time. Hum Brain Mapp 2002;15:216–30.

[3] Virta A, Barnett A, Pierpaoli C. Visualizing and characterizing white matter fiber structure and architecture in the human pyramidal tract using diffusion tensor MRI. Magn Reson Imaging 1999;17:1121–33.

[4] Pfefferbaum A, Sullivan EV, Hedehus M, et al. Age-related decline in brain white matter anisotropy measured with spatially corrected echo-planar diffusion tensor imaging. Magn Reson Med 2000;44:259–68.

[5] Mukherjee P, Miller JH, Shimony JS, et al. Normal brain maturation during childhood: developmental trends characterized with diffusion-tensor MR imaging. Radiology 2001;221:349–58.

[6] Stieltjes B, Kaufmann WE, van Zijl PC, et al. Diffusion tensor imaging and axonal tracking in the human brainstem. Neuroimage 2001;14:723–35.

[7] Bammer R, Auer M, Keeling SL, et al. Diffusion tensor imaging using single-shot SENSE-EPI. Magn Reson Med 2002;48:128–36.

[8] Mukherjee P, Miller JH, Shimony JS, et al. Diffusion-tensor MR imaging of gray and white matter development during normal human brain maturation. AJNR Am J Neuroradiol 2002;23:1445–56.

[9] Hasan KM, Parker DL, Alexander AL. Comparison of gradient encoding schemes for diffusion-tensor MRI. J Magn Reson Imaging 2001;13:769–80.

[10] Papadakis NG, Murrills CD, Hall LD, et al. Minimal gradient encoding for robust estimation of diffusion anisotropy. Magn Reson Imaging 2000;18:671–9.

[11] Skare S, Hedehus M, Moseley ME, Li TQ. Condition number as a measure of noise performance of diffusion tensor data acquisition schemes with MRI. J Magn Reson 2000;147:340–52.

[12] Huppi PS, Maier SE, Peled S, et al. Microstructural development of human newborn cerebral white matter assessed *in vivo* by diffusion tensor magnetic resonance imaging. Pediatr Res 1998;44:584–90.

[13] Bastin ME, Le Roux P. On the application of a non-CPMG single-shot fast spin-echo sequence to diffusion tensor MRI of the human brain. Magn Reson Med 2002;48:6–14.

[14] Pipe JG, Farthing VG, Forbes KP. Multishot diffusion-weighted FSE using PROPELLER MRI. Magn Reson Med 2002;47:42–52.

[15] Shimony JS, McKinstry RC, Akbudak E, et al. Quantitative diffusion-tensor anisotropy imaging: normative human data and anatomic analysis. Radiology 1999;212:770–84.

[16] Pierpaoli C, Jezzard P, Basser PJ, et al. Diffusion tensor MR imaging of the human brain. Radiology 1996;201:637–48.

[17] Guilfoyle DN, Helpern JA, Lim KO. Diffusion tensor imaging in fixed brain tissue at 7.0 T. NMR Biomed 2003;16:77–81.

[18] Sun SW, Neil JJ, Song SK. Relative indices of water diffusion anisotropy are equivalent in live and formalin-fixed mouse brains. Magn Reson Med 2003; 50:743–8.

[19] Pajevic S, Pierpaoli C. Color schemes to represent the orientation of anisotropic tissues from diffusion tensor data: application to white matter fiber tract mapping in the human brain. Magn Reson Med 1999;42:526–40.

[20] Yamada K, Kizu O, Mori S, et al. Brain fiber tracking with clinically feasible diffusion-tensor MR imaging: initial experience. Radiology 2003;227:295–301.

[21] Conturo TE, Lori NF, Cull TS, et al. Tracking neuronal fiber pathways in the living human brain. Proc Natl Acad Sci USA 1999;96:10422–7.

[22] Mori S, Crain BJ, Chacko VP, et al. Three-dimensional tracking of axonal projections in the brain by magnetic resonance imaging. Ann Neurol 1999;45:265–9.

[23] Basser PJ, Pajevic S, Pierpaoli C, et al. In vivo fiber tractography using DT-MRI data. Magn Reson Med 2000;44:625–32.

[24] Wiegell MR, Larsson HB, Wedeen VJ. Fiber crossing in human brain depicted with diffusion tensor MR imaging. Radiology 2000;217:897–903.

[25] Abe O, Aoki S, Hayashi N, et al. Normal aging in the central nervous system: quantitative MR diffusion-tensor analysis. Neurobiol Aging 2002;23:433–41.

[26] Moseley ME, Kucharczyk J, Mintorovitch J, et al. Diffusion-weighted MR imaging of acute stroke: correlation with T2-weighted and magnetic susceptibility-enhanced MR imaging in cats. AJNR Am J Neuroradiol 1990;11:423–9.

[27] Warach S, Chien D, Li W, Ronthal M, et al. Fast magnetic resonance diffusion-weighted imaging of acute human stroke. Neurology 1992;42:1717–23.

[28] Schlaug G, Siewert B, Benfield A, et al. Time course of the apparent diffusion coefficient (ADC) abnormality in human stroke. Neurology 1997;49:113–9.

[29] Huang IJ, Chen CY, Chung HW, et al. Time course of cerebral infarction in the middle cerebral arterial territory: deep watershed versus territorial subtypes on diffusion-weighted MR images. Radiology 2001; 221:35–42.

[30] Schwartz RB, Mulkern RV, Gudbjartsson H, Jolesz F. Diffusion-weighted MR imaging in hypertensive encephalopathy: clues to pathogenesis. AJNR Am J Neuroradiol 1998;19:859–62.

[31] Mukherjee P, McKinstry RC. Reversible posterior leukoencephalopathy syndrome: evaluation with diffusion-tensor MR imaging. Radiology 2001;219: 756–65.

[32] Yang Q, Tress BM, Barber PA, et al. Serial study of apparent diffusion coefficient and anisotropy in patients with acute stroke. Stroke 1999;30:2382–90.

[33] Mukherjee P, Bahn MM, McKinstry RC, et al. Differences between gray matter and white matter water diffusion in stroke: diffusion-tensor MR imaging in 12 patients. Radiology 2000;215:211–20.

[34] Munoz Maniega S, Bastin ME, Armitage PA, Farrall AJ, Carpenter TK, Hand PJ, et al. Temporal evolution of water diffusion parameters is different in grey and white matter in human ischaemic stroke. J Neurol Neurosurg Psychiatry 2004;75:1714–8.

[35] Sorensen AG, Wu O, Copen WA, et al. Human acute cerebral ischemia: detection of changes in water diffusion anisotropy by using MR imaging. Radiology 1999;212:785–92.

[36] Armitage PA, Bastin ME, Marshall I, Wardlaw JM, Cannon J. Diffusion anisotropy measurements in ischaemic stroke of the human brain. MAGMA 1998;6:28–36.

[37] Zelaya F, Flood N, Chalk JB, et al. An evaluation of the time dependence of the anisotropy of the water diffusion tensor in acute human ischemia. Magn Reson Imaging 1999;17:331–48.

[38] Ozsunar Y, Grant PE, Huisman TA, et al. Evolution of water diffusion and anisotropy in hyperacute stroke: significant correlation between fractional anisotropy and T2. AJNR Am J Neuroradiol 2004;25:699–705.

[39] Harris AD, Pereira RS, Mitchell JR, et al. A comparison of images generated from diffusion-weighted and diffusion-tensor imaging data in hyper-acute stroke. J Magn Reson Imaging 2004;20:193–200.

[40] Yoshikawa T, Aoki S, Masutani Y, et al. Diffusion tensor imaging of cerebral infarction: analysis of ADC and DTI scalar metrics (fractional anisotropy and eigenvalues). Radiology 2002;225(Suppl):278–9.

[41] Lie C, Hirsch JG, Rossmanith C, et al. Clinicotopographical correlation of corticospinal tract stroke: a color-coded diffusion tensor imaging study. Stroke 2004;35:86–92.

[42] Sea Lee J, Han MK, Hyun Kim S, et al. Fiber tracking by diffusion tensor imaging in corticospinal tract stroke: topographical correlation with clinical symptoms. Neuroimage 2005;26:771–6.

[43] Yamada K, Ito H, Nakamura H, et al. Stroke patients' evolving symptoms assessed by tractography. J Magn Reson Imaging 2004;20:923–9.

[44] Gillard JH, Papadakis NG, Martin K, et al. MR diffusion tensor imaging of white matter tract disruption in stroke at 3 T. Br J Radiol 2001;74:642–7.

[45] Buffon F, Molko N, Herve D, et al. Longitudinal diffusion changes in cerebral hemispheres after MCA infarcts. J Cereb Blood Flow Metab 2005;25: 641–50.

[46] Werring DJ, Toosy AT, Clark CA, et al. Diffusion tensor imaging can detect and quantify corticospinal tract degeneration after stroke. J Neurol Neurosurg Psychiatry 2000;69:269–72.

[47] Pierpaoli C, Barnett A, Pajevic S, et al. Water diffusion changes in wallerian degeneration and their dependence on white matter architecture. Neuroimage 2001; 13:1174–85.

[48] Thomalla G, Glauche V, Koch MA, et al. Diffusion tensor imaging detects early Wallerian degeneration of the pyramidal tract after ischemic stroke. Neuroimage 2004;22:1767–74.

[49] Seghier ML, Lazeyras F, Vuilleumier P, et al. Functional magnetic resonance imaging and diffusion tensor imaging in a case of central poststroke pain. J Pain 2005;6:208–12.

[50] Chabriat H, Pappata S, Poupon C, et al. Clinical severity in CADASIL related to ultrastructural damage in white matter: in vivo study with diffusion tensor MRI. Stroke 1999;30:2637–43.

[51] Molko N, Pappata S, Mangin JF, et al. Monitoring disease progression in CADASIL with diffusion magnetic resonance imaging: a study with whole brain histogram analysis. Stroke 2002;33:2902–8.

[52] Molko N, Pappata S, Mangin JF, et al. Diffusion tensor imaging study of subcortical gray matter in CADASIL. Stroke 2001;32:2049–54.

[53] McKinstry RC, Miller JH, Snyder AZ, et al. A prospective, longitudinal diffusion tensor imaging study of brain injury in newborns. Neurology 2002; 59:824–33.

[54] Miller SP, Vigneron DB, Henry RG, et al. Serial quantitative diffusion tensor MRI of the premature brain: Development in newborns with and without injury. J Magn Reson Imaging 2002;16:621–32.

[55] Huppi PS, Murphy B, Maier SE, et al. Microstructural brain development after perinatal cerebral white matter injury assessed by diffusion tensor magnetic resonance imaging. Pediatrics 2001;107:455–60.

[56] Glenn OA, Henry RG, Berman JI, et al. DTI-based three-dimensional tractography detects differences in the pyramidal tracts of infants and children with congenital hemiparesis. J Magn Reson Imaging 2003;18:641–8.

[57] Hoon Jr AH, Lawrie Jr WT, Melhem ER, et al. Diffusion tensor imaging of periventricular leukomalacia shows affected sensory cortex white matter pathways. Neurology 2002;59:752–6.

ELSEVIER
SAUNDERS

Neuroimag Clin N Am 15 (2005) 667 – 680

NEUROIMAGING
CLINICS OF
NORTH AMERICA

Functional Cerebrovascular Imaging in Brain Ischemia: Permeability, Reactivity, and Functional MR Imaging

David J. Mikulis, MD[a,b,]*

[a]*Division of Neuroradiology, Department of Medical Imaging,
Toronto Western Hospital of the University Health Network and University of Toronto, Toronto, ON, Canada*
[b]*Toronto Western Hospital Research Institute and Institute of Medical Science, University of Toronto, Toronto, ON, Canada*

The brain and the computer chip can be thought of as information processors that operate through electrical signaling over "wired" networks. They require energy to function, but the source and distribution of that energy vary greatly between the two systems. The computer chip is much simpler because it derives its energy from an external source and does not require additional systems for generating energy locally. The brain, conversely, generates energy within the electrical network itself and has therefore evolved a spatially colocalized "subsystem" for generating this energy. A major component of this subsystem involves the delivery, distribution, and removal of metabolites. These requirements have led to the evolution of a sophisticated plumbing system, namely, the cerebral vasculature.

The cerebral vasculature has two primary features that are unique within the body. The first is the blood-brain barrier (BBB). This barrier has evolved pre-

sumably to protect the delicate homeostasis of the synaptic junction and neuronal membrane from unwanted substances that could disrupt proper network function. Note the effect of a simple molecule like ethanol, which readily crosses this barrier. The primary feature of the BBB is the tight adherence of endothelial cells to each other. Gaps between these cells develop during acute ischemic injury, ultimately leading to extravasation of red cells into the brain interstitium. The degree of extravasation can vary from insignificant to lethal. Permeability imaging using MR imaging during gadolinium administration can be used to assess the state of the BBB in acute ischemic stroke (AIS), a parameter that could have considerable relevance in assessing the safety of thrombolytic treatment.

The second unique feature of the cerebral vasculature is its ability to control blood flow locally. Other organs, such as the skin, gut, and musculature, can control flow regionally but not on the same spatial (millimeter) scale as the brain. This control mechanism evolved presumably in response to the high-energy requirements associated with neural transmission, even in the resting or baseline awake state of the brain. The need for this control mechanism can be demonstrated by considering the following argument. High-energy requirements are reflected in the proportion of cardiac output received by the brain compared with other organs. The brain, representing only 2% of body weight, receives 20% of the cardiac

* Division of Neuroradiology, Department of Medical Imaging, Toronto Western Hospital of the University Health Network and University of Toronto, 399 Bathurst Street, Room MP3-404, Toronto, ON, Canada M5T 2S8.

E-mail address: mikulis@uhnres.utoronto.ca

output. In general, neuronal activation is associated with a 50% increase in blood flow. Without a mechanism to control flow locally, a global blood flow response to neuronal activation would result in redistribution of cardiac output to the brain from 20% to 30%, or because some part of the brain is always active, baseline cardiac output would have to be increased. Tight coupling of brain blood flow with local neuronal activation is therefore energy conserving for the organism. Imaging the changes in blood flow and deoxyhemoglobin concentration ensuing from the response of this control mechanism to neuronal activation forms the basis of MR imaging mapping of neural networks (function MR imaging [fMR imaging]). This mechanism also serves to protect the brain under stressful conditions that compromise blood flow or oxygen delivery. It does this by preserving blood flow through vasodilation in response to a decrease in blood pressure or an increase in carbon dioxide (CO_2) caused by reduced ventilation.

Manipulation of inhaled CO_2 can be performed to determine the state, or test the capacity, of this "autoregulatory" mechanism (ie, cerebrovascular reactivity [CVR]) testing. CVR can be used to validate the ability of the system to respond under those conditions in which proximal large vessel obstruction limits any further vasodilation (exhaustion of autoregulation) in response to stimuli. We have termed this the *brain stress test*, analogous to the well-known cardiac stress test used to assess the impact of coronary lesions on cardiac blood flow.

Permeability imaging in acute ischemic stroke

Permeability MR imaging measures the integrity of the BBB by tracking the entry of intravenously administered contrast into the extravascular space. When combined with pharmacokinetic modeling, permeability can provide quantitative information about defects in the BBB. Permeability imaging has most frequently been applied to the study of brain tumors, where angiogenesis leads to the formation of microvessels with defective endothelial function and organization, and hence a compromised BBB. Dynamic contrast-enhanced (DCE) MR imaging using a bidirectional two-compartment model of permeability has shown that the transendothelial transfer "permeability" constant, k^{PS}, is highly correlated with tumor grade [1]. Because it is well known that high-grade tumors have an increased risk of hemorrhage, it would seem likely that this risk is inversely related to the quality of the BBB in these tumors.

Defects in the BBB are known to occur in most patients with AIS, because gadolinium (Gd)-enhanced T1-weighted imaging typically shows evidence of contrast enhancement within days of stroke ictus. Extravasation of red cells into the tissue is also quite common and, when extreme, can produce symptomatic and potentially lethal hemorrhage. It is therefore tempting to use the brain tumor model in relating the risk of hemorrhage to the degree and extent of the BBB defect. Although the exact site of hemorrhagic transformation (HT) in AIS is debatable, there is mounting evidence that it indeed occurs at the microvascular level [2]. Prediction of HT using dynamic T1-weighted Gd-diethylenetriamine penta-acetic acid (DTPA)–enhanced MR imaging in a rat stroke model has also shown that progressive tissue enhancement is highly correlated with the presence of HT after reperfusion [3]. These findings suggest the potential benefit of assessing permeability in AIS patients, especially because some are candidates for thrombolysis, a therapy that carries a 10-fold increased risk of HT [4].

We have therefore added a DCE MR imaging permeability acquisition to our acute stroke MR imaging protocol that uses a two-compartment model to assess BBB defects in AIS patients. Our preliminary results in 10 subjects assessed within 24 hours from onset of symptoms have shown that k^{PS} can be measured in the acute stroke setting and that significant elevations are present in infarcts that progress to hemorrhage ($k^{PS} = 3.10$ mL per 100 g/min ± 0.44 in the hemorrhage group compared with $k^{PS} = 0.123$ mL per 100 g/min ± 0.10 in the nonhemorrhage group; $P < .02$) [5]. This 25-fold increase in permeability was found within the central core of the diffusion abnormality and likely reflects the most severely injured and/or ischemic tissue in the developing infarct. Fig. 1 shows an example of a permeability defect observed in an acute stroke case that later progressed to hemorrhage after treatment with tissue thromboplastin activator (tPA). Clearly, more work needs to be performed in a much larger cohort.

Nevertheless, these initial findings raise several important issues concerning the management of patients with thrombolytic agents. Current strategies for selecting appropriate candidates are based on time windows derived from epidemiologic studies. These guidelines are generally applicable but may not necessarily be optimal for individual patients. For example, some patients, despite having tissue at risk, are not eligible for thrombolysis because they have presented outside the acceptable time window. If it can be shown that permeability in the region of their infarct has not yet become elevated, it may be safe to

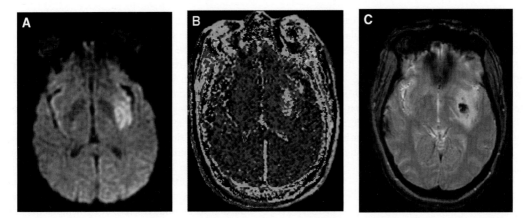

Fig. 1. Permeability imaging. (*A*) Diffusion MR imaging showing ischemic injury involving the left inferior striatum and subinsular region 4 hours 45 minutes after onset of hemiparesis with inability to speak. (*B*) Permeability image obtained during the same imaging session shows a region of increased permeability within the core of the developing infarct. (*C*) MR imaging on day 3 after ictus shows hemorrhage in the same region as the permeability defect. Patient had been treated with tissue thromboplastin activator on admission based on a normal CT study (not shown).

institute thrombolytic treatment. Conversely, if they present within the appropriate time window for thrombolysis but have a considerable increase in permeability, treatment may need to be reconsidered, or perhaps treatment with BBB stabilizers before thrombolytics would be required. This concept of a fixed therapeutic time window in acute stroke has been questioned by many authors [6], and there is an increasing demand to base therapy on physiologic criteria. Permeability mapping may be able to provide a crucial piece of this physiologic information, potentially increasing the safety of thrombolytic therapy and increasing the number of patients who could benefit from it.

Cerebrovascular reactivity

The functional site of cerebrovascular autoregulation is at the level of the arterioles, particularly the precapillary sphincter. It is the tone of the smooth muscle comprising this sphincter that regulates flow to the capillary bed. The tone of the sphincter can be influenced by a number of agents, including blood pressure, oxygen (a vasoconstrictor), and CO_2 (a vasodilator), but signaling from locally active neurons also controls it. The exact nature of the neuronal signaling pathway is still under investigation.

It is clear, however, that there is a delay of several seconds between neuronal activation and local increases in blood flow, suggesting that the mediating agent is probably a diffusible molecule. This coupling between neuronal activation and blood flow, first described by Roy and Sherrington [7] at the end of the nineteenth century, forms the basis of functional brain mapping.

Cerebrovascular autoregulation serves to maintain cerebral homeostasis by ensuring adequate blood flow, and thus constant delivery of oxygen and glucose to the brain under varying physiologic conditions. It can maintain cerebral blood flow (CBF) within the range of blood pressure from 80 to 160 mm Hg. If acute pressures fall outside this range, failure of CVR ensues. Pressures greater than 160 mm Hg overwhelm the ability of the sphincter to contract, exposing the microcirculation to elevated pressures leading to perfusion breakthrough with the development of vasogenic edema and hypertensive encephalopathy or, in extreme cases, intracerebral hemorrhage. At pressures less than 80 mm Hg, the ability of the sphincter to decrease flow resistance through further relaxation reaches it limit. No further vasodilation is possible, and CBF becomes directly dependent on perfusion pressure. Further lowering of blood pressure leads to ischemia.

In general, vascular diseases impair the ability of the feeding vasculature to deliver adequate flow to the microcirculation. Autoregulation can compensate for supply deficits through vasodilation and decreased vascular resistance. From a clinical perspective, it would be helpful to know if the limits of autoregulation have been reached to determine the source of symptoms in patients with severe carotid stenosis. For example, are the transient ischemic attacks (TIAs) in such patients caused by a low-flow condition with exhaustion of CVR or by emboli?

Several methods exist for assessing CVR, which is defined in Eq. 1:

$$CVR = \frac{\Delta \text{ blood flow}}{\Delta \text{ stimulus}} \qquad (1)$$

CO_2 and acetazolamide are the most commonly used agents for manipulating vascular tone. Several imaging tools are available for measuring the blood flow changes induced by the applied stimuli. Transcranial Doppler (TCD) ultrasound can quantitate the flow in the circle of Willis vessels, is readily available, and is inexpensive. It cannot, however, map reactivity at the tissue level because it is not a cross-sectional imaging technique when used for this purpose. Positron emission tomography (PET) and single photon emission computed tomography (SPECT) can map CVR spatially, with PET providing true quantitative analysis. The major disadvantage of PET is that oxygen-15 is needed to measure flow, and it must be generated in a cyclotron. Clinical availability is therefore severely limited. Although SPECT and xenon CT are viable options, we prefer an MR imaging solution that can be added to conventional clinical MR imaging protocols.

At our institution, we have co-opted fMR imaging methodology for this purpose. Blood oxygen level–dependent (BOLD) imaging is used, because, as in fMR imaging, the goal is to observe changes in deoxyhemoglobin concentration produced by changing blood flow. The main difference between BOLD fMR imaging and BOLD CVR is that the latter measures global changes in signal that occur in the setting of constant oxygen use by the tissue. BOLD fMR imaging measures local changes in deoxyhemoglobin concentration induced by locally active neurons that increase their consumption of oxygen. As an aside, changes in oxygen use by the tissue can be measured by applying both methods (see section on MR imaging horizons).

The disadvantage of the BOLD MR imaging method in assessing CVR is that BOLD cannot measure flow directly. BOLD images measure flow-induced changes in deoxyhemoglobin. Increased flow in the setting of constant oxygen use results in a reduction of intravoxel deoxyhemoglobin, producing an increase in signal. The BOLD signal itself is a function of the deoxyhemoglobin concentration in the imaging voxel as well as its intravascular volume of distribution; the latter is primarily a function of the size of the microvessels.

Deoxyhemoglobin is paramagnetic, and when it is compartmentalized within the microvasculature, local magnetic field distortion occurs in the diamagnetic tissue surrounding the vessels. This magnetic field distortion leads to incoherence, and hence reduction in the BOLD signal. As noted previously, the magnitude and location of this field distortion are a function of the intravascular deoxyhemoglobin concentration and the size of the microvessels. Because blood flow and volume are proportional [8], increased flow produced by increasing end-tidal partial pressure of CO_2 ($P_{ET}CO_2$) during constant oxygen use results in deoxyhemoglobin washout in the presence of increased blood volume. Although the end result of these factors on the BOLD signal is not immediately obvious, the signal increase associated with decreased deoxyhemoglobin concentration more than compensates for the signal decrease caused by the increased volume over which the field distor-

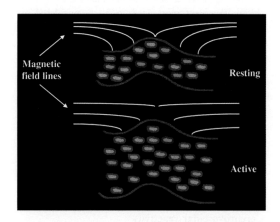

Fig. 2. The physical basis of the BOLD effect. The effect of increased blood flow on deoxyhemoglobin concentration in the microcirculation (capillaries and small venules) and on the magnetic field in the tissue adjacent to the vessels is shown in this cartoon. Increased flow (in the lower vessel) results in a washout of deoxyhemoglobin (blue-red cells) even if neuronal activation is present. Blood volume also increases. The paramagnetic effects from deoxyhemoglobin diminish, and the magnetic field lines (*white*) become more homogeneous. Because BOLD intensity is directly related to field homogeneity, signal intensity on BOLD images increases.

tion can act. There is thus an overall increase in the BOLD signal (Fig. 2).

Because the magnitude of the signal changes induced by CO_2 manipulation is similar to that seen with neuronal activation (approximately 4%), further adaptation of fMR imaging methodology is warranted, including statistical averaging of the signal. We therefore manipulate CO_2 in a "block" fashion and process the data with the BOLD signal, shifted by the lung-to-brain transit time, as the regressor [9]. The ability to control CO_2 rapidly and precisely is required to produce the desired square-wave changes in $PETCO_2$. These effects cannot be produced using simple mask inhalation of CO_2, because subjects hyperventilate during administration in an attempt to "blow off" CO_2.

We have therefore developed a continuous breathing rebreather mask and gas sequencer that can rapidly and precisely control $PETCO_2$. Fig. 3 shows the square-wave transitions of $PETCO_2$ that can be obtained with this device. The ability to provide rapid

transitions between extended steady-state levels of PCO_2 optimizes the efficiency of image acquisition, requiring 12 minutes or less of imaging time. The "flat tops" of the $PETCO_2$ curve allow stabilization of the vascular response to a steady-state PCO_2, eliminating the uncertainty arising from a lag in vasomotor response to incremental changes in PCO_2.

Fig. 4 shows the result of CVR mapping in a patient with moyamoya disease. This patient as well as others with moyamoya disease and carotid stenosis and/or occlusion has shown unexpected regions with a negative correlation to the $PETCO_2$ waveform (increased CO_2 associated with a decrease in BOLD signal, colored in blue). We currently do not know if this paradoxically represents a reduction in blood flow with increased CO_2 or simply increased CBV. It seems to identify areas that have the greatest vascular deficit. We have currently implemented MR imaging arterial spin labeling (ASL) methods that can make quantitative flow measurements in an attempt to answer this question. It would be desirable, from a

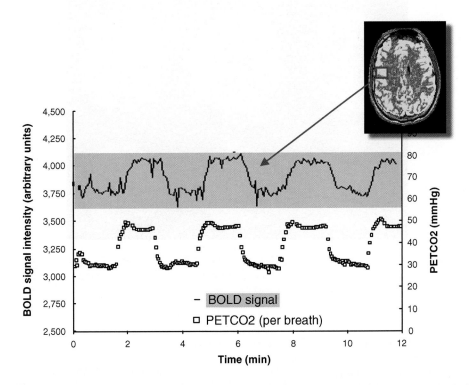

Fig. 3. BOLD CVR mapping. The lower curve shows the square-wave transitions that can be obtained in PCO_2 with the in-house developed rebreathing mask and gas sequencer. The transitions between $PETCO_2$ levels of 30 and 50 mm Hg are achieved in five breaths or less. The upper curve shows the tight correlation of the BOLD signal, which has been phase shifted to account for lung-to-brain blood transit time. Note that each cycle lasts 90 seconds, for a total of 12 minutes (whole-brain coverage).

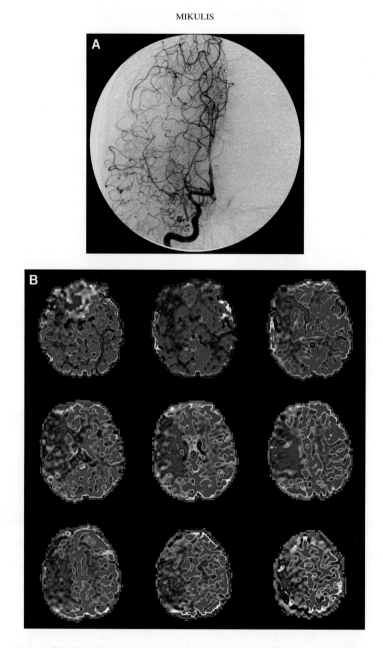

Fig. 4. Clinical application of BOLD CVR mapping in a patient with moyamoya disease. (*A*) Conventional angiogram shows occlusion of the right middle cerebral artery (*red arrow*). (*B*) CVR map shows "paradoxic reactivity" in the right middle cerebral artery territory indicating exhaustion of autoregulation (*blue*). The BOLD signal decreased with increased CO_2.

research perspective, to replace BOLD techniques with ASL for measuring "true" CVR. Because ASL is insensitive to deoxyhemoglobin, however, it may not replace BOLD for clinical assessments of CVR, because these blue or "paradoxic" areas may ultimately identify those regions in the brain suffering from the greatest oxygen delivery deficit.

Functional MR imaging

Another application of CVR testing is validation of the integrity of neurovascular coupling. We assume that autoregulation and neurovascular coupling are mediated through the same control system (ie, arteriolar smooth muscle). It is therefore inferred that neurons are unable to mediate local increases in blood flow if autoregulation is exhausted, because arteriolar smooth muscle is in a maximally relaxed state.

Although a common control system is a reasonable assumption, it has not been confirmed, especially because the exact mechanism of neurovascular coupling remains to be determined. Newell and Aaslid [10] first hypothesized identical mechanisms for neurovascular coupling and cerebral autoregulation. Rosengarten and colleagues [11], using a control

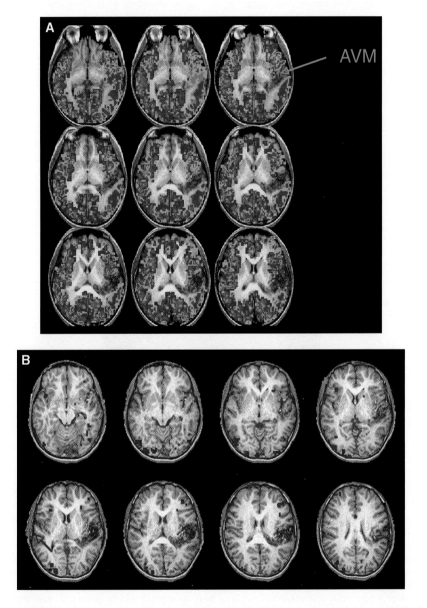

Fig. 5. Unreliable fMR imaging. (*A*) An arteriovenous malformation (AVM; *green arrow*) is present in the left posterior perisylvian region in the area of eloquent language cortex. Paradoxic reactivity (*blue*) is present anterior and posterior to the AVM, indicating exhausted autoregulation, perhaps from a vascular steal phenomenon related to the AVM. This map suggests that language mapping using fMR imaging could lead to false-negative activation. (*B*) Language map obtained from a verb generation paradigm shows an area of activation in the right hemisphere (*blue arrow*), suggestive of Wernicke's area, without activation of the homologous area of the left hemisphere. The CVR map indicates that the fMR imaging map must be interpreted with caution and that it is likely showing false-negative activation in the left hemisphere.

system approach, found support for this theory by comparing flow in the posterior cerebral artery induced by photic stimulation versus sudden deflation of thigh blood pressure cuffs.

This assumption nevertheless forms the basis for CVR validation of fMR imaging mapping. It is not unusual to observe eloquent cortex, the target of most clinical fMR imaging studies, within regions of severely impaired CVR. We have also observed areas of perilesional paradoxic CVR in 20% to 25% of patients with brain arteriovenous malformations, with nidus dimensions between 3 and 6 cm in diameter (Fig. 5A). Adequate knowledge of the state of CVR in an eloquent region is required to avoid adverse

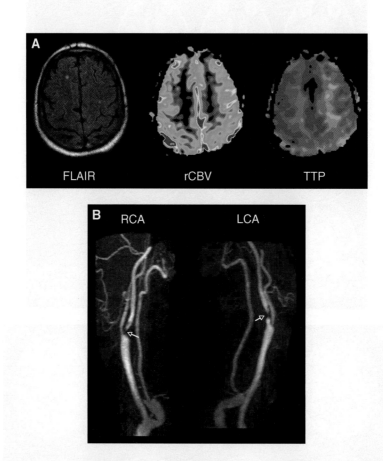

Fig. 6. Patient with shaking hand syndrome. (*A*) Fluid-attenuated inversion recovery (FLAIR) image and surrogate blood volume map (*middle*) show no abnormalities. The slightly paler blue–appearing left hemisphere on the time to peak image (TTP) suggests that there is a minimal flow delay. rCBV, regional cerebral blood volume. (*B*) MR angiography shows 90% or greater stenosis of both proximal internal carotid arteries (*arrows*). Although the TTP map suggests that the left lesion is more significant, it is a relative map and cannot distinguish bilaterally significant disease. In fact, both sides may be abnormal in this patient. TTP simply indicates that the left side is slightly worse relative to the right. (*C*) Pre-endarterectomy CVR map shows absence of reactivity in much of the left hemisphere, including the primary motor cortex controlling right hand function. The right hemisphere is normal, indicating that the left carotid stenosis is hemodynamically significant. The advantage of BOLD CVR is that the maps are not scaled against normal areas in the brain. Its accuracy is independent of disease distribution. (*D*) Pre-endarterectomy fMR imaging map obtained with a right finger-tapping paradigm shows no activation in the left hemisphere, implying that motor control of the right hand has been transferred to the right hemisphere. The CVR map suggests that fMR imaging is unreliable for assessing the left hemisphere, however. (*E*) Post-endarterectomy (day 6) CVR map shows normalization of CVR in the left hemisphere. (*F*) Post-endarterectomy (day 6) fMR imaging map surprisingly shows persistent right hemisphere and absent left hemisphere activation during right hand finger tapping. This may represent a delay in normalization of neurovascular coupling, despite normal CO_2 reactivity to stimuli (see text). (*G*) Postendarterectomy (5 months) fMR imaging map now shows the normal pattern of left hemisphere activation during right hand finger tapping.

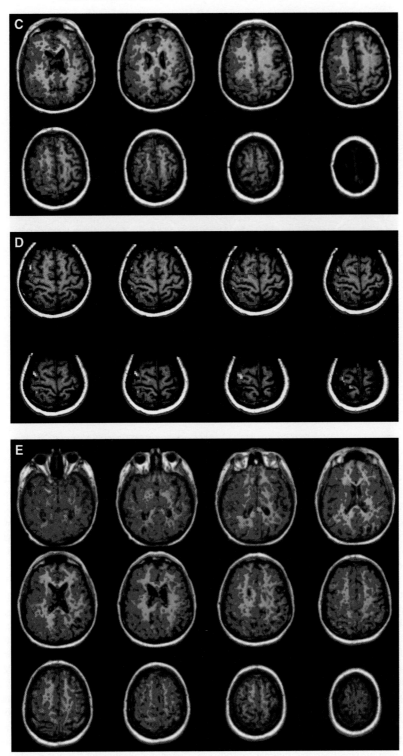

Fig. 6 (*continued*).

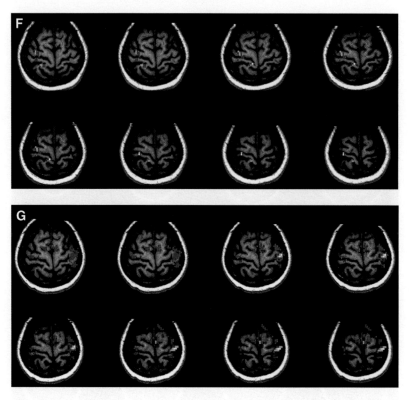

Fig. 6 (*continued*).

management decisions secondary to false-negative activation. These errors can even lead to the impression that the remaining areas of brain activation seen in the fMR imaging map are the result of cortical plasticity (see Fig. 5B).

The following case addresses some of these issues and is a fascinating demonstration of false-negative activation in the setting of severe carotid stenosis with delayed recovery of neurovascular coupling after carotid endarterectomy. A 70-year-old man presented with "shaking hand syndrome," consisting of a progressive use-dependent inability to control his right hand. He would begin writing and lose the ability to control his hand within seconds. He underwent preoperative conventional MR imaging, MR angiography, dynamic susceptibility perfusion MR imaging, BOLD CVR, and motor fMR imaging (Fig. 6).

These studies showed greater than or equal to 90% short segment proximal cervical internal carotid artery stenoses bilaterally. Conventional images were unremarkable, with no abnormality visible in the left corticospinal tract from the primary motor cortex to the brain stem. The time to peak perfusion map, a surrogate of transit time, suggested a minimal delay in the left hemisphere, which was most apparent in the hemispheric white matter. CVR was normal in the right hemisphere despite the presence of severe right carotid stenosis, which matched that seen on the left. CVR in the left hemisphere was clearly abnormal, indicating that the symptoms were probably related to impaired energy metabolism in the setting of an inadequate vascular supply (see Fig. 6C).

Left finger tapping fMR imaging (not shown) showed a normal pattern in the right hemisphere, with activation in the hand area of the primary motor cortex, primary sensory cortex, parietal cortex, premotor cortex, and supplementary motor areas (SMAs). There was a striking difference in cortical activation with right finger tapping. Except for the SMAs, no activation was seen in the expected motor network in the left hemisphere. Activation was distributed throughout the motor network in the right hemisphere, however (see Fig. 6D). Although the images are convincing for motor plasticity with transference of right hand control to the right hemisphere, why was there progressive deterioration of right hand control with use? Was false-negative activation present? The pattern was consistent with that reported in patients within the early recovery phase (first few weeks) of acute ischemic injury to the motor cortex [12,13], but we must now interpret these findings in light of the severe CVR deficit in the left motor cortex. This raises serious methodologic issues in those studies that have examined "plasticity" after ischemic stroke, in which the integrity of autoregulation was not assessed.

Six days after carotid endarterectomy, right hand function normalized, as did the repeat CVR study (see Fig. 6E). The fMR imaging study, however, showed failure of activation in the left hemisphere during right finger tapping (see Fig. 6F). The interpretation of these results is not straightforward. Perhaps true adaptive plasticity had occurred, or perhaps there was a delay in the recovery of neurovascular coupling. The latter is more likely when the physiology of autoregulation is considered in light of perfusion breakthrough evidence.

It is well known that a small percentage of patients (0.6%) develop postendarterectomy parenchymal brain hemorrhage, which is thought to be the result of failure of autoregulatory adaptation to the sudden and much higher postendarterectomy pressures [14]. In effect, the arterioles and precapillary sphincters must be "retrained" to manage higher pressures. This does not fully explain the lack of fMR imaging activation in the presence of recovered CO_2 responsivity seen in this case. If, in the preoperative state, the neurovascular signaling mechanism is saturated, there may be a delay in resetting the gain in this coupling mechanism after surgical restoration of the blood supply. Follow-up fMR imaging studies at 5 months showed recovery of the normal pattern of activation in the left hemisphere in response to right finger tapping, indicating that the coupling mechanism has been restored (see Fig. 6G).

This case illustrates, from a clinical perspective, the risk of false-negative fMR imaging activation in the setting of obstructive lesions of major feeding vessels. It also emphasizes the complexity of performing plasticity research in the setting of acute and sub-AIS, where there is a high incidence of vascular disease.

MR imaging horizons: oxygen delivery and use

The brain depends on a continuous supply of oxygen to meet metabolic demands. As has been discussed in the preceding sections, MR imaging is a useful tool for measuring the capacity of the vasculature to regulate the delivery of oxygen. There are disorders, however, such as anemia and lung disease, in which the vasculature is normal but there is impairment of delivery because of decreased blood oxygen content. Measuring flow alone cannot assess the impact that these diseases have on the brain. We can measure flow reductions or increases in transit time in patients with occlusive cerebrovascular diseases, but these parameters are also inadequate in determining the impact on the tissue, especially as it relates to the risk of irreversible injury.

In the population of patients with occlusion of the carotid arteries, tissue oxygen extraction fraction (OEF), as measured by PET, has been shown to be an independent predictor of subsequent ipsilateral stroke [15]. Clearly, knowledge of OEF and oxygen use by tissue ($CMRO_2$) could be useful in assessing the metabolic impact of oxygen delivery. Traditionally, the ability to measure these parameters has been solely in the realm of PET imaging, using oxygen-15–labeled tracers. A more expedient, available, and tantalizing tool, such as MR imaging, would be welcomed; the possibility is tantalizing, because much has already been done in examining the effect of blood oxygenation on tissue signal (BOLD imaging).

A promising method that combines information from MR imaging blood flow and BOLD imaging has been pioneered by Davis and colleagues [16] and Hoge and coworkers [17]. The basic premise of this technique is that the change in tissue $CMRO_2$ produced by neuronal activation can be measured using BOLD MR imaging by matching CBF increases induced by neuronal activation with those produced by CO_2 manipulation. The following describes the basic principle of this method.

BOLD signal and ASL blood flow are measured at rest and after neuronal activation using, for example, a finger-tapping task in a typical block paradigm. CO_2 is then administered at rest to increase CBF to the same level that was achieved with finger tapping. Note that during CO_2 administration, the neurons remain at rest and the increase in CBF is not accompanied by an increase in $CMRO_2$. The change in the BOLD signal is therefore only the result of deoxyhemoglobin washout. During neuronal activation, the change is a function of washout and increased oxygen extraction, which limits the rise in BOLD signal. Finally, the change in $CMRO_2$ produced by the ensemble of task active neurons can be determined from a ratio comparing the change in BOLD signal caused by neuronal activation with the change in BOLD signal caused by CO_2 inhalation.

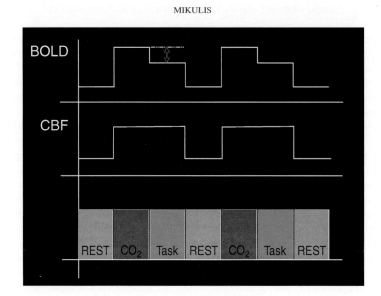

Fig. 7. Mapping the relative increase in tissue use of oxygen. The BOLD signal is measured under two conditions in which the change in blood flow over baseline is equivalent: in the first condition (CO_2), end-tidal CO_2 is increased to match the increase in blood flow produced by the second condition (task), which uses neuronal activation during the performance of a task to increase blood flow. The difference in BOLD signal between the two conditions indicated by the red arrows is proportional to the change in oxygen used by the neurons involved in the task.

Fig. 7 is a working diagram that shows the basic structure of the acquisition paradigm. Fig. 8 shows the $\Delta CMRO_2$ map obtained in a volunteer during bimanual finger tapping in our laboratory. The display is thresholded to show pixels that have a greater than 10% increase in $\Delta CMRO_2$ during the task. As expected, bilateral primary motor and sensory regions show task-related increases in oxygen use. We

measured a 22% increase in $\Delta CMRO_2$ in the motor cortex during this task, similar to the 16% and 25% increases observed by Davis and colleagues [16] and Hoge and coworkers [17], respectively, during visual stimulation tasks.

Measuring these changes in oxygen use with MR imaging is an exceptional advance; however, the method cannot measure $CMRO_2$ quantitatively. It can only measure relative changes, requires a cooperative subject, and is only sensitive to brain regions involved in task performance. Global measurements are not possible, and clinical applications have yet to be implemented or reported. Nevertheless, there is considerable optimism that further refinement of these methods could lead to clinically feasible tools that would enable global mapping of oxygen delivery and/or use in various disease states.

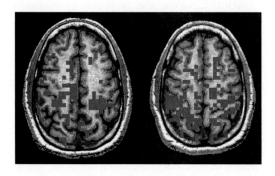

Fig. 8. Current state of the art in MR imaging mapping of brain oxygen use. Red pixels thresholded to show a greater than 10% increase in $\Delta CMRO_2$ are clustered in the motor cortices of both hemispheres during bimanual finger tapping.

Summary

Considerable progress has been made in the imaging assessment of acute stroke over the last 15 years. At that time, the standard of care was anatomic imaging consisting of noncontrast CT and conventional angiography. Since that time, MR imaging and

CT have evolved to the point where they are capable of providing important physiologic information that can guide acute stroke management. As a result, a healthy and robust debate has developed over which of the two is better able to provide the needed information in a timely fashion. There is growing unease concerning the low numbers of patients who meet the nonindividualized epidemiologically derived enrollment criteria for thrombolytic treatment, however. This is especially a problem for those patients in whom time of onset of the ischemic event is unclear (eg, those waking up from sleep with a stroke). Individualized assessment using physiologic parameters, such as permeability, could ultimately improve the manner in which these patients are triaged as well as increasing enrollment.

Imaging can also play a vital role in stroke prevention and rehabilitation. CVR analysis, or brain stress testing, could improve the management of patients with carotid stenosis and/or occlusion who are having TIAs. Detection of impaired or exhausted autoregulation would favor surgical or endovascular intervention as opposed to medical management in these patients. Similarly, significant numbers of coronary artery bypass (CABG) candidates have coexisting high-grade carotid stenosis with or without symptoms. Identification of CVR deficits in this population could help to select those patients who should undergo pre-CABG endarterectomy or stenting to reduce the risk of perioperative stroke.

Assessment of brain plasticity using fMR imaging after AIS is beginning to influence rehabilitation strategies, with observations and findings hinting at the presence of adaptive and maladaptive patterns. The ability to detect unfavorable or maladaptive patterns is leading to the development and testing of new rehabilitation strategies. The major caveat, as has already been discussed, is the danger of performing fMR imaging studies in this population of patients who have major occlusive disease as a cause of their stroke. Confirmation of intact autoregulation is mandatory if erroneous results are to be avoided. This validation is rarely performed but is highly recommended in this setting.

Evolution of imaging technology continues, together with the ability to perform more sophisticated functional and physiologic imaging. It would not be surprising to find that information concerning the metabolic condition of the tissue through measurement of oxygen delivery and use is routinely available by MR imaging within the next several years. On the horizon are molecular imaging techniques promising to provide smart contrast agents that can further advance our ability to visualize physiologic processes and perhaps track stem cells administered for brain repair. These methods are undoubtedly going to play an important role in the assessment of neurovascular disorders in the future and may even become part of routine clinical imaging.

References

[1] Roberts HC, Roberts TP, Brasch RC, et al. Quantitative measurement of microvascular permeability in human brain tumors achieved using dynamic contrast-enhanced MR imaging: correlation with histologic grade. AJNR Am J Neuroradiol 2000;21(5):891–9.

[2] Hamann GF, Okada Y, del Zoppo GJ. Hemorrhagic transformation and microvascular integrity during focal cerebral ischemia/reperfusion. J Cereb Blood Flow Metab 1996;16:1373–8.

[3] Knight RA, Barker PB, Fagan SC, et al. Prediction of impending hemorrhagic transformation in ischemic stroke using MRI in rats. Stroke 1998;29:144–51.

[4] The National Institute of Neurological Disorders and Stroke rt-PA Stroke Study Group. Tissue plasminogen activator for acute ischemic stroke. N Engl J Med 1995;333:1581–7.

[5] Kassner A, Roberts TP, Taylor K, et al. Prediction of hemorrhagic transformation in acute ischemic stroke using dynamic contrast-enhanced permeability MRI. In: 43rd Annual Meeting Proceedings of the American Society of Neuroradiology. Oakbrook (IL): American Society of Neuroradiology; 2005. p. 57.

[6] Baron JC, von Kummer R, del Zoppo GJ. Treatment of acute ischemic stroke. Challenging the concept of a rigid and universal time window. Stroke 1999;30(1):180–2.

[7] Roy C, Sherrington C. On the regulation of the blood supply of the brain. J Physiol 1890;11:85–108.

[8] Rostrup E, Knudsen GM, Law I, et al. The relationship between cerebral blood flow and volume in humans. Neuroimage 2005;24(1):1–11.

[9] Vesely A, Sasano H, Volgyesi G, et al. MRI mapping of cerebrovascular reactivity using square wave changes in end tidal P_{CO_2}. Magn Reson Med 2001;45:1011–3.

[10] Aaslid R. Cerebral hemodynamics. In: Newell DW, Aaslid R, editors. Transcranial Doppler. New York: Raven Press; 1992. p. 49–52.

[11] Rosengarten B, Huwendiek O, Kaps M. Neurovascular coupling and cerebral autoregulation can be described in terms of a control system. Ultrasound Med Biol 2001;27(2):189–93.

[12] Jaillard A, Martin CD, Garambois K, et al. Vicarious function within the human primary motor cortex? A longitudinal fMRI stroke study. Brain 2005;128(Pt 5):1122–38.

[13] Feydy A, Carlier R, Roby-Brami A, et al. Longitudinal study of motor recovery after stroke: recruitment

and focusing of brain activation. Stroke 2002;33(6): 1610–7.

[14] Piepgras DG, Morgan MK, Sundt Jr TM, et al. Intracerebral hemorrhage after carotid endarterectomy. J Neurosurg 1988;68(4):532–6.

[15] GrubbJr RL, Derdeyn CP, Fritsch SM, et al. Importance of hemodynamic factors in the prognosis of symptomatic carotid occlusion. JAMA 1998;280(12): 1055–60.

[16] Davis TL, Kwong KK, Weisskoff RM, et al. Calibrated functional MR. I: Mapping the dynamics of oxidative metabolism. Proc Natl Acad Sci USA 1998;95(4): 1834–9.

[17] Hoge RD, Atkinson J, Gill B, et al. Investigation of BOLD signal dependence on cerebral blood flow and oxygen consumption: the deoxyhemoglobin dilution model. Magn Reson Med 1999;42(5):849–63.

ELSEVIER
SAUNDERS

Neuroimag Clin N Am 15 (2005) 681 – 695

Stroke Recovery and Its Imaging

Craig D. Takahashi, PhD[a], Lucy Der Yeghiaian, MA, OTR/L[b],
Steven C. Cramer, MD[a,c],*

[a]Department of Neurology, University of California at Irvine, Irvine, CA, USA
[b]Department of Occupational Therapy, University of California at Irvine, Irvine, CA, USA
[c]Department of Anatomy and Neurobiology, University of California at Irvine, Irvine, CA, USA

Stroke perennially is a major source of human morbidity and mortality. Approximately 1 in 15 deaths in the United States is attributable to stroke. Stroke is the third leading cause of death after heart disease and cancer in the United States, and the second leading cause worldwide. Approximately 85% of United States patients survive an acute stroke, living an average of 7 years thereafter. Most are left with significant disability [1,2] that reduces activities and participation.

All aspects of brain function can be affected by stroke. The nature and severity of poststroke deficits vary widely. In the weeks and months after a stroke, most patients show spontaneous improvement in behaviors affected by stroke [3–5]. This recovery, however, is highly variable and generally incomplete. As a result, stroke is the leading cause of adult disability in the United States and many other countries.

Several investigations have examined the brain events that underlie spontaneous recovery of function after stroke and, more recently, studies have examined the brain events underlying experimentally derived poststroke gains. The majority of these studies focus on motor or language recovery. Several brain-mapping techniques are used to investigate recovery, each with its strengths. Functional MRI (fMRI) is the

tool for many of these, given the safety and accessibility of MRI machines and this method's good temporal and excellent spatial resolution. Other investigative approaches have a separate profile of strengths. Transcranial magnetic stimulation (TMS) is easier to use with patients but has reduced spatial resolution versus fMRI. Positron emission tomography (PET) scanning has reduced temporal resolution and generally is less accessible but can measure many aspects of brain physiology.

This review focuses on fMRI. The emphasis is on recovery of motor function, one of the major sources of impairment in stroke patients. Findings in motor recovery, however, overlap substantially with investigations of recovery in other brain systems, such as language [6].

The overall goal of these studies is to understand reorganization of brain function better to improve patient outcomes. Such a goal might be realized by better prediction of outcomes, patient triage, defining duration and intensity of restorative therapy, and measuring treatment effects. Several restorative interventions are under study, including cells, selective serotonin reuptake inhibitors, catecholaminergics, brain stimulation, robotic and other device-based interventions, imagery-based protocols, and constraint-induced and other intensive physical therapy regimens, although currently none is approved for enhancing outcome after central nervous system injury, such as stroke. The maximum value of functional neuroimaging methods, such as fMRI, will be appreciated when used in the context of an established restorative intervention.

* Corresponding author. Department of Neurology, University of California Irvine Medical Center, 101 The City Drive South, Building 53, Room 203, Orange, CA 92868-4280.
  E-mail address: scramer@uci.edu (S.C. Cramer).

1052-5149/05/$ – see front matter © 2005 Elsevier Inc. All rights reserved.
doi:10.1016/j.nic.2005.08.006

The biology of spontaneous recovery after stroke

Several changes arise in the brain during the weeks after a stroke. These are described at multiple levels. Cellular and molecular studies in animals undergoing an experimental unilateral infarction characterize neurogenesis, angiogenesis, inflammation, excitability, and cellular growth, many of which evolve bilaterally during the days to weeks after a unilateral insult. A body of evidence suggests that many of these events contribute to spontaneous recovery of function after a stroke [7].

In animal studies, exogenous interventions are found that amplify these molecular events and simultaneously improve behavioral outcome. Examples include amphetamine [8], growth factors [9,10], cellular therapies [11,12], brain stimulation [13–15], increased environmental complexity [16,17], and physical activity level [18].

Thus, there are discrete molecular brain events that arise days and weeks after an infarction; these brain events likely underlie spontaneous recovery and can be augmented therapeutically in association with improved behavioral outcome in animals. Stroke deficits remain the most common cause of disability in adults living in the United States and many other countries.

There is a great need to translate results of animal studies into improved therapeutics for human patients who have stroke. To do so requires an understanding of the biology of recovery in humans. The cellular-molecular measurements obtained in animal studies are not duplicated easily in human patients, where brain tissue is not commonly available for examination. Human brain mapping with techniques, such as fMRI, however, are providing insights important to this goal. Human studies also are of value because of the limitations of animal models in this context [19]. For example, rodent studies are of limited value because most of these creatures are quadrupeds with vastly different brain organization from humans, including relative size of basal ganglia and white matter. Primate studies are instructive; however, size and pathogenesis of brain injury has limited overlap with spontaneous human cerebrovascular disease. Animal models often lack the heterogeneity of injury found in the human condition; animals generally have a more uniform preinfarction behavioral status; animals generally are at a much younger point in the life span; most, if not all, human stroke risk factors are absent in animal models; cognitive/affective features important to all aspects of recovery usually have limited correspondence with the human condition; and medical complications that in combination affect a majority of human stroke patients generally are absent in animal studies. There are no humans like humans to understand humans.

Functional imaging in human subjects may be of value in the area of stroke recovery, because these data provide biologic insights that sometimes otherwise are not available. Molecular events generally are difficult to obtain in humans. Behavioral changes are easier to measure but do not consistently correspond tightly with the molecular/physiologic events that comprise therapeutic targets. For example, a range of brain events and behavioral strategies can produce the same behavioral phenotype. Also, behavioral assessments generally do not provide mechanistic insights or distinguish patient subgroups with biologically distinct therapeutic targets. Functional imaging, which exists between the molecular and behavioral levels, provides insights into brain changes at the systems level.

For example, functional imaging can provide improved insight into anatomic measures. Human [20,21] and experimental animal [22,23] studies of brain infarction consistently find that behavioral deficits correlate significantly with acute or chronic measurement of infarction volume. These correlations, however, sometimes are limited, especially chronically, as this approach to understanding brain injury assumes an equivalency of cortical function akin to theories of cerebral mass action [24]. Introduction of fMRI measures into analysis of injury can improve the correlation between injury and behavioral effects [25]; thus, this approach may have improved value for predicting stroke outcome versus using anatomic scans to measure total stroke volume (Fig. 1). Use of a method, such as structural or perfusion imaging, characterizes injury but provides limited insight as to how this injury influences final behavioral deficits from injury.

There is a broad range of neurologic settings in which functional imaging is useful when behavioral examination or anatomic brain imaging provides limited insight. For example, when neurologic examination is normal, expression of genetic risk for Alzheimer's disease [26] nevertheless can be measured when a memory task is performed during fMRI. When neuropsychologic testing is normal, fMRI frontal lobe activation during a memory task performance describes effects of HIV status on the brain [27]. Decreases in cortical metabolism by PET scanning are linked with cognitive deficits in patients who have traumatic brain injury, even when anatomic MRI is unrevealing [28]. When stroke renders a patient hemiplegic, and examination, thus, is silent, fMRI permits measurement of activity across brain motor networks [29]. Even in patients who do not have a

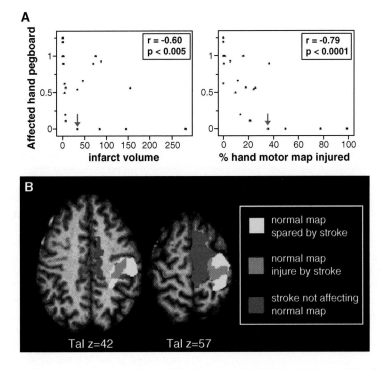

Fig. 1. (*A*) Infarction volume (*top left*) and fraction of hand motor map injured by stroke (*top right*) each show a significant inverse relationship with pegboard performance by the affected hand (normalized to pegboard results for the unaffected hand). Correlation is stronger and more significant, however, in the latter case. Note that injury to more than 37% of the hand motor map is associated with total loss of hand motor function. The arrow indicates the patient whose images are displayed below. (*B*) Images from a patient whose stroke was mild to moderate in size (33 cm^3) but injured 35% of the hand motor area. This stroke was associated with total loss of hand motor function. (*From* Crafton K, Mark A, Cramer S. Improved understanding of cortical injury by incorporating measures of functional anatomy. Brain 2003;126:1650–9; with permission.)

neurologic diagnosis, functional brain imaging studies suggest that the same behavioral phenotype can arise from varying patterns of brain activity; for example, some elderly patients might activate a greater fraction of their cognitive reserve to maintain normal function [30].

Human brain mapping with fMRI and other techniques, therefore, hold great potential for implementation of therapeutics that target stroke recovery. Potential roles for functional imaging include gaining insights into the nature of the biologic targets for individual patients who have stroke, triaging patients according to features of brain function, and providing a surrogate marker of treatment effects. The goal is to use brain mapping to extract key neurophysiologic data for improved clinical decision making. This goal has precedence in medical practice. For example, when a patient presents with a ventricular tachyarrhythmia or a refractory epileptic disorder, current practice often incorporates electrophysiologic data to guide specific decisions in treatment [31,32]. With

further study, brain-mapping techniques, such as fMRI, might provide information useful for decision making in treatment of stroke recovery for individual patients. Examples of using brain mapping for improved decision making are emerging. In one study [33], fMRI was used to localize the stroke hemisphere's hand motor area in patients who had chronic stroke. This information then was used to guide targeted subthreshold cortical stimulation.

When considering clinical measures for the study of stroke recovery, it is important to remember that restorative neurotherapeutics emphasizes specific brain systems. This is true at the behavioral level, where reinforcing specific behaviors is critical to successful therapeutic effect on outcome [34]. This also is true for functional imaging, where a specific behavior is used to activate the brain. Thus, the global clinical measures used in acute stroke trials by themselves are insufficient to capture system-directed therapies or to interpret many studies of functional activation after stroke.

Methodologic considerations and sources of bias

Many patterns of altered brain function are described during the study of patients who have stroke. These are compiled exhaustively elsewhere [6,35–38].

Initial functional imaging studies were cross-sectional and observational in nature. Subsequent studies examined stroke patient subpopulations, increased sample size, correlated features of brain activation with clinical measures, and performed serial studies during the period of behavioral gains post stroke. The overall understanding of changes in brain function after stroke, however, and the relationship between these changes and clinical measures, remain limited. This is in part because of the relative dearth of such investigations.

At least three groups of issues limit current understanding of brain events underlying spontaneous return of function after a stroke. The first is the heterogeneity of stroke—its causes, injury patterns, effects, and therapies. There are many variables that

---

Box 1. Clinical variables that potentially influence stroke recovery and its measurement by functional imaging

Stroke topography
Time post stroke
Age
Hemispheric dominance
Side of brain affected
Depression
Injury to other brain network nodes
Infarction volume
Initial stroke deficits
Arterial patency
Prestroke disability
Medical comorbidities
Prestroke experience and education
Type of poststroke therapy
Amount poststroke therapy
Acute stroke interventions
Medications during stroke recovery period
Medications at time of brain mapping
Final clinical status
Stroke mechanism

Data from Cramer S. Functional imaging in stroke recovery. Stroke 2004;35: 2695–8.

---

likely modify brain function after stroke (Box 1). Some of these also are important to the study of brain function in health, such as age, hemispheric dominance, and medical comorbidity. Others are important to the study of brain function in the setting of acute stroke, such as infarction volume, concomitant depression, and prestroke disability. Each is a source of variance that can reduce power in functional imaging studies of stroke recovery.

A second group of issues pertains to the divergence of investigative approaches. Currently, there is a lack of standardized methods for studying and reporting brain function across studies. Indeed, small differences in data acquisition methods can have significant effects on results. For example squeezing versus finger-tapping activates different motor circuits [39,40]. Differences in force [41–43], frequency [44–47], amplitude [48], or complexity [49–51] of finger movements can have a substantial impact on activation in multiple brain sensorimotor areas. A similar degree of variability exists in clinical assessments used to measure stroke recovery [52,53]. This situation in stroke recovery contrasts with that found in multiple sclerosis, where the Multiple Sclerosis Functional Composite [54] routinely is included, and in spinal cord injury, where the American Spinal Injury Association (ASIA) motor score, ASIA pinprick sensory score, ASIA light touch sensory score, and ASIA impairment scale [55] routinely are reported. Adoption of a standardized approach to be included in studies of stroke recovery might reduce the impact of this issue.

A third group of issues pertains to brain and vascular changes common in patients who have stroke. Vascular disease can modify neuronal-vascular coupling. Available data suggest this is most important with highly advanced stenosis or occlusion of the cerebral arteries [56–61]. Moreover, advanced large cerebral artery narrowing itself can be associated with reorganization of brain function [62]. Further studies are needed in this area. Also, brain injury, such as stroke, can affect the intrinsic T2* property of brain tissue, the underlying measurement in blood oxygenation level–dependent (BOLD) fMRI. Recent data from the authors' laboratory (discussed below) suggest that this may be important. Multimodal assessment of brain function may be useful in addressing these concerns in contexts where they are most significant. Methods, such as electroencephalography and magnetoencephalography, have reduced spatial resolution compared with fMRI, but temporal resolution is improved, and these vascular issues might not have the same impact on findings with these methods.

Spontaneous changes in brain function after stroke

Despite current limitations, functional imaging studies examining spontaneous events related to stroke recovery converge on several findings.

Changes in networks

The earliest study emphasized altered function within multiple nodes of relevant distributed networks [63]. This finding has been replicated repeatedly. Clearly, altered function within one area changes function within interconnected areas within a distributed brain network after stroke, similar to multifocal, distant changes in brain function reported after a focal brain perturbation in the motor system of healthy subjects [64–66]. Animal studies are concordant with results in humans [67–74]. Fig. 2 presents a model that compiles these findings [75–79].

Changes in laterality

One commonly reported effect of stroke on brain function in humans is a reduction in the laterality of activity [80–86]. This issue also has received consid-

erable attention in the study of normal aging [87] and, furthermore, is described in other neurologic contexts, including epilepsy [88], traumatic brain injury [89], and multiple sclerosis [90]. Early reports emphasized a less lateralized pattern of activation after stroke than normal (ie, the effect of stroke on motor system function is to increase the extent to which both hemispheres are recruited rather than just the hemisphere contralateral to movement). For example, a language task or a right-hand motor task that activates the left hemisphere in healthy controls activates relevant regions within the right and left hemispheres in patients who have a left hemisphere stroke.

Several factors modify the extent to which stroke is associated with reduced laterality. Examples include time after stroke (laterality often increases toward normal as patients recover) [91–96], hemispheric dominance (motor task performance with the nondominant hand is less lateralized than with the dominant hand in health and after stroke) [82,97,98], and topography of injury (reduced laterality may be more common with a cortical, rather than subcortical, infarction) [92,99]. Other factors relevant to laterality in normal subjects also likely are important to the experience of stroke recovery, such as task complexity (more complex tasks are a more bilaterally or-

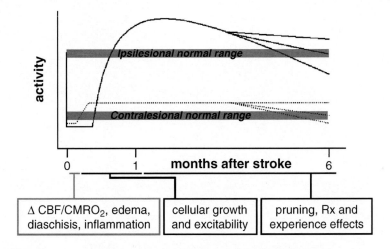

Fig. 2. Changes in bilateral brain areas after unilateral stroke have been grouped into three time periods. Time period 1: in the initial hours to days after a stroke, brain function and behavior can be deranged globally , and few restorative structural changes have started. Time period 2: a period of growth then begins lasting several weeks. Structural and functional changes in the contralesional hemisphere precede those of the ipsilesional hemisphere and at such times activity in relevant contralesional areas can even exceed activity in the lesion hemisphere. This growth-related period may be a key target for certain restorative therapies. Time period 3: subsequently, there is pruning, reduction in functional overactivations, and establishment of a static pattern of brain activity and behavior. The final pattern, nevertheless, may remain accessible to plasticity-inducing, clinically meaningful, interventions. An excess of growth followed by pruning has precedence in human neurobiology, being a recapitulation of normal developmental events. Supra- and subnormal activity levels in the ipsilesional and contralesional hemispheres correlate with features of behavioral outcome in specific patient populations (described previously). (*From* Cramer S. Functional imaging in stroke recovery. Stroke 2004;35:2695–8; with permission.)

ganized brain event) [100–102], subject age (reduced laterality with increased age) [87], task familiarity (repeating the same behavior can reduce laterality) [103], proximal versus distal (more proximal motor tasks show reduced laterality compared with distal tasks) [39,104,105], and perhaps gender [106]. The motor cortex site of activation during movement of the ipsilateral hand is different from that activated during movement of the contralateral hand, the latter possibly representing premotor cortex activity, often on anterior precentral gyrus [107].

Studies suggest that the spontaneous increase in activity within the nonstroke hemisphere after stroke (ie, reduced laterality) reflects greater injury or deficits. This is emphasized particularly in the serial fMRI study by Fujii and coworkers [93] and by TMS studies [108,109]. TMS studies suggest further possible mechanisms for this finding. In primary motor cortex, stroke hemisphere inhibition on the nonstroke hemisphere is reduced [110], and nonstroke hemisphere inhibition on the stroke hemisphere is increased [111], although this phenomenon might vary with level of deficits [112].

Some studies suggest that changes in laterality of brain function might be important to whatever behavioral recovery is achieved after stroke [85,94, 113–115], even if the final behavior is less than normal. Cases are published wherein brain activation is restricted mostly or completely to the nonstroke hemisphere, contralateral to results in controls [82,107, 116,117]. Reduced laterality has behavioral significance, in at least some cases, and, therefore, does not reflect merely more severe stroke or passive changes in inhibition.

Changes in activation site

A spontaneous shift in the site of activation also is reported after stroke, in all manner of direction, by fMRI, PET, and TMS. The most common changes described are a ventral or a posterior shift in the contralateral (stroke hemisphere) activation site during unilateral motor task performance by the stroke-affected hand. Weiller and colleagues describe a ventral shift in the center of activation during motor task performance in recovered patients whose stroke

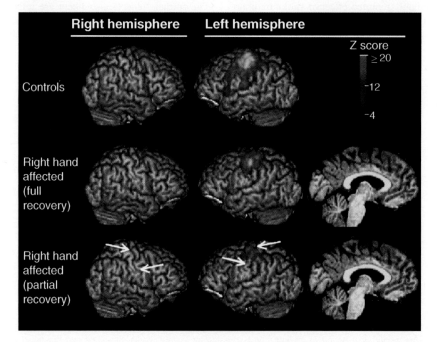

Fig. 3. Group maps from patients who had stroke affecting the right arm (left brain) show a difference in activation site and size varying with level of recovery. The Talairach coordinates for center of activation for the activation cluster in left primary sensorimotor cortex in those who had complete recovery was (31, −21, 50), which was ventral as versus those who had partial recovery, among whom the center of activation was located at (30, −19, 54). In addition, patients who had full recovery, versus partial recovery, showed 2.7-fold larger contralateral sensorimotor activation, with negligible differences in the supplementary motor area, despite no differences in finger tapping force or in surface EMG recordings. (*From* Zemke A, Heagerty P, Lee C, et al. Motor cortex organization after stroke is related to side of stroke and level of recovery. Stroke 2003;34:E23–8; with permission.)

affected the posterior aspect of the internal capsule, suggesting that topographic shifts in cortical activation site might reflect survival of selected corticospinal tract fibers [86]. An fMRI study also reports the same finding in patients who have complete motor recovery compared with patients who have partial recovery (Fig. 3) [36,39,42,80,81,98,118]. This suggests that, at least for hand motor recovery, a ventral shift might be associated with better recovery of function. A posterior shift in activation site is described in motor studies of stroke recovery across multiple imaging modalities [118–121] and is described in the motor system of patients who have multiple sclerosis [90] or spinal cord injury [122,123]. In most studies of patients who have stroke, a posterior shift does not correlate with clinical status; however, a recent study suggests that degree of posterior shift is related linearly to degree of recovery, at least for proximal movements [105].

Changes in activation size

Studies describe changes in activation size in many brain areas in the setting of stroke recovery. Several studies emphasize increased activation over time within several areas within the stroke-affected hemisphere, accompanied by decreased activation over time in several areas, particularly within the nonstroke hemisphere [94–96,124,125], consistent with TMS studies [126,127]. TMS studies converge on the conclusion that progressive expansion in the area of excitable primary motor cortex within the stroke hemisphere during the period of stroke recovery is a feature of patients who have superior motor outcomes [126,128]. Although clinical status reaches a plateau in 3 months or less for many functions, such as motor status [3,129], brain reorganization might continue to evolve for months beyond this [125,127].

The task used to probe activation can influence the volume of activation significantly. For example, contralateral activation volume during right-hand squeezing is significantly larger than the volume during right index-finger tapping [39]. This illustrates one of the important principles of brain mapping of stroke recovery, that the results are influenced highly by the nature of the fMRI task used to address the questions.

Correlations between behavior and changes in brain activation

In some serial functional imaging studies, the correlate of better clinical outcome is increased acti-

vation in key stroke-hemisphere areas [93–96,98], but in other studies, the correlate is reduction in such activation [91,130]. These differences across fMRI studies might arise from several sources. Several methodologic issues might contribute, such as divergence in time after stroke at which investigations are performed, the task used to activate the brain, the patient populations enrolled, the nature of therapy given to patients after stroke, or other variables. A single fMRI probe can yield different results across different populations. For example, using a single probe consisting of tapping the affected index finger at 2 Hz (driven by auditory metronome) across a 25°–range of motion with eyes closed, shoulder adducted, and elbow extended, at 1.5 Tesla field strength, the authors found that, compared with age-matched controls, activation volume is decreased after stroke [98] and increased after spinal cord injury [131]. These observations suggest that a particular brain-mapping method has the best clinical validity when applied to a specific patient population and clinical context.

Across studies, certain relationships between behavior and brain function seem likely. First, for behaviors arising from a lateralized, primary cortex–driven brain area, increased activation in the primary cortex correlates with better outcome (see Fig. 3) [94,98,126], indicating preservation of key substrate with optimal connections for supporting the behavior of interest. Second, in other brain areas, such as association cortex (eg, secondary motor areas) greater activation correlates with poorer outcome, as, in this case, greater activation represents a compensatory event that generally is not able to support full return of behavior because of the nature of anatomic connections in these areas [132]. Best outcomes are associated with the greatest return to the normal state of brain function [132].

Changes along infarction rim

Increased activity along the rim of a cortical infarction is described in fMRI and PET studies [82,99,133]. Butz and coworkers [134] find peri-infarction, low-frequency activity in the majority of patients who have cortical stroke, although the functional significance of this finding was unclear. These observations might correspond to the increased levels of growth-related proteins found along the rim of experimental infarctions introduced into animals [8,135]. The intrinsic T2* property of brain tissue, changes in which underlie activation in BOLD fMRI, however, can be altered by stroke. Recent data from the authors' laboratory suggest that the area surrounding an infarction might have increased T2* signal versus normal brain tissue, the impact of which on BOLD fMRI could be important.

Diaschisis

Diaschisis also may be an important process related to behavioral recovery after stroke. Brain areas connected to, but spatially distant from, the region of infarction show many changes post stroke [96,136–138]. For example, the authors found several patients who had a behavioral deficit early after stroke among whom areas that normally showed activation were near silent. These areas with reduced brain activation had no injury from stroke and showed normal resting cerebral blood flow. Behavioral recovery was associated with restitution of brain activity in these areas [96]. In several cases, an area of the brain had normal perfusion, was inactive early after stroke, was highly active months later, and was sufficiently distant from the infarction so as to be in a separate vascular territory. Although many methods are used to describe diaschisis, this process may be measured directly using fluorodeoxyglucose–PET [113,139]. Further studies in humans are needed to understand this spontaneous, distant suppression of function and the extent to which it might be a therapeutic target.

Recovery resulting from therapeutic intervention

fMRI and other brain-mapping methods provide insights into the brain events underlying spontaneous return of function after stroke. These methods also are useful for understanding how iatrogenic interventions improve behavioral outcome. The promise of these methods extends beyond neurobiologic insight. Measures of brain function might provide useful information on prognosis, triage, and as a surrogate marker [140]. Such usefulness could vastly enhance the extent to which restorative therapies effectively change the face of stroke recovery.

Several examples of brain-mapping treatment effects on stroke recovery are published. Animal studies provide useful lessons in this regard [14,16,18,67,73]. Many human studies to date have focused on effects of increased physical activity [76,141–145]. Effects of pharmacologic [78] and other [33,146] interventions also have been studied.

Reorganization of brain motor function after stroke and its treatment is related to repetitiveness of intervention, learning, sensorimotor integration, complexity, and attention. Restorative therapy likely needs to be graded to patient status with regard to such issues, such as by altering dose, context, de-

mand level, and complexity of intervention. Such dosing adjustments might be based on features of behavior or perhaps of functional brain organization. In light of these issues, adjuvant aspects of therapeutic intervention warrant consideration.

Active, intense, repetitive content of therapy

Active repetitive movement practice [147] can enhance the strength and functional use of affected limbs in patients who have chronic stroke. For instance, repetitive practice of hand and finger flexion and extension movements result in significant motor performance improvements during the therapy period [148]. Intensity of therapy might be an important factor in the level of functional improvement [149]; in this regard, repetitive therapy in part may be based on events related to normal learning [150–152]. Active participation is more effective in improving motor performance improvement compared with passive training [153]. Constraint-induced movement therapy includes intense, active training. Changes in brain function are described after constraint-induced movement therapy, with the divergence in results possibly reflecting differences in patients and study methods [142,144,145,154,155].

Sensorimotor integration

Motor gains can be demonstrated when impaired voluntary movements are supplemented with some form of assistance, either through neuromuscular stimulation [156–158] or by mechanical assistance [159,160]. Studies that use techniques to enhance somatosensory input show effectiveness at improving motor function in healthy [158] and paretic limbs [161]. Sensorimotor integration theory might provide insight into the basis for these motor gains: motor output is inextricably linked to sensory input, and those unable to complete movements voluntarily cannot produce appropriate sensory patterns associated with motor effort [162,163]. This theory provides a rationale for active assistive therapy [164]. Implementation of sensorimotor integration theory might be improved with measurement of function in key brain functional areas for integration [165,166].

Environmental complexity and context

Environmental complexity or enrichment alters brain function and structure in normal [167–169] and neurologically impaired [67,170,171] animals. Animals with experimental stroke have improved functional outcomes when exposed to enriched environments that allow social interaction and a variety of activities [172,173]. Similarly, poststroke experience influences the functional outcome in humans. Specialized multidisciplinary stroke units show improved patient outcomes compared with that of general wards [174,175].

Computer, robotics, and motion tracking technology recently have been used to produce rich virtual reality environments [176–178]. This technology can be used in a variety of settings and can influence environment in many ways, such as by augmenting sensory feedback [179]. Deriving maximum clinical gains from implementing environmental complexity into restorative therapies might be achieved by incorporating findings from brain-mapping studies on the neurobiology of complexity [49,100,180–182]. In addition, virtual reality approaches lend themselves readily to incorporation into most brain-mapping protocols.

The context in which restorative therapy is administered influences clinical gains. Task-specific training [158,183–187], use of a functionally rich task ecology [188–190], and increased purpose of practiced exercise [191] can improve clinical gains. Functional imaging can contribute to implementation of these observations by providing insight into their mechanism of effect on the injured brain.

Attention

Practice conditions that make performance more difficult, relative to less difficult, enhance the cognitive and motor processes involved in long-term performance [192]. For instance, contextual interference, which incorporates random practice conditions, is known to stimulate attention and cognition. This pattern of practice conditions is shown to enhance retention and transfer of motor skill learning [192–197]. Associative plasticity also depends on attention [198]. Simply looking at one's tapping finger, versus looking away, increases the volume of motor cortex activated by 50% [199]. Studies examining the effect of attention on brain function in healthy subjects [194,198,200] may be of guiding value in understanding how to manipulate attention to maximize therapeutic gains in patients who have stroke.

Summary

Functional imaging of stroke recovery is a unique source of information that might be useful in the development of restorative treatments. Several features of brain function change spontaneously after stroke. Current studies define many of the most common events. Key challenges for the future are to develop standardized approaches to help address certain questions, determine the psychometric qualities of these measures, and define the clinical usefulness of these methods.

References

[1] Gresham G, Duncan P, Stason W, et al. Post-stroke rehabilitation. Rockville (MD): US Department of Health and Human Services. Public Health Service, Agency for Health Care Policy and Research; 1995.

[2] Rathore S, Hinn A, Cooper L, et al. Characterization of incident stroke signs and symptoms: findings from the atherosclerosis risk in communities study. Stroke 2002;33:2718–21.

[3] Duncan P, Goldstein L, Matchar D, et al. Measurement of motor recovery after stroke. Stroke 1992; 23:1084–9.

[4] Hier D, Mondlock J, Caplan L. Recovery of behavioral abnormalities after right hemisphere stroke. Neurology 1983;33:345–50.

[5] Kertesz A, McCabe P. Recovery patterns and prognosis in aphasia. Brain 1977;100(Pt 1):1–18.

[6] Baron J, Cohen L, Cramer S, et al. Neuroimaging in stroke recovery: a position paper from the First International Workshop on Neuroimaging and Stroke Recovery. Cerebrovasc Dis 2004;18:260–7.

[7] Cramer S, Chopp M. Recovery recapitulates ontogeny. Trends Neurosci 2000;23:265–71.

[8] Stroemer R, Kent T, Hulsebosch C. Enhanced neocortical neural sprouting, synaptogenesis, and behavioral recovery with D-amphetamine therapy after neocortical infarction in rats. Stroke 1998;29: 2381–95.

[9] Kawamata T, Dietrich W, Schallert T, et al. Intracisternal basic fibroblast growth factor (bFGF) enhances functional recovery and upregulates the expression of a molecular marker of neuronal sprouting following focal cerebral infarction. Proc Natl Acad Sci USA 1997;94:8179–84.

[10] Ren J, Kaplan P, Charette M, et al. Time window of intracisternal osteogenic protein-1 in enhancing functional recovery after stroke. Neuropharmacology 2000;39:860–5.

[11] Chen J, Li Y, Katakowski M, et al. Intravenous bone marrow stromal cell therapy reduces apoptosis and promotes endogenous cell proliferation after stroke in female rat. J Neurosci Res 2003;73:778–86.

[12] Mahmood A, Lu D, Chopp M. Intravenous administration of marrow stromal cells (MSCs) increases the expression of growth factors in rat brain after traumatic brain injury. J Neurotrauma 2004;21:33–9.

[13] Adkins-Muir D, Jones T. Cortical electrical stimulation combined with rehabilitative training: enhanced functional recovery and dendritic plasticity following

focal cortical ischemia in rats. Neurol Res 2003;25: 780–8.

[14] Kleim J, Bruneau R, VandenBerg P, et al. Motor cortex stimulation enhances motor recovery and reduces peri-infarct dysfunction following ischemic insult. Neurol Res 2003;25:789–93.

[15] Plautz E, Barbay S, Frost S, et al. Post-infarct cortical plasticity and behavioral recovery using concurrent cortical stimulation and rehabilitative training: a feasibility study in primates. Neurol Res 2003;25:801–10.

[16] Johansson B, Belichenko P. Neuronal plasticity and dendritic spines: effect of environmental enrichment on intact and postischemic rat brain. J Cereb Blood Flow Metab 2002;22:89–96.

[17] Johansson B, Ohlsson A. Environment, social interaction, and physical activity as determinants of functional outcome after cerebral infarction in the rat. Exp Neurol 1996;139:322–7.

[18] Jones T, Chu C, Grande L, et al. Motor skills training enhances lesion-induced structural plasticity in the motor cortex of adult rats. J Neurosci 1999;19: 10153–63.

[19] Cramer S. Clinical issues in animal models of stroke and rehabilitation. ILAR J 2003;44:83–4.

[20] Brott T, Marler J, Olinger C, et al. Measurements of acute cerebral infarction: lesion size by computed tomography. Stroke 1989;20:871–5.

[21] Saver J, Johnston K, Homer D, et al. Infarct volume as a surrogate or auxiliary outcome measure in ischemic stroke clinical trials. The RANTTAS Investigators. Stroke 1999;30:293–8.

[22] Lyden P, Lonzo L, Nunez S, et al. Effect of ischemic cerebral volume changes on behavior. Behav Brain Res 1997;87:59–67.

[23] Rogers D, Campbell C, Stretton J, et al. Correlation between motor impairment and infarct volume after permanent and transient middle cerebral artery occlusion in the rat. Stroke 1997;28:2060–5 [discussion: 2066].

[24] Lashley K. In search of the engram. Symposia of the Society of Experimental Biology. Cambridge (England): Cambridge University Press; 1950. p. 454–82.

[25] Crafton K, Mark A, Cramer S. Improved understanding of cortical injury by incorporating measures of functional anatomy. Brain 2003;126:1650–9.

[26] Bookheimer S, Strojwas M, Cohen M, et al. Patterns of brain activation in people at risk for Alzheimer's disease. N Engl J Med 2000;343:450–6.

[27] Ernst T, Chang L, Jovicich J, et al. Abnormal brain activation on functional MRI in cognitively asymptomatic HIV patients. Neurology 2002;59:1343–9.

[28] Fontaine A, Azouvi P, Remy P, et al. Functional anatomy of neuropsychological deficits after severe traumatic brain injury. Neurology 1999;53:1963–8.

[29] Cramer S, Mark A, Barquist K, et al. Motor cortex activation is preserved in patients with chronic hemiplegic stroke. Ann Neurol 2002;52:607–16.

[30] Scarmeas N, Zarahn E, Anderson K, et al. Cognitive reserve modulates functional brain responses during

memory tasks: a PET study in healthy young and elderly subjects. Neuroimage 2003;19:1215–27.

[31] Sheth R. Epilepsy surgery. Presurgical evaluation. Neurol Clin 2002;20:1195–215.

[32] Wetzel U, Hindricks G, Dorszewski A, et al. Electroanatomic mapping of the endocardium. Implication for catheter ablation of ventricular tachycardia. Herz 2003;28:583–90.

[33] Cramer S, Benson R, Himes D, et al. Use of functional MRI to guide therapy in a clinical stroke trial. Stroke 2005;36(5):e50–2.

[34] Feeney D, Gonzalez A, Law W. Amphetamine, Halperidol, and experience interact to affect the rate of recovery after motor cortex injury. Science 1982; 217:855–7.

[35] Calautti C, Baron J. Functional neuroimaging studies of motor recovery after stroke in adults: a review. Stroke 2003;34:1553–66.

[36] Chen R, Cohen L, Hallett M. Nervous system reorganization following injury. Neuroscience 2002; 111:761–73.

[37] Cramer S, Bastings E. Mapping clinically relevant plasticity after stroke. Neuropharmacology 2000;39: 842–51.

[38] Rijntjes M, Weiller C. Recovery of motor and language abilities after stroke: the contribution of functional imaging. Prog Neurobiol 2002;66: 109–22.

[39] Cramer S, Nelles G, Schaechter J, et al. A functional MRI study of three motor tasks in the evaluation of stroke recovery. Neurorehabil Neural Repair 2001; 15:1–8.

[40] Ehrsson H, Fagergren A, Jonsson T, et al. Cortical activity in precision- versus power-grip tasks: an fMRI study. J Neurophysiol 2000;83:528–36.

[41] Cramer S, Weisskoff R, Schaechter J, et al. Motor cortex activation is related to force of squeezing. Hum Brain Mapp 2002;16:197–205.

[42] Dettmers C, Fink G, Lemon R, et al. Relation between cerebral activity and force in the motor areas of the human brain. J Neurophysiol 1995;74:802–15.

[43] Ward N, Frackowiak R. Age-related changes in the neural correlates of motor performance. Brain 2003; 126:873–88.

[44] Blinkenberg M, Bonde C, Holm S, et al. Rate dependence of regional cerebral activation during performance of a repetitive motor task: a PET study. J Cereb Blood Flow Metab 1996;16:794–803.

[45] Rao S, Bandettini P, Binder J, et al. Relationship between finger movement rate and functional magnetic resonance signal change in human primary motor cortex. J Cereb Blood Flow Metab 1996;16: 1250–4.

[46] Schlaug G, Sanes J, Thangaraj V, et al. Cerebral activation covaries with movement rate. Neuroreport 1996;7:879–83.

[47] VanMeter J, Maisog J, Zeffiro T, et al. Parametric analysis of functional neuroimages: application to a variable-rate motor task. Neuroimage 1995;2:273–83.

[48] Waldvogel D, van Gelderen P, Ishii K, et al. The effect of movement amplitude on activation in functional magnetic resonance imaging studies. J Cereb Blood Flow Metab 1999;19:1209–12.

[49] Gerloff C, Corwell B, Chen R, et al. The role of the human motor cortex in the control of complex and simple finger movement sequences. Brain 1998; 121(Pt 9):1695–709.

[50] Rao S, Binder J, Bandettini P, et al. Functional magnetic resonance imaging of complex human movements. Neurology 1993;43:2311–8.

[51] Sadato N, Campbell G, Ibanez V, et al. Complexity affects regional cerebral blood flow change during sequential finger movements. J Neurosci 1996;16: 2691–700.

[52] Duncan P, Jorgensen H, Wade D. Outcome measures in acute stroke trials: a systematic review and some recommendations to improve practice. Stroke 2000; 31:1429–38.

[53] Uchino K, Billheimer D, Cramer S. Entry criteria and baseline characteristics predict outcome in acute stroke trials. Stroke 2001;32:909–16.

[54] Cutter G, Baier M, Rudick R, et al. Development of a multiple sclerosis functional composite as a clinical trial outcome measure. Brain 1999;122:871–82.

[55] Ditunno J, Young W, Donovan W. The international standards booklet for neurological and functional classification of spinal cord injury. American Spinal Injury Association. Paraplegia 1994;32:70–80.

[56] Bilecen D, Radu E, Schulte A, et al. fMRI of the auditory cortex in patients with unilateral carotid artery steno-occlusive disease. J Magn Reson Imaging 2002;15:621–7.

[57] Carusone L, Srinivasan J, Gitelman D, et al. Hemodynamic response changes in cerebrovascular disease: implications for functional MR imaging. AJNR Am J Neuroradiol 2002;23:1222–8.

[58] Cramer S, Mark A, Maravilla K. Preserved cortical function with reduced cerebral blood flow after stroke. Stroke 2002;33:418.

[59] Hamzei F, Knab R, Weiller C, et al. The influence of extra- and intracranial artery disease on the BOLD signal in FMRI. Neuroimage 2003;20:1393–9.

[60] Hund-Georgiadis M, Mildner T, Georgiadis D, et al. Impaired hemodynamics and neural activation? A fMRI study of major cerebral artery stenosis. Neurology 2003;61:1276–9.

[61] Rossini P, Altamura C, Ferretti A, et al. Does cerebrovascular disease affect the coupling between neuronal activity and local haemodynamics? Brain 2004;127:99–110.

[62] Krakauer JW, Radoeva PD, Zarahn E, et al. Hypoperfusion without stroke alters motor activation in the opposite hemisphere. Ann Neurol 2004;56:796–802.

[63] Brion J-P, Demeurisse G, Capon A. Evidence of cortical reorganization in hemiparetic patients. Stroke 1989;20:1079–84.

[64] Ilmoniemi R, Virtanen J, Ruohonen J, et al. Neuronal responses to magnetic stimulation reveal cortical reactivity and connectivity. Neuroreport 1997;8: 3537–40.

[65] Lee L, Siebner H, Rowe J, et al. Acute remapping within the motor system induced by low-frequency repetitive transcranial magnetic stimulation. J Neurosci 2003;23:5308–18.

[66] Siebner H, Peller M, Willoch F, et al. Lasting cortical activation after repetitive TMS of the motor cortex: a glucose metabolic study. Neurology 2000;54: 956–63.

[67] Biernaskie J, Corbett D. Enriched rehabilitative training promotes improved forelimb motor function and enhanced dendritic growth after focal ischemic injury. J Neurosci 2001;21:5272–80.

[68] Dijkhuizen R, Singhal A, Mandeville J, et al. Correlation between brain reorganization, ischemic damage, and neurologic status after transient focal cerebral ischemia in rats: a functional magnetic resonance imaging study. J Neurosci 2003;23:510–7.

[69] Jones T, Kleim J, Greenough W. Synaptogenesis and dendritic growth in the cortex opposite unilateral sensorimotor cortex damage in adult rats: a quantitative electron microscopic examination. Brain Res 1996;733:142–8.

[70] Jones T, Schallert T. Overgrowth and pruning of dendrites in adult rats recovering from neocortical damage. Brain Res 1992;581:156–60.

[71] Kolb B. Plasticity and recovery in adulthood. In: Kolb B, editor. Brain plasticity and behavior. Mahwah (NJ): Lawrence Erlbaum Associates Publishers; 1995. p. 95–112.

[72] Liu Y, Rouiller E. Mechanisms of recovery of dexterity following unilateral lesion of the sensorimotor cortex in adult monkeys. Exp Brain Res 1999;128:149–59.

[73] Nudo R, Wise B, SiFuentes F, et al. Neural substrates for the effects of rehabilitative training on motor recovery after ischemic infarct. Science 1996;272: 1791–4.

[74] Xerri C, Merzenich M, Peterson B, et al. Plasticity of primary somatosensory cortex paralleling sensorimotor skill recovery from stroke in adult monkeys. J Neurophysiol 1998;79:2119–48.

[75] Grotta J, Bratina P. Subjective experiences of 24 patients dramatically recovering from stroke. Stroke 1995;26:1285–8.

[76] Carey J, Kimberley T, Lewis S, et al. Analysis of fMRI and finger tracking training in subjects with chronic stroke. Brain 2002;125:773–88.

[77] Liepert J, Bauder H, Wolfgang H, et al. Treatment-induced cortical reorganization after stroke in humans. Stroke 2000;31:1210–6.

[78] Pariente J, Loubinoux I, Carel C, et al. Fluoxetine modulates motor performance and cerebral activation of patients recovering from stroke. Ann Neurol 2001; 50:718–29.

[79] Chugani H, Phelps M, Mazziotta J. Positron emission tomography study of human brain functional development. Ann Neurol 1987;22:487–97.

[80] Cao Y, D'Olhaberriague L, Vikingstad E, et al. Pilot study of functional MRI to assess cerebral activation of motor function after poststroke hemiparesis. Stroke 1998;29:112–22.

[81] Chollet F, DiPiero V, Wise R, et al. The functional anatomy of motor recovery after stroke in humans: a study with positron emission tomography. Ann Neurol 1991;29:63–71.

[82] Cramer S, Nelles G, Benson R, et al. A functional MRI study of subjects recovered from hemiparetic stroke. Stroke 1997;28:2518–27.

[83] Hamdy S, Aziz Q, Rothwell J, et al. Recovery of swallowing after dysphagic stroke relates to functional reorganization in the intact motor cortex. Gastroenterology 1998;115:1104–12.

[84] Seitz R, Hoflich P, Binkofski F, et al. Role of the premotor cortex in recovery from middle cerebral artery infarction. Arch Neurol 1998;55:1081–8.

[85] Thulborn K, Carpenter P, Just M. Plasticity of language-related brain function during recovery from stroke. Stroke 1999;30:749–54.

[86] Weiller C, Ramsay S, Wise R, et al. Individual patterns of functional reorganization in the human cerebral cortex after capsular infarction. Ann Neurol 1993;33:181–9.

[87] Cabeza R. Hemispheric asymmetry reduction in older adults: the HAROLD model. Psychol Aging 2002; 17:85–100.

[88] Detre J. fMRI: applications in epilepsy. Epilepsia 2004;45(Suppl 4):26–31.

[89] Christodoulou C, DeLuca J, Ricker J, et al. Functional magnetic resonance imaging of working memory impairment after traumatic brain injury. J Neurol Neurosurg Psychiatry 2001;71:161–8.

[90] Lee M, Reddy H, Johansen-Berg H, et al. The motor cortex shows adaptive functional changes to brain injury from multiple sclerosis. Ann Neurol 2000;47: 606–13.

[91] Calautti C, Leroy F, Guincestre J, et al. Dynamics of motor network overactivation after striatocapsular stroke: a longitudinal PET study using a fixed-performance paradigm. Stroke 2001;32:2534–42.

[92] Feydy A, Carlier R, Roby-Brami A, et al. Longitudinal study of motor recovery after stroke: recruitment and focusing of brain activation. Stroke 2002; 33:1610–7.

[93] Fujii Y, Nakada T. Cortical reorganization in patients with subcortical hemiparesis: neural mechanisms of functional recovery and prognostic implication. J Neurosurg 2003;98:64–73.

[94] Heiss W, Kessler J, Thiel A, et al. Differential capacity of left and right hemispheric areas for compensation of poststroke aphasia. Ann Neurol 1999;45: 430–8.

[95] Marshall R, Perera G, Lazar R, et al. Evolution of cortical activation during recovery from corticospinal tract infarction. Stroke 2000;31:656–61.

[96] Nhan H, Barquist K, Bell K, et al. Brain function early after stroke in relation to subsequent recovery. J Cereb Blood Flow Metab 2004;24: 756–63.

[97] Kim S-G, Ashe J, Hendrich K, et al. Functional magnetic resonance imaging of motor cortex: hemispheric asymmetry and handedness. Science 1993; 261:615–7.

[98] Zemke A, Heagerty P, Lee C, et al. Motor cortex organization after stroke is related to side of stroke and level of recovery. Stroke 2003;34:E23–8.

[99] Luft A, Waller S, Forrester L, et al. Lesion location alters brain activation in chronically impaired stroke survivors. Neuroimage 2004;21:924–35.

[100] Just M, Carpenter P, Keller T, et al. Brain activation modulated by sentence comprehension. Science 1996;274:114–6.

[101] Shibasaki H, Sadato N, Lyshkow H, et al. Both primary motor cortex and supplementary motor area play an important role in complex finger movement. Brain 1993;116:1387–98.

[102] Wexler B, Fulbright R, Lacadie C, et al. An fMRI study of the human cortical motor system response to increasing functional demands. Magn Reson Imaging 1997;15:385–96.

[103] Lohmann H, Deppe M, Jansen A, et al. Task repetition can affect functional magnetic resonance imaging-based measures of language lateralization and lead to pseudoincreases in bilaterality. J Cereb Blood Flow Metab 2004;24:179–87.

[104] Colebatch J, Deiber M-P, Passingham R, et al. Regional cerebral blood flow during voluntary arm and hand movements in human subjects. J Neurophysiol 1991;65:1392–401.

[105] Cramer S, Crafton K. Somatotopy and movement representation sites following stroke. Exp Brain Res, in press.

[106] Vikingstad EM, George KP, Johnson AF, et al. Cortical language lateralization in right handed normal subjects using functional magnetic resonance imaging. J Neurol Sci 2000;175:17–27.

[107] Cramer S, Finklestein S, Schaechter J, et al. Distinct regions of motor cortex control ipsilateral and contralateral finger movements. J Neurophysiol 1999;81: 383–7.

[108] Netz J, Lammers T, Homberg V. Reorganization of motor output in the non-affected hemisphere after stroke. Brain 1997;120:1579–86.

[109] Turton A, Wroe S, Trepte N, et al. Contralateral and ipsilateral EMG responses to transcranial magnetic stimulation during recovery of arm and hand function after stroke. Electroencephalogr Clin Neurophys 1996;101:316–28.

[110] Shimizu T, Hosaki A, Hino T, et al. Motor cortical disinhibition in the unaffected hemisphere after unilateral cortical stroke. Brain 2002;125: 1896–907.

[111] Murase N, Duque J, Mazzocchio R, et al. Influence of interhemispheric interactions on motor function in chronic stroke. Ann Neurol 2004;55:400–9.

[112] Butefisch C, Netz J, Wessling M, et al. Remote

changes in cortical excitability after stroke. Brain 2003; 126:470–81.

[113] Cappa S, Perani D, Grassi F, et al. A PET follow-up study of recovery after stroke in acute aphasics. Brain Lang 1997;56:55–67.

[114] Cardebat D, Demonet J, De Boissezon X, et al. Behavioral and neurofunctional changes over time in healthy and aphasic subjects: a PET Language Activation Study. Stroke 2003;34:2900–6.

[115] Johansen-Berg H, Rushworth M, Bogdanovic M, et al. The role of ipsilateral premotor cortex in hand movement after stroke. Proc Natl Acad Sci USA 2002;99:14518–23.

[116] Buckner R, Corbetta M, Schatz J, et al. Preserved speech abilities and compensation following prefrontal damage. Proc Natl Acad Sci USA 1996;93: 1249–53.

[117] Gold B, Kertesz A. Right hemisphere semantic processing of visual words in an aphasic patient: an fMRI study. Brain Lang 2000;73:456–65.

[118] Calautti C, Leroy F, Guincestre J, et al. Displacement of primary sensorimotor cortex activation after subcortical stroke: a longitudinal PET study with clinical correlation. Neuroimage 2003;19:1650–4.

[119] Cramer S, Moore C, Finklestein S, et al. A pilot study of somatotopic mapping after cortical infarct. Stroke 2000;31:668–71.

[120] Pineiro R, Pendlebury S, Johansen-Berg H, et al. Functional mri detects posterior shifts in primary sensorimotor cortex activation after stroke: evidence of local adaptive reorganization? Stroke 2001;32: 1134–9.

[121] Rossini PM, Caltagirone C, Castriota-Scanderbeg A, et al. Hand motor cortical area reorganization in stroke: a study with fMRI, MEG and TCS maps. Neuroreport 1998;9:2141–6.

[122] Green J, Sora E, Bialy Y, et al. Cortical sensorimotor reorganization after spinal cord injury: an electroencephalographic study. Neurology 1998;50: 1115–21.

[123] Turner J, Lee J, Schandler S, et al. An fMRI investigation of hand representation in paraplegic humans. Neurorehabil Neural Repair 2003;17:37–47.

[124] Nelles G, Spiekermann G, Jueptner M, et al. Evolution of functional reorganization in hemiplegic stroke: a serial positron emission tomographic activation study. Ann Neurol 1999;46:901–9.

[125] Tombari D, Loubinoux I, Pariente J, et al. A longitudinal fMRI study: in recovering and then in clinically stable sub-cortical stroke patients. Neuroimage 2004;23:827–39.

[126] Traversa R, Cicinelli P, Bassi A, et al. Mapping of motor cortical reorganization after stroke. A brain stimulation study with focal magnetic pulses. Stroke 1997;28:110–7.

[127] Traversa R, Cicinelli P, Oliveri M, et al. Neurophysiological follow-up of motor cortical output in stroke patients. Clin Neurophysiol 2000;111: 1695–703.

[128] Cicinelli P, Traversa R, Rossini P. Post-stroke reorganization of brain motor output to the hand: a 2–4 month follow-up with focal magnetic transcranial stimulation. Electroencephalogr Clin Neurophysiol 1997;105:438–50.

[129] Nakayama H, Jorgensen H, Raaschou H, et al. Recovery of upper extremity function in stroke patients: the Copenhagen Stroke Study. Arch Phys Med Rehabil 1994;75:394–8.

[130] Ward N, Brown M, Thompson A, et al. Neural correlates of motor recovery after stroke: a longitudinal fMRI study. Brain 2003;126:2476–96.

[131] Cramer S, Fray E, Tievsky A, et al. Changes in motor cortex activation after recovery from spinal cord inflammation. Mult Scler 2001;7:364–70.

[132] Ward N, Brown M, Thompson A, et al. Neural correlates of outcome after stroke: a cross-sectional fMRI study. Brain 2003;126:1430–48.

[133] Rosen H, Petersen S, Linenweber M, et al. Neural correlates of recovery from aphasia after damage to left inferior frontal cortex. Neurology 2000;55: 1883–94.

[134] Butz M, Gross J, Timmermann L, et al. Perilesional pathological oscillatory activity in the magnetoencephalogram of patients with cortical brain lesions. Neurosci Lett 2004;355:93–6.

[135] Li Y, Jiang N, Powers C, et al. Neuronal damage and plasticity identified by MAP-2, GAP-43 and cyclin D1 immunoreactivity after focal cerebral ischemia in rat. Stroke 1998;29:1972–81.

[136] Baron J, D'Antona R, Pantano P, et al. Effects of thalamic stroke on energy metabolism of the cerebral cortex. A positron tomography study in man. Brain 1986;109:1243–59.

[137] Seitz R, Azari N, Knorr U, et al. The role of diaschisis in stroke recovery. Stroke 1999;30:1844–50.

[138] Witte O, Stoll G. Delayed and remote effects of focal cortical infarctions: secondary damage and reactive plasticity. Adv Neurol 1997;73:207–27.

[139] Heiss W, Emunds H, Herholz K. Cerebral glucose metabolism as a predictor of rehabilitation after ischemic stroke. Stroke 1993;24:1784–8.

[140] Dobkin B. The clinical science of neurologic rehabilitation. New York: Oxford University Press; 2003.

[141] Johansen-Berg H, Dawes H, Guy C, et al. Correlation between motor improvements and altered fMRI activity after rehabilitative therapy. Brain 2002;125: 2731–42.

[142] Liepert J, Miltner W, Bauder H, et al. Motor cortex plasticity during constraint-induced movement therapy in stroke patients. Neurosci Lett 1998;250: 5–8.

[143] Luft A, McCombe-Waller S, Whitall J, et al. Repetitive bilateral arm training and motor cortex activation in chronic stroke: a randomized controlled trial. JAMA 2004;292:1853–61.

[144] Schaechter J, Kraft E, Hilliard T, et al. Motor recovery and cortical reorganization after constraint-induced movement therapy in stroke patients: a pre-

liminary study. Neurorehabil Neural Repair 2002;16: 326–38.

[145] Wittenberg G, Chen R, Ishii K, et al. Constraint-induced therapy in stroke: magnetic-stimulation motor maps and cerebral activation. Neurorehabil Neural Repair 2003;17:48–57.

[146] Meinzer M, Elbert T, Wienbruch C, et al. Intensive language training enhances brain plasticity in chronic aphasia. BMC Biol 2004;2:20–8.

[147] Woldag H, Hummelsheim H. Evidence-based physiotherapeutic concepts for improving arm and hand function in stroke patients: a review. J Neurol 2002; 249:518–28.

[148] Butefisch C, Hummelsheim H, Denzler P, et al. Repetitive training of isolated movements improves the outcome of motor rehabilitation of the centrally paretic hand. J Neurol Sci 1995;130:59–68.

[149] Kwakkel G, Wagenaar RC, Twisk JW, et al. Intensity of leg and arm training after primary middle-cerebral-artery stroke: a randomised trial. Lancet 1999;354: 191–6.

[150] Karni A, Meyer G, Jezzard P, et al. Functional MRI evidence for adult motor cortex plasticity during motor skill learning. Nature 1996;377:155–8.

[151] Kleim J, Barbay S, Cooper N, et al. Motor learning-dependent synaptogenesis is localized to functionally reorganized motor cortex. Neurobiol Learn Mem 2002; 77:63–77.

[152] Nudo R, Plautz E, Frost S. Role of adaptive plasticity in recovery of function after damage to motor cortex. Muscle Nerve 2001;24:1000–19.

[153] Lotze M, Braun C, Birbaumer N, et al. Motor learning elicited by voluntary drive. Brain 2003;126:866–72.

[154] Kopp B, Kunkel A, Muhlnickel W, et al. Plasticity in the motor system related to therapy-induced improvement of movement after stroke. Neuroreport 1999; 10:807–10.

[155] Park SW, Butler AJ, Cavalheiro V, et al. Changes in serial optical topography and TMS during task performance after constraint-induced movement therapy in stroke: a case study. Neurorehabil Neural Repair 2004;18:95–105.

[156] Cauraugh J, Light K, Kim S, et al. Chronic motor dysfunction after stroke: recovering wrist and finger extension by electromyography-triggered neuromuscular stimulation. Stroke 2000;31:1360–4.

[157] Cauraugh JH, Kim S. Two coupled motor recovery protocols are better than one: electromyogram-triggered neuromuscular stimulation and bilateral movements. Stroke 2002;33:1589–94.

[158] Muellbacher W, Richards C, Ziemann U, et al. Improving hand function in chronic stroke. Arch Neurol 2002;59:1278–82.

[159] Lum PS, Burgar CG, Shor PC, et al. Robot-assisted movement training compared with conventional therapy techniques for the rehabilitation of upper-limb motor function after stroke. Arch Phys Med Rehabil 2002;83:952–9.

[160] Volpe BT, Krebs HI, Hogan N, et al. A novel approach to stroke rehabilitation: robot-aided sensorimotor stimulation. Neurology 2000;54:1938–44.

[161] Floel A, Nagorsen U, Werhahn KJ, et al. Influence of somatosensory input on motor function in patients with chronic stroke. Ann Neurol 2004;56:206–12.

[162] Bornschlegl M, Asanuma H. Importance of the projection from the sensory to the motor cortex for recovery of motor function following partial thalamic lesion in the monkey. Brain Res 1987;437:121–30.

[163] Pavlides C, Miyashita E, Asanuma H. Projection from the sensory to the motor cortex is important in learning motor skills in the monkey. J Neurophysiol 1993;70:733–41.

[164] Reinkensmeyer DJ, Emken JL, Cramer SC. Robotics, motor learning, and neurologic recovery. Annu Rev Biomed Eng 2004;6:497–525.

[165] Huttunen J, Wikstrom H, Korvenoja A, et al. Significance of the second somatosensory cortex in sensorimotor integration: enhancement of sensory responses during finger movements. Neuroreport 1996; 7:1009–12.

[166] Thickbroom G, Byrnes M, Archer S, et al. Differences in sensory and motor cortical organization following brain injury early in life. Ann Neurol 2001; 49:320–7.

[167] Diamond MC, Johnson RE, Gold MW. Changes in neuron number and size and glia number in the young, adult, and aging rat medial occipital cortex. Behav Biol 1977;20:409–18.

[168] Kempermann G, Kuhn HG, Gage FH. More hippocampal neurons in adult mice living in an enriched environment. Nature 1997;386:493–5.

[169] van Praag H, Kempermann G, Gage FH. Neural consequences of environmental enrichment. Nat Rev Neurosci 2000;1:191–8.

[170] Kolb B, Gibb R. Environmental enrichment and cortical injury: behavioral and anatomical consequences of frontal cortex lesions. Cereb Cortex 1991;1:189–98.

[171] Kolb B, Holmes C, Whishaw IQ. Recovery from early cortical lesions in rats. III. Neonatal removal of posterior parietal cortex has greater behavioral and anatomical effects than similar removals in adulthood. Behav Brain Res 1987;26:119–37.

[172] Johansson BB. Environmental influence on recovery after brain lesions–experimental and clinical data. J Rehabil Med 2003;41(Suppl):11–6.

[173] Will BE, Rosenzweig MR, Bennett EL, et al. Relatively brief environmental enrichment aids recovery of learning capacity and alters brain measures after postweaning brain lesions in rats. J Comp Physiol Psychol 1977;91:33–50.

[174] Langhorne P, Williams BO, Gilchrist W, et al. Do stroke units save lives? Lancet 1993;342:395–8.

[175] Ottenbacher KJ, Jannell S. The results of clinical trials in stroke rehabilitation research. Arch Neurol 1993;50:37–44.

[176] Holden MK, Dettwiler A, Dyar T, et al. Retraining movement in patients with acquired brain injury using

a virtual environment. Stud Health Technol Inform 2001;81:192–8.

[177] Jack D, Boian R, Merians AS, et al. Virtual reality-enhanced stroke rehabilitation. IEEE Trans Neural Syst Rehabil Eng 2001;9:308–18.

[178] Ku J, Mraz R, Baker N, et al. A data glove with tactile feedback for FMRI of virtual reality experiments. Cyberpsychol Behav 2003;6:497–508.

[179] Sisto SA, Forrest GF, Glendinning D. Virtual reality applications for motor rehabilitation after stroke. Top Stroke Rehabil 2002;8:11–23.

[180] Dhamala M, Pagnoni G, Wiesenfeld K, et al. Neural correlates of the complexity of rhythmic finger tapping. Neuroimage 2003;20:918–26.

[181] Stowe L, Broere C, Paans A, et al. Localizing components of a complex task: sentence processing and working memory. Neuroreport 1998;9:2995–9.

[182] Verstynen T, Diedrichsen J, Albert N, et al. Ipsilateral motor cortex activity during unimanual hand movements relates to task complexity. J Neurophysiol 2005;93:1209–22.

[183] Alon G, Sunnerhagen KS, Geurts AC, et al. A home-based, self-administered stimulation program to improve selected hand functions of chronic stroke. NeuroRehabilitation 2003;18:215–25.

[184] Carey JR, Kimberley TJ, Lewis SM, et al. Analysis of fMRI and finger tracking training in subjects with chronic stroke. Brain 2002;125:773–88.

[185] Nelson DL, Konosky K, Fleharty K, et al. The effects of an occupationally embedded exercise on bilaterally assisted supination in persons with hemiplegia. Am J Occup Ther 1996;50:639–46.

[186] Schaechter JD. Motor rehabilitation and brain plasticity after hemiparetic stroke. Prog Neurobiol 2004; 73:61–72.

[187] Trombly CA, Wu CY. Effect of rehabilitation tasks on organization of movement after stroke. Am J Occup Ther 1999;53:333–44.

[188] Ma HI, Trombly CA, Robinson-Podolski C. The effect of context on skill acquisition and transfer. Am J Occup Ther 1999;53:138–44.

[189] Wu C, Trombly CA, Lin K, et al. Effects of object affordances on reaching performance in persons with and without cerebrovascular accident. Am J Occup Ther 1998;52:447–56.

[190] Wu C, Trombly CA, Lin K, et al. A kinematic study of contextual effects on reaching performance in persons with and without stroke: influences of object availability. Arch Phys Med Rehabil 2000;81: 95–101.

[191] Hsieh CL, Nelson DL, Smith DA, et al. A comparison of performance in added-purpose occupations and rote exercise for dynamic standing balance in persons with hemiplegia. Am J Occup Ther 1996;50: 10–6.

[192] Lee TD, Swanson LR, Hall AL. What is repeated in a repetition? Effects of practice conditions on motor skill acquisition. Phys Ther 1991;71:150–6.

[193] Hall KG, Magill RA. Variability of practice and contextual interference in motor skill learning. J Mot Behav 1995;27:299–309.

[194] Immink MA, Wright DL. Motor programming during practice conditions high and low in contextual interference. J Exp Psychol Hum Percept Perform 2001;27:423–37.

[195] Shea CH, Lai Q, Wright DL, et al. Consistent and variable practice conditions: effects on relative and absolute timing. J Mot Behav 2001;33:139–52.

[196] Ste-Marie DM, Clark SE, Findlay LC, et al. High levels of contextual interference enhance handwriting skill acquisition. J Mot Behav 2004;36:115–26.

[197] Wulf G, Schmidt RA. Variability in practice: facilitation in retention and transfer through schema formation or context effects? J Mot Behav 1988;20: 133–49.

[198] Stefan K, Wycislo M, Classen J. Modulation of associative human motor cortical plasticity by attention. J Neurophysiol 2004;92:66–72.

[199] Baker J, Donoghue J, Sanes J. Gaze direction modulates finger movement activation patterns in human cerebral cortex. J Neurosci 1999;19:10044–52.

[200] Li Y, Wright DL. An assessment of the attention demands during random- and blocked-practice schedules. Q J Exp Psychol [A] 2000;53:591–606.

ELSEVIER
SAUNDERS

Neuroimag Clin N Am 15 (2005) 697 – 720

NEUROIMAGING
CLINICS OF
NORTH AMERICA

Advances in Stroke Neuroprotection: Hyperoxia and Beyond

Aneesh B. Singhal, MD[a,b],*, Eng H. Lo, PhD[a,c], Turgay Dalkara, MD, PhD[d], Michael A. Moskowitz, MD[a,e]

[a]*Harvard Medical School, Boston, MA, USA*
[b]*Stroke Service, Department of Neurology, Massachusetts General Hospital, Boston, MA, USA*
[c]*Neuroprotection Research Laboratory, Department of Radiology, Massachusetts General Hospital, Charlestown, MA, USA*
[d]*Faculty of Medicine, Hacettepe University, Ankara, Turkey*
[e]*Stroke and Neurovascular Regulation Laboratory, Neuroscience Center, Departments of Radiology and Neurology,*
Massachusetts General Hospital, Charlestown, MA, USA

The field of ischemic stroke therapy is evolving rapidly. During the past 2 decades, several mechanisms of cell death after stroke have been delineated, yielding multiple molecular and biochemical targets for stroke treatment, and numerous neuroprotective drugs have been developed. Several of these drugs have proved effective in reducing infarction size and functional deficits in animal models of stroke. Although no neuroprotective drug has shown efficacy in clinical trials, much knowledge has been gained. Now there is a better understanding of factors, such as the therapeutic time window and optimal patient selection, that are critical for success. Neuroimaging simultaneously has advanced—at an astonishing pace—and now it is possible to determine ischemic lesion size and stroke mechanism accurately within minutes of symptom onset and perhaps identify patients who have a higher likelihood of response to acute stroke therapy. Preliminary results of ongoing stroke trials are promising, suggesting that successful stroke neuroprotection will be achieved in the near future. This article provides an overview of the major mechanisms of neuronal injury and the status of neuroprotective drug trials and reviews emerging strategies for treatment of acute ischemic stroke, including

normobaric hyperoxia, hypothermia, and the application of neuroimaging in stroke neuroprotection.

Basic mechanisms of ischemic cell death

The major mechanisms of ischemic cell death include excitotoxicity, oxidative/nitrative stress, inflammation, apoptosis, and perinfarction depolarization (Fig. 1). These fundamental mechanisms are interdepedendent, have several overlapping features, and evolve over time to mediate injury in neuronal cells, glial cells, and vascular elements (Fig. 2). The individual contribution of each mechanism toward the net stroke-related injury varies with time, the degree of ischemia, and the timing of reperfusion. In areas of severely reduced blood flow or the "core" of the ischemic territory, excitotoxic cell death plays a dominant role and cell death occurs within minutes. In the peripheral zones that are supported by collateral circulation (the "ischemic penumbra"), cell death occurs relatively slowly via mechanisms, such as inflammation, apoptosis, and peri-infarction depolarization.

Excitotoxicity and ionic imbalance

Interruption of blood flow leads to deprivation of oxygen and glucose supply to the cell, resulting in failure of energy-dependent processes, such as the sodium-potassium adenosine triphosphatase. Energy

* Corresponding author. VBK-802, Stroke Service, Department of Neurology, Massachusetts General Hospital, Boston, MA 02114.
E-mail address: asinghal@partners.org (A.B. Singhal).

neuroimaging.theclinics.com

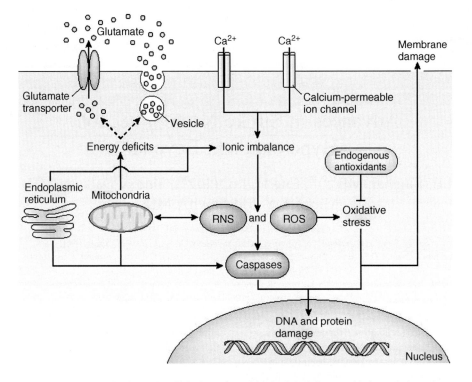

Fig. 1. Major pathways implicated in ischemic cell death: excitotoxicity, ionic imbalance, oxidative and nitrosative stresses, and apoptotic-like mechanisms. There is extensive interaction and overlap between multiple mediators of cell injury and cell death. After ischemic onset, loss of energy substrates leads to mitochondrial dysfunction and generation of reactive oxygen species (ROS) and reactive nitrogen species (RNS). Additionally, energy deficits lead to ionic imbalance, excitotoxic glutamate efflux, and build-up of intracellular calcium. Downstream pathways ultimately include direct free radical damage to membrane lipids, cellular proteins, DNA, and calcium-activated proteases plus caspase cascades that dismantle a wide range of homeostatic, reparative and cytoskeletal proteins. (*Reprinted from* Lo EH, Dalkara T, Moskowitz MA. Mechanisms, challenges and opportunities in stroke. Nature Nat Rev Neurosci 2003;4:399–415; with permission.)

loss causes ionic imbalance and neurotransmitter release and inhibits the reuptake of neurotransmitters, such as glutamate [1,2]. Excessive glutamate binding to ionotropic N-methyl-D-aspartate (NMDA) and alpha-amino-3-hydroxy-5-methyl-4-isoxazole-propionic acid (AMPA) receptors promotes the influx of calcium, with activation of downstream phospholipases and proteases that degrade membranes and proteins that are essential for cellular integrity. Ionotropic glutamate receptors also promote perturbations in ionic homeostasis that play a critical role in cerebral ischemia. Pharmaceutical agents that block the glutamate, NMDA, AMPA, and the metabotropic subfamily of receptors attenuate stroke lesion volumes in experimental models of stroke [3,4].

Oxidative and nitrosative stress

Reactive oxygen species, such as superoxide and hydroxyl radicals, normally are produced by mito-chondria during electron transport. These toxic free radicals are scavenged routinely by endogenous antioxidant enzymes, including superoxide dismutase (SOD), catalase and glutathione, and antioxidant vitamins (eg, α-tocopherol and ascorbic acid). Oxidative and nitrosative stresses are modulated by enzyme systems, such as SOD and the nitric oxide synthase (NOS) family. Mice with enhanced SOD expression show reduced injury after cerebral ischemia [5–8]. Similarly, mice with deficient expression of the neuronal and inducible NOS (iNOS) isoforms show reduced stroke-induced injury [9,10]. Ischemia-induced accululation of intracellular Ca^{++}, Na^+, and adenosine 5c-diphosphate (ADP) stimulates excessive mitochondrial, oxygen-free radical production, which overwhelms endogenous scavenging mechanisms and directly damages lipids, proteins, nucleic acids, and carbohydrates [11]. Oxygen radicals also are produced during enzymatic conversions, such as the cyclooxygenase-dependent conversion of arachidonic acid to prostanoids and

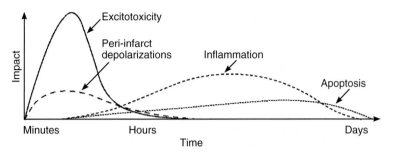

Fig. 2. Putative cascade of damaging events in focal cerebral ischaemia: early after the onset of the focal perfusion deficit, excitotoxic mechanisms can damage neurones and glia lethally. In addition, excitotoxicity triggers events that can contribute further to the demise of the tissue. Such events include PIDs and the more-delayed mechanisms of inflammation and programmed cell death. The *x* axis reflects the evolution of the cascade over time, whereas the *y* axis aims to illustrate the impact of each element of the cascade on final outcome. (*Reprinted from* Dirnagl U, Iadecola C, Moskowitz MA. Pathobiology of ischemic stroke: an integrated view. Trends Neurosci 1999;22:391–7; with permission.)

degradation of hypoxanthine, especially upon reperfusion, and substantial amounts of free radicals are generated during the inflammatory response after ischemia. Oxygen radicals and oxidative stress facilitate mitochondrial transition pore formation, which dissipates the proton motive force required for oxidative phosphorylation and adenosine triphosphate (ATP) generation [12]. As a result, mitochondria release apoptosis-related proteins and other constituents within the inner and outer mitochondrial membranes [13]. Thus, oxidative stress, excitotoxicity, apoptosis, and inflammation are linked closely and together contribute to ischemic cell death.

Apoptosis

Apoptosis, or programmed cell death [14], is characterized histologically by terminal dUTP nick-end labeling (TUNEL)–positive cells that exhibit DNA laddering. Cell type, cell age, and brain location render cells more or less resistant to apoptosis or necrosis. Because apoptptic pathways require energy in the form of ATP, apoptosis occurs predominantly in the ischemic penumbra (which sustains milder injury) rather than in the ischemic core, where ATP levels are depleted rapidly [15].

Apoptogenic triggers [16] include oxygen free radicals [17], Bid cleavage, death receptor ligation [18], DNA damage, and, possibly, lysosomal protease activation [19]. Apoptosis occurs via caspase-dependent and caspase-independent mechanisms. Caspases are protein-cleaving enzymes (zymogens) that belong to a family of cysteine aspartases constitutively expressed in adult and especially newborn brain cells, particularly neurons. The normal human brain expresses caspases 1, 3, 8, and 9; apoptosis protease-activating factor 1 (Apaf-1); death receptors; P53; and

several Bcl2 family members, all of which are implicated in apoptosis. The tumor necrosis factor (TNF) superfamily of death receptors regulates upstream caspase processes powerfully. Emerging data suggests that the nucleus is involved in releasing signals for apoptosis and the mitochondrion plays a central role in mediating apoptosis [20,21]. At least four mitochondrial molecules mediate downstream cell-death pathways: cytochrome *c,* secondary mitochondria-derived activator of caspase (Smac/DIABLO), apoptosis-inducing factor, and endonuclease G [22]. Apoptosis-inducing factor and endonuclease G mediate caspase-independent apoptosis. Cytochrome *c* and Smac/DIABLO mediate caspase-dependent apoptosis. Cytochrome *c* binds to Apaf-1, which, together with procaspase 9, forms the "apoptosome" that activates caspase 9. In turn, caspase 9 activates caspase 3. Smac/DIABLO binds to inhibitors of activated caspases and causes further caspase activation. Upon activation, executioner caspases (caspase 3 and 7) target and degrade many substrate proteins, including gelsolin, actin, poly ADP-ribose polymerase (PARP-1), inhibitor of caspase-activated DNase (ICAD) and other caspases, ultimately leading to DNA fragmentation and cell death (Fig. 3). Caspase-3 inhibitors [23], gene deletions of Bid or caspase-3 [24], and the use of peptide inhibitors, viral vector-mediated gene transfer, and antisense oligonucleotides that suppress the expression and activity of apoptosis genes all are neuroprotective [25]. Caspase inhibitors do not, however, reduce infarction size in all brain ischemia models, perhaps because of the greater severity of ischemia, limited potency or inability of the agent to cross the blood-brain barrier, relatively minor impact of apoptosis on stroke outcome, and upregulation of caspase-independent or redundant cell death pathways.

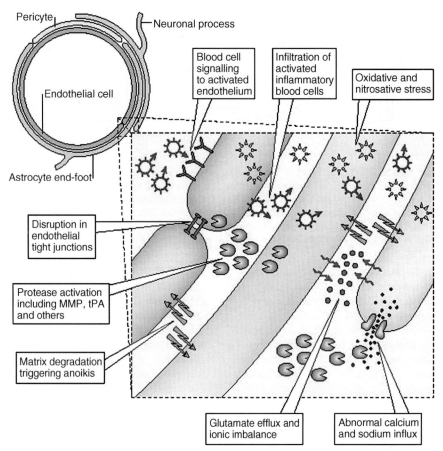

Fig. 3. Schematic view of the neurovascular unit or module and some of its components: circulating blood elements, endothelial cells, astrocytes, extracellular matrix, basal lamina, adjacent neurons, and pericytes. After ischemia, perturbations in neurovascular functional integrity initiate multiple cascades of injury. Upstream signals, such as oxidative stress together with neutrophil or platelet interactions with activated endothelium, upregulate MMPs, PAs, and other proteases, which degrade matrix and lead to blood-brain barrier leakage. Inflammatory infiltrates through the damaged blood-brain barrier amplify brain tissue injury. Additionally, disruption of cell-matrix homeostasis also may trigger anoikis-like cell death in vascular and parenchymal compartments. Overlaps with excitotoxicity also are documented via tPA-mediated interactions with the NMDA receptor that augment ionic imbalance and cell death. (*Reprinted from* Lo EH, Dalkara T, Moskowitz MA. Mechanisms, challenges and opportunities in stroke. Nature Nat Rev Neurosci 2003;4:399–415; with permission.)

Inflammation

Inflammation is related intricately to atherosclerosis, stroke onset [26,27], and subsequent stroke-related tissue damage. Elevated stroke risk is linked to high levels of serologic markers of inflammation, such as C-reactive protein [28], erythrocyte sedimentation rate, interleukin (IL)-6, TNF-α, and soluble intercellular adhesion molecule [29]. Arterial thrombosis associated with plaque ulceration is triggered by multiple processes involving endothelial activation and proinflammatory and prothrombotic interactions between vessel wall and circulating blood elements. Ischemic stroke-related brain injury itself triggers in-

flammatory cascades within the parenchyma that amplify tissue damage further [30,31]. As reactive microglia, macrophages, and leukocytes are recruited into ischemic brain, inflammatory mediators are generated by these cells and by neurons and astrocytes. iNOS, cyclooxygenase-2 (COX-2), IL-1, and monocyte chemoattractant protein-1 (MCP-1) are key inflammatory mediators, as evidenced by attenuated ischemic injury in mutant mice with targeted disruption of these genes [31–35]. Initially after occlusion, there is a transient upregulation of immediate early genes encoding transcription factors (eg, *c-fos* and *c-jun*) that occurs within minutes. This is followed by a second wave of heat shock genes (eg, HSP70 and

HSP72) that increase within 1 to 2 hours and then decrease by 1 to 2 days. Approximately 12 to 24 hrs after stroke, a third wave comprised of chemokines and cytokines is expressed (IL-1, IL-6, IL-8, TNF-α, MCP-1, and so forth). Whether or not these 3 waves are related causally is not known.

Peri-infarction depolarizations

Brain tissue depolarizations after ischemic stroke are believed to play a vital role in recruiting adjacent penumbral regions of reversible injury into the core area of infarction. In penumbral regions after stroke, where blood supply is compromised, waves of spreading depression (peri-infarction depolarizations [PIDs]) exacerbate tissue damage, perhaps as a result of the increased energy requirements for re-establishing ionic equilibrium in the metabolically compromised ischemic tissues [3]. PIDs have been demonstrated in mice, rat, and cat stroke models [36,37]; however, their relevance to human stroke pathophysiology remains unclear. In the initial 2 to 6 hours after experimental stroke, PIDs result in a step-wise increase in the region of core-infarcted tissue into adjacent penumbral regions [38,39], and the incidence and total duration of spreading depression correlates with infarction size [40]. Recent evidence suggests that PIDs contribute to the expansion of the infarction core throughout the period of infarction maturation [41]. Inhibition of spreading depression using pharmaceutical agents, such as NMDA or glycine antagonists [41,42], or physiologic approaches, such as hypothermia [43], could be an important strategy to suppress the expansion of an ischemic lesion.

White matter ischemia and the neurovascular unit

In addition to stroke size, the location of the stroke and the relative involvement of gray versus white matter are key determinants of outcome. Cells within the gray and white matter have different susceptibilities to ischemic injury. Among neurons, the CA1 hippocampal pyramidal neurons, cortical projection neurons in layer 3, neurons in dorsolateral striatum, and cerebellar Purkinje cells, particularly are susceptible and undergo selective death after transient global cerebral ischemia [44]. Among the cell types comprising the white matter, oligodendrocytes are more vulnerable than astroglial or endothelial cells. White matter ischemia typically is severe, with rapid cell swelling and tissue edema, because there is little collateral blood supply in deep white matter. Cell death mechanisms, such as excitotoxicity, have different

pathophysiology in white matter ischemia compared with gray matter [45].

Tissue injury after stroke is not restricted to the cellular components of the gray and white matter but involves the endothelial and vascular smooth muscle cells, the astro- and microglia, and associated tissue matrix proteins (ie, the neurovascular unit) (see Fig. 3) [46]. Endothelial-astrocyte-matrix interactions are vital in protecting the integrity of brain tissue [47]. Disruption of the neurovascular matrix, which includes basement membrane components, such as type IV collagen, heparan sulfate proteoglycan, laminin, and fibronectin, upsets cell-matrix and cell-cell signaling that maintains neurovascular homeostasis. Although many proteases, including cathepsins and heparanases, contribute to extracellular matrix proteolysis, in the context of stroke, plasminogen activator (PA) and matrix metalloproteinases (MMPs) probably are the two most important [46]. This is because tissue PA (tPA) is used successfully as a stroke therapy and because emerging data show important links between tPA, MMPs, edema, and hemorrhage after stroke [48]. The potential efficacy of MMP inhibitors in ameliorating ischemic damage after stroke is being actively investigated [46,49–52].

Neuroprotection

Neuroprotection can be defined as the protection of cell bodies and neuronal and gial processes by strategies that interrupt the cellular processes involved in the development of irreversible ischemic injury. Neuroprotection after stroke can be achieved using pharmaceutical or physiologic therapies that inhibit biochemical, metabolic, cellular consequences of ischemic injury directly or by using indirect approaches, such as tPA and mechanical devices, that restore blood flow promptly to ischemic tissues. The complex and overlapping pathways involving excitotoxicity, ionic imbalance, oxidative and nitrosative stress, and apoptotic-like mechanisms are discussed previously. Each of these pathways offers several potential therapeutic targets, several of which have proved successful in reducing ischemic injury in animal models.

Prior stroke neuroprotective trials

Despite promise in animal studies, no neuroprotective agent (with the exception of rtPA in the National Institute of Neurological Disorders and Stroke trial) [53] has proved efficacious in phase III randomized clinical trials. The single agent that came close was cytidine-5′-diphosphocholine or CDP-choline (citicoline), an intermediate in the biosynthesis of phosphatidylcholine. Citicoline showed promise in animal studies and in several phase II clinical trials. A phase III efficacy trial failed to show benefit in the primary analysis; however, post-hoc secondary analysis indicates modest efficacy. Citicholine also reduced the growth of lesions on diffusion-weighted MR imaging. Other agents that have been tested but failed to prove effective include the lipid peroxidation inhibitor tirilazad mesylate [54], the intercellular adhesion molecule (ICAM)-1 antibody enlimomab [55], the calcium channel blocker nimodipine [56], the γ-aminobutyric acid (GABA) agonist clomethiazole [57,58], the glutamate antagonist and sodium channel blocker lubeluzole [59], the competitive NMDA antagonist selfotel [60], and several noncompetitive NMDA antagonists (dextrorphan, gavestinel, aptiganel, and eliprodil) [61–63].

The lack of efficacy can be related to several factors, some relating to the preclinical stage of drug development and others to clinical trial design and methodology. Nevertheless, much knowledge has been gained through past failures, laying a strong foundation for the possibility of success. It is becoming clear that factors, such as the therapeutic time window, stroke location and mechanism, and choice of endpoint measures, are critical for trial design. The focus has shifted toward expanding the therapeutic time window, improved patient selection, the use of brain imaging as a selection criterion, combination acute stroke treatments, use of validated rating scales to assess functional endpoints, and improved stroke trial design and organization [64,65].

Ongoing neuroprotective drug trials

Several new neuroprotection trials currently are underway or in the planning stages. These include trials of the free radical spin trap agent NXY-059; intravenous (IV) magnesium; the antioxidant, Ebselen; the AMPA antagonist, YM872; and the serotonin antagonist, Repinotan [66–68]. In addition, a phase III trial of the novel thromboltyic agent desmoteplase and several phase II/III studies of non-pharmacologic strategies, such as hyperoxia, induced hypertension, and hypothermia, currently are underway. With the insights gained from prior neuroprotective trials, it is anticipated one or more of the impending trials will prove successful. A brief review of some of the ongoing trials is provided.

NXY-059: Stroke-Acute Ischemic-NXY Treatment trials

Disodium 4-[(*tert*-butylimino) methyl] benzene-1,3-disulfonate *N*-oxide (NXY-059 [Cerovive]), is a nitrone-based free radical scavenger. Experimental studies in rodent, rabbit, and primate stroke models show that NXY-059 is an effective neuroprotective agent in transient (reperfusion) and permanent focal ischaemia, has a relatively long therapeutic time window, improves histologic and neurobehavioral outcomes after stroke, and can be combined safely with tPA [69–73]. NXY-059 also shows promise in reducing tPA-associated brain hemorrhage [74]. Based on these promising preclinical results and the results of tolerability and pharmacokinetic studies in humans [68,75,76], AstraZeneca Pharmaceuticals has initiated phase II/III clinical trials of NXY-059 in ischemic and hemorrhagic stroke. Preliminary results of the Stroke-Acute Ischemic-NXY Treatment (SAINT) trial, conducted in more than 200 centers across Europe, Asia, Australia, and South Africa, were presented in May 2005. In this study, 1772 patients who had acute ischemic stroke less than 6 hours and National Institutes of Health stroke scale score (NIHSSS) greater than or equal to 6 (including limb weakness) were randomized to 72-hour IV infusions of either placebo or NXY-059. The coprimary outcome measures were a significant difference in modified Rankin scale scores at 3 months and an improvement in NIHSSS from baseline to 3 months. The group treated with NXY-059 showed a significant improvement in modified Rankin scale at 3 months ($P = 0.038$, intention-to-treat analysis); however, there was no significant improvement in NIHSSS ($P = 0.86$). There was no significant difference in secondary outcome measures, such as the Barthel Index, at 3 months ($P = 0.18$). Subgroup analysis did not show any significant clinical benefit of NXY-059 in patients who were treated with tPA ($P = 0.93$ versus patients treated with placebo and tPA); however, the incidence of thrombolysis-associated hemorrhage was lower in the NXY-059 group (6.4% versus 2.5%). Although these results seem encouraging, the results of SAINT-II, a similar study currently being conducted in North America, will help clarify whether or not this drug has promise as an acute stroke therapy.

Desmoteplase trials and the usefulness of neuroimaging

Several investigators hypothesize that neuroimaging tools, such as MR imaging and CT, can help optimize the selection of candidates for thrombolytic therapy or for adjunctive therapy many hours after stroke onset and also provide quantitative surrogate endpoints for clinical trials. With MR imaging, there often is a volume mismatch between tissue showing reduced water molecule diffusion (a signature for cell swelling and ischemic tissue) and a larger area of tissue hypoperfusion early after stroke onset—the so-called "perfusion-diffusion mismatch." The difference, at least for practical purposes, is believed to reflect the ischemic penumbra or tissue more likely to be salvaged with acute intervention [77–81]. Perfusion MR imaging currently affords a relative, rather than absolute, quantitative measure of cerebral tissue perfusion. Recent studies indicate that perfusion CT also can be used to identify regions of ischemic, noninfarcted tissue after stroke and that perfusion CT may be comparable to MR imaging for this purpose [82–84]. The main advantage of perfusion CT is that it allows rapid data acquisition and postprocessing and can be performed in conjunction with CT angiography to complete the initial evaluation of stroke [85].

The Desmoteplase in Acute Ischemic Stroke trial (DIAS) is the first published acute stroke thrombolysis trial using MR imaging for patient selection and as a primary efficacy endpoint [86]. In this trial, patients were selected on basis of greater than 20% perfusion-diffusion mismatch on the admission MR and treated as late as 3 to 9 hours after stroke symptom onset with 3 doses of IV desmoteplase, a newer PA with high fibrin specificity. Patients who were treated with desmoteplase had significantly higher rates of reperfusion, as defined by MR perfusion, and improved 90-day clinical outcome. The results of the Dose Escalation Study of Desmoteplase in Acute Ischemic Stroke (DEDAS) recently have become available. This study was performed in the United States with a study design similar to DIAS. Thirty-eight patients who had NIHSSS between 4 and 20 and at least 20% perfusion-diffusion mismatch on MR imaging were treated with one of two doses of desmoteplase (90 μg/kg and 120 μg/kg) or placebo. Clinical improvement, as assessed by a combined endpoint of NIHSSS, modifed Rankin scale, and Barthel Index scores, was achieved in 60% of patients treated with 125 μg/kg desmoteplase, 29% of patients treated with 90 μg/kg desmoteplase, and 25% of those treated with placebo. Reperfusion within 8 hours of treatment was achieved in 53% of patients in the 125-μg/kg dose group, 18% of patients in 90-μg/kg dose group, and in 38% of the placebo group. These results replicate closely the findings in the 125-μg/kg group from DIAS trial.

The DIAS/DEDAS and the Normobaric Hyperoxia in Acute Ischemic Stroke pilot study [87] (discussed later) are the first clinical trials to demonstrate the advantages of using MR imaging to improve patient selection and reduce the sample size required for stroke clinical trials. Similar to the citicholine study, these studies suggest that MR imaging is a useful surrogate outcome measure. The positive results of these studies support the concept that tissue viability is heterogeneous distal to an occluded brain blood vessel. Although positron emission tomography arguably is the most accurate method of detecting ischemic but viable tissue, the experience with MR imaging gained in these studies indicates that the greatest promise lies with multimodal MR imaging. It is possible that multimodal CT, because of its widespread availability, lower cost, and shorter imaging times, similarly will prove to be a useful tool to select patients who are more likely to benefit from thrombolytic therapy. The DIAS investigators have launched a second randomized clinical trial wherein patients are selected based on the presence of mismatch on either diffusion-perfusion MR imaging or perfusion-CT studies.

Intravenous magnesium trials

Magnesium has several potentially beneficial effects: it inhibits presynaptic glutamate release [88], blocks NMDA receptors [89], antagonizes calcium channels, and maintains cerebral blood flow [90]. In animal models, administration of IV magnesium as late as 6 hours after stroke onset reduces infarction volumes [91,92]. In pilot clinical studies, magnesium is found to reduce death and disability from stroke, raising expectations that magnesium could be a safe and inexpensive treatment [93]. Intravenous Magnesium Efficacy in Stroke (IMAGES) was a large multicenter trial involving 2589 patients treated with IV magnesium or normal saline (placebo) within 12 hours after acute stroke. The primary clinical outcome (death or disability at 3 months) was not improved by magnesium, although some benefit was documented in subcortical (lacunar) strokes [66]. MR-IMAGES is an ongoing substudy designed to assess whether or not magnesium reduces the frequency of infarction growth on serial MR imaging studies. Field Administration of Stroke Therapy—Magnesium (FAST-MAG) is a phase III trialdesigned to determine whether or not paramedic initiation of magnesium, by reducing the time to treatment, yields benefit in stroke patients [94].

Albumin: the Albumin in Acute Stroke trial

Ginsberg's group has shown that albumin infusions enhance red cell perfusion and suppress thrombosis and leucocyte adhesion within the brain microcirculation, particularly during the early reperfusion phase after experimental focal ischemia [95]. Albumin also lowers the hematocrit significantly and by so doing improves microcirculatory flow, viscosity of plasma and cell deformability, and oxygen transport capacity. Albumin reduces infarction size, improves neurologic scores, and reduces cerebral edema in experimental animals [96]. These effects may reflect a combination of therapeutic properties, including its antioxidant effects, antiapoptotic effects on the endothelium, and effects on reducing blood stasis within the microcirculation. The safety of IV human serum albumin in patients who have acute (<16 hours) ischemic stroke is being tested in the Albumin in Acute Stroke trial, an open-labeled, dose-escalation, nonrandomized pilot clinical trial being conducted at two centers in North America.

Statins

3-Hydroxy-3-methylglutaryl coenzyme A reductase inhibitors (statins) are shown to improve vascular outcomes as a result of their cholesterol-lowering effects and multiple pleiotrophic effects [97]. Pretreatment with statins reduces infarction volumes and improve outcomes in rodent stroke studies [98,99]. In high-risk populations, statin therapy is known to reduce the risk of vascular events, such as myocardial infarction (MI) and stroke. A meta-analysis of 10 trials involving 79,494 subjects [100] shows that statin therapy reduces the incidence of stroke by 18%, major coronary events by 27%, and all-cause mortality by 15%. Several studies show that prior statin

treatment reduces the severity of acute ischemic stroke and MI [101–104].

Recent studies indicate that benefit can be achieved even when treatment is initiated after the onset of symptoms. In rodents, atorvastatin and simvastatin reduce the growth of ischemic lesions, enhance functional outcome, and induce brain plasticity when administered after stroke onset [105,106]. A retrospective analysis of the population-based Northern Manhattan Stroke Study [107] shows that patients using lipid-lowering agents (mainly statins) at the time of ischemic stroke have a lower incidence of clinical worsening during hospitalization and reduced 90-day mortality rates. Retrospective multivariable analysis of data from 852 patients enrolled in the phase III citicoline trial shows that poststroke statin use (123 patients) predicts good functional outcome on the modified Rankin scale and NIHSSS at 3 months [108]. In support of these data, several groups report that statins reduce the incidence and severity of vasospasm after subarachnoid hemorrhage [109,110]. Furthermore, recent animal and human studies indicate that withdrawal of statins after subarachnoid hemorrhage and ischemic stroke may have deleterious effects [111,112]. Clinical trials also provide some evidence of improved poststroke outcomes with statin use. A small pilot study from Spain (Markers of Inflammation after Simvastatin in Ischemic Cortical Stroke) shows significant improvement in the 3-day and 90-day NIHSSS in patients treated with simvastatin 3 to 12 hours after stroke onset compared with patients treated with placebo [113]. Based on

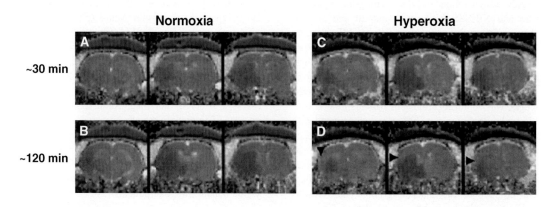

Fig. 4. Trace ADC maps of adjacent coronal rat brain slices at approximately 30 minutes (*A* and *C*) and approximately 120 minutes (*B* and *D*) after MCA occlusion. Note the increase in lesion size between the approximately 30-minute (*A*) and approximately 120-minute (*B*) scans in the normoxic animal. In the hyperoxic animal, who received 100% oxygen from approximately 45 minutes after MCA occlusion, the lesion reduced in size between the 30-minute (*C*) and 120-minute (*D*) scans, particularly in cortical borderzone regions (*black arrowheads*). (*Reprinted from* Singhal AB, Dijkhuizen RM, Rosen BR, et al. Normobaric hyperoxia reduces MR imaging diffusion abnormalities and infarct size in experimental stroke. Neurology 2002; 58:945–52; with permission.)

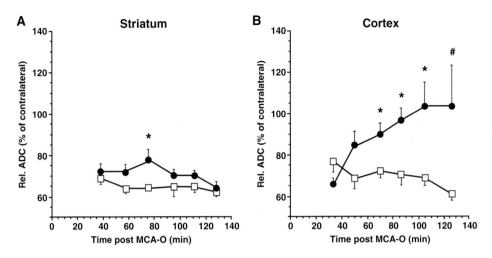

Fig. 5. Temporal changes in relative ADC (% of contralateral) in the ischemic striatum (*A*) and cortical borderzone (*B*) in the MR imaging–normoxia (*white boxes*) and MR imaging–hyperoxia (*black circles*) groups: The MR imaging–hyperoxia group received 100% oxygen from approximately 45 minutes after MCA occlusion. *, $P < 0.05$; #, $P = 0.057$ versus MRI-normoxia group). (*Reprinted from* Singhal AB, Dijkhuizen RM, Rosen BR, et al. Normobaric hyperoxia reduces MRI diffusion abnormalities and infarct size in experimental stroke. Neurology 2002;58:945–52; with permission.)

these preliminary data, clinical trials of statin therapy in acute stroke have been initiated.

Physiologic strategies: hypothermia, induced hypertension, and hyperoxia

Hypothermia

Because temperature modulates nearly all biochemical and molecular pathways, cerebroprotection from hypothermia is believed to increase resistance against multiple deleterious pathways, including oxidative stress and inflammation [114–120]. Generally, a 1°C reduction in temperature reduces the rate of cellular respiration, oxygen demand, and carbon dioxide production by approximately 10% [121]. Reduced temperature also slows the rate of pathologic processes, such as lipid peroxidation, and the activity of certain cysteine or serine proteases. Although the net outcome may be complex because detoxification and repair processes also are slowed, the preclinical and clinical results are encouraging, making hypothermia an attractive physiologic therapy that targets multiple injury mechanisms.

Brain cooling can be achieved more rapidly (and spontaneously) when blood flow to the entire brain ceases after cardiac arrest. In the case of focal ischemia, the noninjured brain remains a metabolically active heat source. Although moderate hypothermia (28°–32°C) technically is difficult and fraught with complications, recent experimental studies show that small decreases in core temperature (from normother-

mia to 33°–36°C) are sufficient to reduce neuronal death. The consensus from preclinical data suggests that the therapeutic time window for hypothermia is narrow [122]. In a global model of ischemia, hypothermia proves beneficial if initiated within 30 minutes

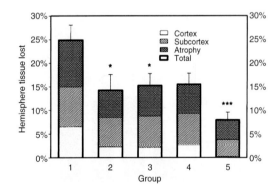

Fig. 6. Volume of necrosis in cortex and subcortical regions, plus atrophy, gives total tissue loss at 2 weeks' survival, expressed as percentage of the hemisphere (see text). There is no dose-response relation between low levels (group 2) and high levels (group 3) of arterial hyperoxemia nor is there a difference between these groups and reperfusion hyperoxemia (group 4). Continuous arterial hyperoxygenation during and after ischemia (group 5), however, shows marked reduction in necrosis, suggesting duration, not degree of hyperoxygenation, is the important factor. *, $P < 0.05$; ***, $P < 0.001$. (*Reprinted from* Flynn EP, Auer RN. Eubaric hyperoxemia and experimental cerebral infarction. Ann Neurol 2002;52:566–72; with permission.)

before stroke onset but not 10 minutes after stroke onset [123]. With prolonged cooling (12–48 hours), substantial neuroprotection can be achieved in focal and global cerebral ischemia [124,125]. In humans, positive results were obtained in two randomized clinical trials of mild hypothermia in survivors of out-of-hospital cardiac arrest [126,127]. Cooling significantly improved outcomes despite a relatively delayed interval (105 minutes) from ischemic onset until the initiation of cooling. Based on these results, additional controlled trials are underway to test the thera-

peutic impact of hypothermia in focal ischemia and embolic stroke when combined with thrombolysis. Preliminary data justify enthusiasm. In a study of 25 patients who had acute, large, complete middle cerebral artery (MCA) infarction, mild hypothermia (33°C maintained for 48 to 72 hours) significantly reduced morbidity and improved long-term neurologic outcome. [128]. The results of a recent trial (Cooling for Acute Ischemic Brain Damage) [129] suggest that the combination of intra-arterial thrombolysis and mild hypothermia is safe; however, complications, such as

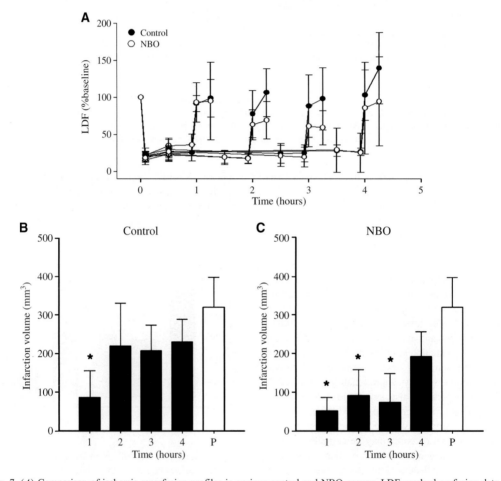

Fig. 7. (A) Comparison of ischemia-reperfusion profiles in various control and NBO groups. LDF cerebral perfusion data are calculated as a percentage of preischemic baselines (mean ± SD). NBO did not lead to any statistically significant differences in ischemia or reperfusion. (B) Forty-eight hour infarction volumes (mean ± SD) in control transient ischemia rats compared with untreated permanent focal cerebral ischemia. In this model, the reperfusion window is approximately 1 to 2 hours. *, $P < 0.05$ versus permanent ischemia. (C) Forty-eight hour infarction volumes (mean ± SD) in NBO-treated transient ischemia rats compared with untreated permanent focal cerebral ischemia. NBO increased the reperfusion window to approximately 3 to 4 hours. *, $P < 0.05$ versus permanent ischemia. (D) Representative ischemic lesions in NBO and control rats. NBO dramatically reduces ischemic injury, especially in the cortex. Scale bar = 10 mm. (E, F) Neurologic deficit scores (mean ± SD) show that NBO significantly improves outcomes compared with untreated controls. *, $P < 0.05$; **, $P < 0.01$ versus permanent ischemia. (Reprinted from Kim HY, Singhal AB, Lo EH. Normobaric hyperoxia extends the reperfusion window in focal cerebral ischemia. Ann Neurol 2005;57:571–5; with permission.)

cardiac arrhythmia, deep vein thrombosis, and pneumonia, are known to occur [130]. Several single and multicenter randomized trials are underway in patients who have ischemic and hemorrhagic stroke.

Induced hypertension

The ischemic penumbra is sensitive particularly to blood pressure manipulation because of impaired autoregulation. Raising mean arterial pressure results in improved cerebral perfusion within the penumbra and a concomitant return of electrical activity. In animal models of focal cerebral ischemia, induced hypertension therapy is found to augment cerebral blood flow, attenuate brain injury, and improve neurologic function [131,132]. In humans who have acute ischemic stroke, spontaneous hypertension is not uncommon, and neurologic deterioration can occur with "excessive" antihypertensive therapy [133]. Furthermore, a paradigm for induced hypertension for

cerebral ischemia exists in the treatment of vasospasm after subarachnoid hemorrhage [134].

Based on this rationale, recent trials have studied the effect of pharmacologically induced hypertension (using IV phenylephrine) on clinical and imaging outcomes in patients who have acute stroke [135–137]. Patients who have significant perfusion-diffusion mismatch on MR imaging, large vessel occlusive disease, and fluctuating neurologic deficits were found to be more likely to respond, and improvement in tests of cortical function correlated with improved perfusion of corresponding cortical regions [138,139]. A multicenter randomized trial of induced hypertension is ongoing. The main concerns with induced hypertension therapy include the risk of precipitating intracerebral hemorrhage and worsening cerebral edema, particularly in patients with lesions that reperfuse, and systemic complications, such as MI, cardiac arrhythmias, and ischemia from phenylephrine-

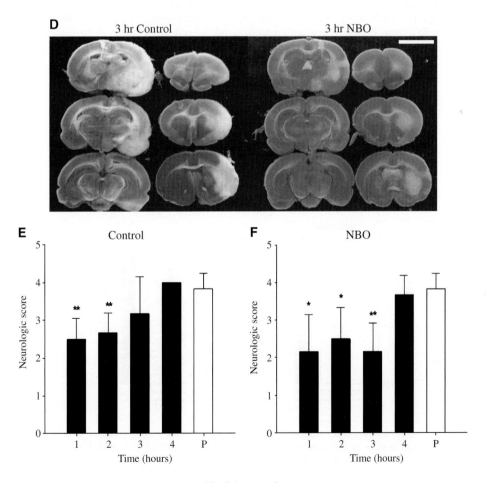

Fig. 7 (*continued*).

induced vasoconstriction. A major limitation of in-duced hypertension as an acute stroke treatment is that it cannot be combined with thrombolysis because of the danger of precipitating serious brain hemorrhage.

Hyperoxia

Tissue hypoxia plays a critical role in the primary and secondary events leading to cell death after is-chemic stroke; therefore, increasing brain oxygena-tion long has been considered a logical stroke treatment strategy. Theoretically, oxygen should be an excellent drug for treating stroke because it has distinct advantages over pharmaceutical agents: it diffuses across the blood-brain barrier easily; has multiple beneficial biochemical, molecular, and he-modynamic effects; is well tolerated; and can be deliv-ered in high doses without dose-limiting side effects (except in patients who have chronic obstructive pul-monary disease).

Because the rationale for oxygen in stroke is so compelling, many groups have focused on it as a potential therapy. The methods of oxygen delivery include hyperbaric oxygen (HBO), normobaric oxy-gen (NBO), and use of perfluorocarbons, synthetic henoglobins, and aqueous oxygen solutions. HBO has been studied widely because it raises brain tissue PO_2 (brain $PtiO_2$) significantly, a factor believed criti-cal for effective neuroprotection. Clinical improve-ment during exposure to HBO was observed nearly 40 years ago [140]. HBO proved effective in animal stroke studies [141–149]; however, it failed three clinical trials [150–152], resulting in reduced interest in HBO. There is growing recognition that factors, such as barotrauma from excessive chamber pres-sures, delayed time to therapy (2–5 days after stroke), and poor patient selection, may have led to the failure of previous HBO clinical trials. Although the results of recent animal studies provide strong evidence that early HBO therapy attenuates stroke-related injury [143,153–155], the limitations of HBO, such as limited availability of HBO chambers, poor patient tolerance because of claustrophobia, and the difficulties of administering HBO to patients receiv-ing thrombolysis, threaten to render it an impractical stroke therapy.

In light of the difficulties of HBO, there is grow-ing interest in investigating the therapeutic potential of NBO or the administration of high concentrations

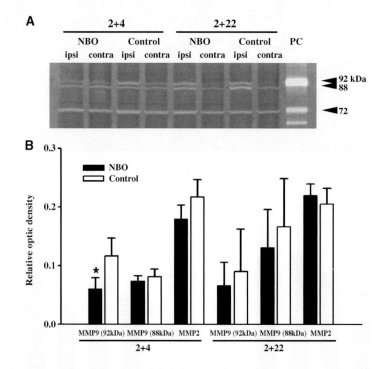

Fig. 8. MMP-2 and MMP-9 levels at 4 and 22 hours after 2-hour transient MCA occlusion in control versus NBO–treated rats. (*A*) Representative gelatin zymogram. (*B*) Quantitative analysis of MMP-9 and -2. Pro–MMP-9 levels were significantly less in the NBO group compared with control animals at 4 hours (0.06 ± 0.019 versus 0.12 ± 0.031; *, $P = 0.02$). PC, positive controls of human MMP-9 and -2. (*Reprinted from* Kim HY, Singhal AB, Lo EH. Normobaric hyperoxia extends the reperfusion window in focal cerebral ischemia. Ann Neurol 2005;57:571–5; with permission.)

of oxygen via a face mask [156–159]. NBO has several advantages: it is widely available, simple to administer, well tolerated, and inexpensive; it can be started quickly after stroke onset (eg, by paramedics); and it is noninvasive. Unlike other physiologic strategies, such as induced hypertension, NBO potentially can be used in patients undergoing thrombolysis. Data from recent animal and human NBO studies seems highly promising and is reviewed later.

In a rodent model of transient MCA ischemia, NBO therapy during the intraischemic and early reperfusion period resulted in a 70% reduction in hemispheric infarction volumes. The benefit was most pronounced in the cerebral cortex where infarction volumes were reduced by as much as 90% as compared with normoxic controls [160]. As with other neuroprotective agents, the timing of NBO therapy is critical for success. The authors document that the therapeutic time window for NBO in rodents is short (approximately 30–45 minutes); initiating treatment at earlier time points after stroke onset enhances the degree of neuroprotection [161].

In another experiment, rats were subjected to filament occlusion of the MCA and randomized to normoxia (controls) or NBO. Serial diffusion- and perfusion-weighted MR imaging was obtained before and after randomization. Although the volume of hypoperfused tissue remained constant, indicating absence of arterial recanalization in both groups, the NBO-treated rats showed a reduction in the volume of diffusion-MR imaging lesions and an improvement in apparent diffusion coefficient (ADC) values after treatment was initiated (Figs. 4 and 5) [161].

Flynn and Auer document that NBO therapy administered during or after transient focal cerebral ischemia in rodents reduces functional deficits, brain atrophy, and weight loss (Fig. 6) [156]. In their experiments, increasing the PaO_2 levels beyond 200 mm Hg did not result in an incremental benefit, suggesting that HBO therapy (which results in PaO_2 levels greater than 1000 mm Hg) may not offer much advantage over NBO. Although benefit was observed with NBO therapy at any stage of the experimental stroke, maximum benefit was evident with continuous (intraischemic and postischemic) treatment. NBO administered solely during the postreperfusion phase also was found to be neuroprotective. This is an important observation, given the historical fears of exacerbating oxygen free radical–associated reperfusion injury with supplemental oxygen therapy.

Preliminary data suggests that early hyperoxia therapy might be a useful strategy to slow down the process of infarction or "buy time" until reperfusion can be achieved. In a mechanical model of stroke

in rodents, NBO therapy administered shortly after stroke onset extends thereperfusion time window from 1 hour to 3 hours (Fig. 7) [162]. This suggests that by arresting the transition of ischemia to infarction, NBO might be useful in increasing the time window, safety, and efficacy of thrombolytic and other neuroprotective drugs. Because long-term neuroprotection seems unlikely in the absence of timely reperfusion, NBO ultimately may be most useful as an adjunct to reperfusion therapies.

Theoretically, increasing oxygen delivery can increase oxygen free radicals, which could worsen injury by promoting processes, such as lipid peroxidation, inflammation, apoptosis, and glutamate excitotoxicity [11,163–165]. Although these harmful effects of oxygen are documented in in-vitro studies and in animal models of global cerebral ischemia, few studies have examined NBO's effects in transient focal cerebral ischemia. In rodent focal stroke models, NBO did not worsen blood-brain barrier damage significantly and did not increase the levels of

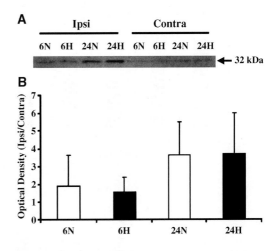

Fig. 9. Western blot analysis of heme oxygenase-1 protein expression at 6 hours and at 24 hours after transient right MCA occlusion in the normoxia group and the hyperoxia group. (*A*) Representative Western blot. (*B*) Ratio of optical density in the ipsilateral versus contralateral hemisphere. There was no significant difference in heme oxygenase-1 levels between the normoxia group and the hyperoxia group, in either the ipsilateral or the contralateral hemisphere, at 6 hours and at 24 hours. Data are expressed as mean ± SD. Contra, contralateral hemisphere; Ipsi, ipsilateral hemisphere; 6N, normoxia group at 6 hours; 6H, hyperoxia group at 6 hours; 24N, normoxia group at 24 hours; 24H, hyperoxia group at 24 hours. (*Reprinted from* Singhal AB, Wang X, Sumii T, et al. Effects of normobaric hyperoxia in a rat model of focal cerebral ischemia-reperfusion. J Cereb Blood Flow Metab 2002;22:861–8; with permission.)

indirect markers of oxidative stress, such as MMP-2 and MMP-9 (Fig. 8), heme oxidase-1 (heat shock protein 32) (Fig. 9), or protein carbonyl formation at acute or subacute time points after stroke. Furthermore, NBO therapy did not increase increase cellular markers of superoxide generation. It remains to be determined whether or not NBO is safe in models of permanent cerebral ischemia and when used in combination with tPA.

In a small pilot clinical trial conducted at Massachusetts General Hospital [87], NBO showed remarkable efficacy in improving neurologic function scores and attenuating MR imaging parameters of cerebral ischemia. In this study, 16 patients who had nonlacunar, hemispheric ischemic stroke were randomized within 12 hours of symptom onset to 8 hours of NBO therapy or room air. Serial diffusion and perfusion MR imaging was performed before treat-

ment (baseline), during treatment, after treatment was stopped, and at more chronic time points (1 week and 3 months). Patients were included if they had a pattern of PWI greater than DWI mismatch on baseline MR imaging. As in DIAS/DEDAS, this imaging pattern was used as a selection criterion because it is believed to indicate the presence of penumbral tissue, which is the target tissue for neuroprotection [166].

As shown in Fig. 10, NBO treatment resulted in an improvement in NIHSSS; reduced growth of DWI lesion volumes; and an increase in the volume of penumbral tissue [167] while therapy was being administered (ie, 4 hours after NBO was initiated). In some patients, areas of DWI abnormalities showed visible improvement during NBO treatment (Fig. 11). These effects were not associated with arterial recanalization. Although DWI reversal is documented after successful early thrombolysis [168], these data

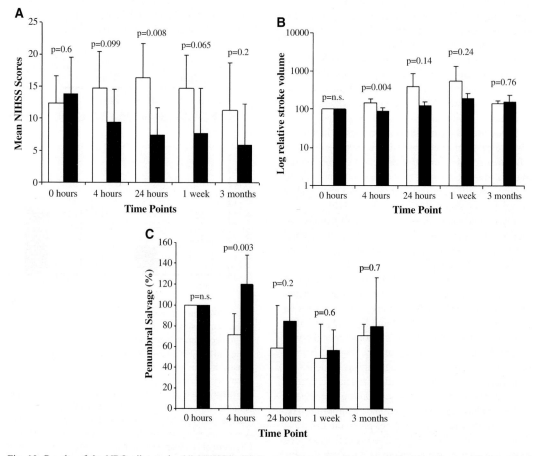

Fig. 10. Results of the NBO pilot study. (*A*) NIHSSS. (*B*) Percent change in relative stroke lesion volumes. (*C*) Penumbral salvage or the ratio of acutely hypoperfused tissue salvaged from infarction [(MTT at time point 1) − (infarction volume at later time point)] to the acute tissue at risk for infarction [(MTT at time point 1) − (DWI at time point 1)]. Controls (*white bars*); NBO (*black bars*); mean ± SD. *, $P < 0.01$ versus Controls. (*Reprinted from* Singhal AB, Benner T, Roccatagliata L, et al. A pilot study of normobaric oxygen therapy in acute ischemic stroke. Stroke 2005;36:797–802; with permission.)

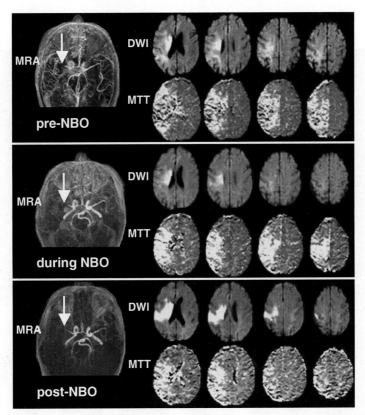

Fig. 11. Serial MR imaging findings in a patient who had cardioembolic right-MCA stroke treated with NBO for 8 hours. (*Top*) Baseline (pre-NBO) MR imaging, 13.1 hours post symptom onset, shows a large DWI lesion, a larger MTT lesion, and MCA occlusion (*arrow*) on head MRA. (*Middle*) A second MR image after 3.75 hours (during NBO) shows 36% reduction in the DWI lesion, stable MTT deficit, and persistent MCA occlusion. (*Bottom*) A third MR imaging after 24 hours (post-NBO) shows reappearance of DWI abnormality in some areas of previous reversal; MTT image shows partial reperfusion (39% MTT volume reduction, mainly in the ACA territory); MRA shows partial MCA recanalization. (*Reprinted from* Singhal AB, Benner T, Roccatagliata L, et al. A pilot study of normobaric oxygen therapy in acute ischemic stroke. Stroke 2005;36:797–802; with permission.)

indicate that NBO can reduce DWI lesions in the absence of arterial recanalization. Some benefit of NBO still was evident at later time points (after NBO was discontinued), perhaps because of spontaneous recanalization in 50% of the patients who were treated with NBO. Automated voxel-by-voxel analysis was performed to determine the fate of individual ADC voxels as per their change in signal intensity above or below an arbitrary threshold of 600×10^{-6} mm^2 per second from the baseline MR imaging to the during-therapy and post-therapy MR imaging scans. The percentage of MR imaging voxels improving from baseline ischemic to 4-hour nonischemic values tended to be higher in patients treated with hyperoxia (Fig. 12). There was no clinical or radiologic evidence of oxygen toxicity in the small number of patients studied. A double-blind randomized controlled trial currently is underway to validate these preliminary results.

The mechanisms of NBO's effects are not understood clearly. Experimental studies with HBO show that hyperoxia favorably alters the levels of glutamate, lactate, bcl-2, manganese SOD, and COX-2 and inhibits cell-death mechanisms, such as apoptosis [141,169–174]. Although NBO is relatively ineffective in raising $PtiO_2$, raising doubts about NBO's potential as a neuroprotectant, the critical mitochondrial oxygen tension is extremely low [175] and even small increases in $PtiO_2$ might suffice to overcome thresholds for neuronal death. Recent studies indicate that brain $PtiO_2$ increases linearly with rising concentrations of inspired oxygen [176], and nearly fourfold increases over baseline are documented in brain trauma patients treated with NBO [172]. A recent in-vivo electron paramagnetic resonance oximetry study shows that NBO increases $PtiO_2$ significantly in penumbral brain tissue [159]. Pre-

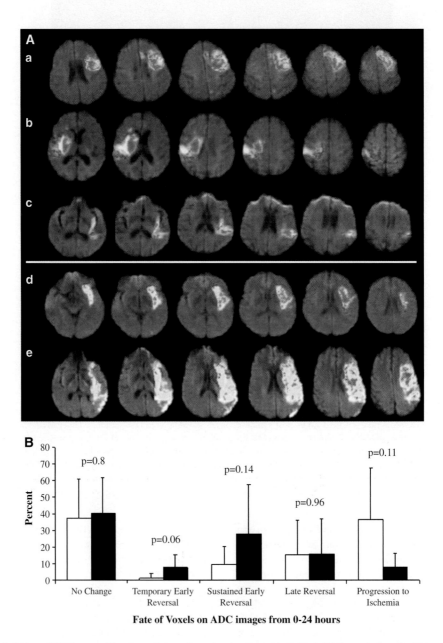

Fig. 12. (*A*) 24-hour DWI image with color-coded overlays showing fate of individual ADC voxels from 0–24 hours, in three NBO (a, b, and c) and two control (d and e) patients. Patient b is the same as in Fig. 2. Voxels undergoing temporary early ADC-reversal (*green*) and sustained early ADC-reversal (*blue*) are present mainly in the lesion periphery and clearly evident in all NBO patients. The few voxels undergoing late ADC-reversal (*cyan*) do not have a distinct distribution pattern. Voxels showing no change (*red*) predominate in the center of the DWI lesions in both groups, and voxels showing progressive ischemia (*yellow*) are most evident in the control patients. (*B*) Bar graph showing the fate of individual voxels (mean ± SD) on ADC maps from 0–24 hours. Controls (*white bars*); NBO (*black bars*). (*Reprinted from* Singhal AB, Benner T, Roccagliata L, et al. A pilot study of normobaric oxygen therapy in acute ischemic stroke. Stroke 2005;36:797–802; with permission.)

liminary data from a subset of patients enrolled in the NBO pilot clinical trial who underwent serial MR spectroscopy show that NBO improves brain lactate levels, perhaps by restoring aerobic metabolism within ischemic brain regions [177]. The most interesting data concerning NBO's mechanism of action comes from perfusion-MR imaging studies. Hyperoxia is known to induce vasoconstriction in normal brain tissue. In rodents, however, NBO increased cerebral blood flow in ischemic brain regions, and in the NBO pilot study, patients who were treated with NBO showed increased cerebral blood flow and blood volume within ischemic regions (Fig. 13). These data suggest that NBO might act by inducing a reverse-steal hemodynamic effect.

Combination therapy for stroke

Given the many cell death pathways activated in cerebral ischemia, it is believed that combining or adding drugs in series that target distinct pathways

during the evolution of ischemic injury enhances the degree of neuroprotection. Various neuroprotective combinations are used with some success in animal models. These include the coadministration of an NMDA receptor antagonist with GABA receptor agonists [178], citicholine [179], free radical scavengers [180], cyclohexamide [181], caspase inhibitors [182], or growth factors, such as basic fibroblast growth factor (bFGF) [183]. Synergy also is observed with two different antioxidants [184] and citicoline plus bFGF [185]. Caspase inhibitors given with bFGF or an NMDA receptor antagonist extend the therapeutic window with lower effective doses [186].

Neuroprotective drugs that decrease reperfusion injury, reduce postischemic hemorrhage, and inhibit downstream targets in cell death cascades may prove useful in increasing the efficacy and safety of thrombolytic drugs, such as tPA. Synergistic or additive effects are reported when thrombolytics are used with neuroprotectants, such as oxygen radical scavengers [187], AMPA [188] receptor antagonists, NMDA

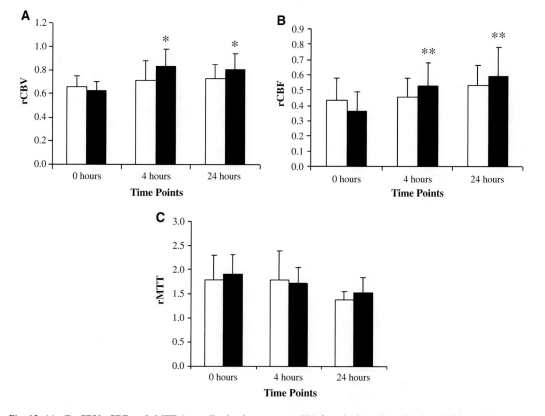

Fig. 13. (*A–C*) rCBV, rCBF, and rMTT (normalized values, mean ± SD) from brain regions showing visible MTT prolongation at baseline. These parameters were not significantly different between groups at any time point; however, in the NBO group, rCBV and rCBF increased significantly. *, $P < 0.01$; **, $P < 0.05$ over baseline values. Controls (*white bars*); NBO (*black bars*). (*Reprinted from* Singhal AB, Benner T, Roccatagliata L, et al. A pilot study of normobaric oxygen therapy in acute ischemic stroke. Stroke 2005;36:797–802; with permission.)

[189] blockers, MMP inhibitors [190], citicoline [191], topiramate [192], antileukocytic adhesion antibodies [193], and antithrombotics [194]. Combination therapies may decrease dosages for each agent, thereby reducing the occurence of adverse events. Two recent clinical trials report the feasibility and safety of treating with IV tPA followed by neuroprotectants, clomethiazole [195], or lubeluzole [196]. As discussed previously, however, in the SAINT-1 trial, the combination of NXY-059 and IV tPA does not yield any clinical benefit over IV tPA treatment alone.

Summary

The pathophysiology of ischemic cell death is complex, with many overlapping pathways. Basic science research has revealed many promising targets for pharmaceutical intervention and several agents show remarkable efficacy in animal models. At present, however, the search for a successful acute stroke neuroprotective drug has not been fruitful. Refinements in patient selection, improved methods of drug delivery, use of more clinically relevant animal stroke models, and the use of combination therapies that target the entire neurovascular unit are warranted to make stroke neuroprotection an achievable goal.

Prior use of statins, thiazide diuretics, and angiotensin-converting enzyme inhibitors reduces the severity of stroke and improve stroke outcomes, which provides a rationale for using neuroprotective agents before stroke, in high-risk populations (such as patients undergoing carotid endarterectomy, carotid angioplasty, or stent placement), in coronary artery bypass grafting, in cardiac valvular surgery, in repair of aortic dissections, and in heart transplants. Recent trial data indicates that the use of neuroimaging tools, such as perfusion MR imaging, can optimize patient selection and that neuroimaging may be useful as a surrogate outcome measure in phase II/III trials.

Ongoing trials of NXY-059 and hyperoxia that are aimed at assessing the efficacy of thrombolysis with neuroprotective agents and at extending the therapeutic window for reperfusion therapy promise to enhance the known benefits of reperfusion therapy. Advances in the fields of stem cell transplantation, stroke recovery, molecular neuroimaging, genomics, and proteomics undoubtedly will provide new therapeutic avenues in the near future. These and other exciting developments over the past decade raise expectations that successful stroke neuroprotection is imminent.

References

[1] Shimizu-Sasamata M, Bosque-Hamilton P, Huang PL, et al. Attenuated neurotransmitter release and spreading depression-like depolarizations after focal ischemia in mutant mice with disrupted type I nitric oxide synthase gene. J Neurosci 1998;18:9564–71.

[2] Wang X, Shimizu-Sasamata M, Moskowitz MA, et al. Profiles of glutamate and gaba efflux in core versus peripheral zones of focal cerebral ischemia in mice. Neurosci Lett 2001;313:121–4.

[3] Hossmann KA. Periinfarct depolarizations. Cerebrovasc Brain Metab Rev 1996;8:195–208.

[4] Bruno V, Battaglia G, Copani A, et al. Metabotropic glutamate receptor subtypes as targets for neuroprotective drugs. J Cereb Blood Flow Metab 2001;21:1013–33.

[5] Kondo T, Reaume AG, Huang TT, et al. Reduction of cuzn-superoxide dismutase activity exacerbates neuronal cell injury and edema formation after transient focal cerebral ischemia. J Neurosci 1997;17:4180–9.

[6] Kinouchi H, Epstein CJ, Mizui T, et al. Attenuation of focal cerebral ischemic injury in transgenic mice overexpressing cuzn superoxide dismutase. Proc Natl Acad Sci USA 1991;88:11158–62.

[7] Sheng H, Bart RD, Oury TD, et al. Mice overexpressing extracellular superoxide dismutase have increased resistance to focal cerebral ischemia. Neuroscience 1999;88:185–91.

[8] Kim GW, Kondo T, Noshita N, et al. Manganese superoxide dismutase deficiency exacerbates cerebral infarction after focal cerebral ischemia/reperfusion in mice: implications for the production and role of superoxide radicals. Stroke 2002;33:809–15.

[9] Huang Z, Huang PL, Panahian N, et al. Effects of cerebral ischemia in mice deficient in neuronal nitric oxide synthase. Science 1994;265:1883–5.

[10] Iadecola C, Zhang F, Casey R, et al. Delayed reduction of ischemic brain injury and neurological deficits in mice lacking the inducible nitric oxide synthase gene. J Neurosci 1997;17:9157–64.

[11] Chan PH. Reactive oxygen radicals in signaling and damage in the ischemic brain. J Cereb Blood Flow Metab 2001;21:2–14.

[12] Kroemer G, Reed JC. Mitochondrial control of cell death. Nat Med 2000;6:513–9.

[13] Bernardi P, Petronilli V, Di Lisa F, et al. A mitochondrial perspective on cell death. Trends Biochem Sci 2001;26:112–7.

[14] Yuan J, Yankner BA. Apoptosis in the nervous system. Nature 2000;407:802–9.

[15] Nicotera P, Leist M, Fava E, et al. Energy requirement for caspase activation and neuronal cell death. Brain Pathol 2000;10:276–82.

[16] Nicotera P, Lipton SA. Excitotoxins in neuronal apoptosis and necrosis. J Cereb Blood Flow Metab 1999;19:583–91.

[17] Budd SL, Tenneti L, Lishnak T, et al. Mitochondrial

and extramitochondrial apoptotic signaling pathways in cerebrocortical neurons. Proc Natl Acad Sci USA 2000;97:6161–6.

[18] Martin-Villalba A, Herr I, Jeremias I, et al. Cd95 ligand (fas-l/apo-1l) and tumor necrosis factor-related apoptosis-inducing ligand mediate ischemia-induced apoptosis in neurons. J Neurosci 1999;19:3809–17.

[19] Salvesen GS. A lysosomal protease enters the death scene. J Clin Invest 2001;107:21–2.

[20] Fiskum G. Mitochondrial participation in ischemic and traumatic neural cell death. J Neurotrauma 2000; 17:843–55.

[21] Leist M, Jaattela M. Four deaths and a funeral: From caspases to alternative mechanisms. Nat Rev Mol Cell Biol 2001;2:589–98.

[22] Friedlander RM. Apoptosis and caspases in neurodegenerative diseases. N Engl J Med 2003;348:1365–75.

[23] Han BH, Xu D, Choi J, et al. Selective, reversible caspase-3 inhibitor is neuroprotective and reveals distinct pathways of cell death after neonatal hypoxic-ischemic brain injury. J Biol Chem 2002; 277:30128–36.

[24] Le DA, Wu Y, Huang Z, et al. Caspase activation and neuroprotection in caspase-3- deficient mice after in vivo cerebral ischemia and in vitro oxygen glucose deprivation. Proc Natl Acad Sci USA 2002;99: 15188–93.

[25] Graham SH, Chen J. Programmed cell death in cerebral ischemia. J Cereb Blood Flow Metab 2001;21: 99–109.

[26] Chamorro A. Role of inflammation in stroke and atherothrombosis. Cerebrovasc Dis 2004;17(Suppl 3): 1–5.

[27] Elkind MS, Cheng J, Boden-Albala B, et al. Tumor necrosis factor receptor levels are associated with carotid atherosclerosis. Stroke 2002;33:31–7.

[28] Ridker PM, Hennekens CH, Buring JE, et al. C-reactive protein and other markers of inflammation in the prediction of cardiovascular disease in women. N Engl J Med 2000;342:836–43.

[29] Tanne D, Haim M, Boyko V, Goldbourt U, et al. Soluble intercellular adhesion molecule-1 and risk of future ischemic stroke: a nested case-control study from the bezafibrate infarction prevention (bip) study cohort. Stroke 2002;33:2182–6.

[30] del Zoppo G, Ginis I, Hallenbeck JM, et al. Inflammation and stroke: putative role for cytokines, adhesion molecules and inos in brain response to ischemia. Brain Pathol 2000;10:95–112.

[31] Barone FC, Feuerstein GZ. Inflammatory mediators and stroke: new opportunities for novel therapeutics. J Cereb Blood Flow Metab 1999;19:819–34.

[32] Hughes PM, Allegrini PR, Rudin M, et al. Monocyte chemoattractant protein-1 deficiency is protective in a murine stroke model. J Cereb Blood Flow Metab 2002;22:308–17.

[33] Iadecola C, Niwa K, Nogawa S, et al. Reduced susceptibility to ischemic brain injury and n-methyl-d-aspartate-mediated neurotoxicity in cyclooxy-genase-2-deficient mice. Proc Natl Acad Sci USA 2001;98:1294–9.

[34] Boutin H, LeFeuvre RA, Horai R, et al. Role of il-1alpha and il-1beta in ischemic brain damage. J Neurosci 2001;21:5528–34.

[35] Schielke GP, Yang GY, Shivers BD, et al. Reduced ischemic brain injury in interleukin-1 beta converting enzyme-deficient mice. J Cereb Blood Flow Metab 1998;18:180–5.

[36] Strong AJ, Smith SE, Whittington DJ, et al. Factors influencing the frequency of fluorescence transients as markers of peri-infarct depolarizations in focal cerebral ischemia. Stroke 2000;31:214–22.

[37] Gill R, Andine P, Hillered L, et al. The effect of mk-801 on cortical spreading depression in the penumbral zone following focal ischaemia in the rat. J Cereb Blood Flow Metab 1992;12:371–9.

[38] Iijima T, Mies G, et al. Repeated negative dc deflections in rat cortex following middle cerebral artery occlusion are abolished by mk-801: Effect on volume of ischemic injury. J Cereb Blood Flow Metab 1992; 12:727–33.

[39] Busch E, Gyngell ML, Eis M, et al. Potassium-induced cortical spreading depressions during focal cerebral ischemia in rats: Contribution to lesion growth assessed by diffusion-weighted nmr and biochemical imaging. J Cereb Blood Flow Metab 1996;16: 1090–9.

[40] Dijkhuizen RM, Beekwilder JP, van der Worp HB, et al. Correlation between tissue depolarizations and damage in focal ischemic rat brain. Brain Res 1999; 840:194–205.

[41] Hartings JA, Rolli ML, Lu XC, et al. Delayed secondary phase of peri-infarct depolarizations after focal cerebral ischemia: Relation to infarct growth and neuroprotection. J Neurosci 2003;23:11602–10.

[42] Tatlisumak T, Takano K, Meiler MR, et al. A glycine site antagonist, zd9379, reduces number of spreading depressions and infarct size in rats with permanent middle cerebral artery occlusion. Stroke 1998; 29:190–5.

[43] Chen Q, Chopp M, Bodzin G, et al. Temperature modulation of cerebral depolarization during focal cerebral ischemia in rats: correlation with ischemic injury. J Cereb Blood Flow Metab 1993;13:389–94.

[44] Petty MA, Wettstein JG. White matter ischaemia. Brain Res Brain Res Rev 1999;31:58–64.

[45] Stys PK. Anoxic and ischemic injury of myelinated axons in cns white matter: from mechanistic concepts to therapeutics. J Cereb Blood Flow Metab 1998;18: 2–25.

[46] Lo EH, Broderick JP, Moskowitz MA. Tpa and proteolysis in the neurovascular unit. Stroke 2004;35: 354–6.

[47] Petty MA, Lo EH. Junctional complexes of the blood-brain barrier: Permeability changes in neuroinflammation. Prog Neurobiol 2002;68:311–23.

[48] Wang X, Lee SR, Arai K, et al. Lipoprotein receptor-mediated induction of matrix metalloprotein-

ase by tissue plasminogen activator. Nat Med 2003; 9:1313–7.

[49] Lee SR, Lo EH. Induction of caspase-mediated cell death by matrix metalloproteinases in cerebral endothelial cells after hypoxia-reoxygenation. J Cereb Blood Flow Metab 2004;24:720–7.

[50] Wang X, Tsuji K, Lee SR, et al. Mechanisms of hemorrhagic transformation after tissue plasminogen activator reperfusion therapy for ischemic stroke. Stroke 2004;35:2726–30.

[51] Lee SR, Wang X, Tsuji K, et al. Extracellular proteolytic pathophysiology in the neurovascular unit after stroke. Neurol Res 2004;26:854–61.

[52] Tsuji K, Aoki T, Tejima E, et al. Tissue plasminogen activator promotes matrix metalloproteinase-9 upregulation after focal cerebral ischemia. Stroke 2005; 36(9):1954–9.

[53] The National Institute of Neurological Disorders and Stroke Rt-Pa Stroke Study Group. Tissue plasminogen activator for acute ischemic stroke. N Engl J Med 1995;333:1581–7.

[54] The Ranttas Investigators. A randomized trial of tirilazad mesylate in patients with acute stroke (ranttas). Stroke 1996;27:1453–8.

[55] Enlimomab Acute Stroke Trial Investigators. Use of anti-icam-1 therapy in ischemic stroke: results of the enlimomab acute stroke trial. Neurology 2001;57: 1428–34.

[56] The American Nimodipine Study Group. Clinical trial of nimodipine in acute ischemic stroke. Stroke 1992;23:3–8.

[57] Wahlgren NG, Ranasinha KW, Rosolacci T, et al. Clomethiazole acute stroke study (class): results of a randomized, controlled trial of clomethiazole versus placebo in 1360 acute stroke patients. Stroke 1999; 30:21–8.

[58] Lyden P, Shuaib A, Ng K, et al. Clomethiazole acute stroke study in ischemic stroke (class-i): final results. Stroke 2002;33:122–8.

[59] Diener HC, Cortens M, Ford G, et al. Lubeluzole in acute ischemic stroke treatment: a double-blind study with an 8-hour inclusion window comparing a 10-mg daily dose of lubeluzole with placebo. Stroke 2000;31:2543–51.

[60] Davis SM, Lees KR, Albers GW, et al. Selfotel in acute ischemic stroke: possible neurotoxic effects of an nmda antagonist. Stroke 2000;31:347–54.

[61] Albers GW, Goldstein LB, Hall D, et al. Aptiganel hydrochloride in acute ischemic stroke: a randomized controlled trial. JAMA 2001;286:2673–82.

[62] Lees KR, Asplund K, Carolei A, et al. Glycine antagonist (gavestinel) in neuroprotection (gain international) in patients with acute stroke: a randomised controlled trial. Gain international investigators. Lancet 2000;355:1949–54.

[63] Sacco RL, DeRosa JT, et al. Glycine antagonist in neuroprotection for patients with acute stroke: gain americas: a randomized controlled trial. JAMA 2001; 285:1719–28.

[64] Fisher M. Recommendations for advancing development of acute stroke therapies: stroke therapy academic industry roundtable 3. Stroke 2003;34: 1539–46.

[65] Kidwell CS, Liebeskind DS, Starkman S, et al. Trends in acute ischemic stroke trials through the 20th century. Stroke 2001;32:1349–59.

[66] Muir KW, Lees KR, Ford I, et al. Magnesium for acute stroke (intravenous magnesium efficacy in stroke trial): randomised controlled trial. Lancet 2004; 363:439–45.

[67] Yamaguchi T, Sano K, Takakura K, et al. Ebselen in acute ischemic stroke: a placebo-controlled, double-blind clinical trial. Ebselen study group. Stroke 1998; 29:12–7.

[68] Lees KR, Barer D, Ford GA, et al. Tolerability of nxy-059 at higher target concentrations in patients with acute stroke. Stroke 2003;34:482–7.

[69] Zhao Z, Cheng M, Maples KR, et al. Nxy-059, a novel free radical trapping compound, reduces cortical infarction after permanent focal cerebral ischemia in the rat. Brain Res 2001;909:46–50.

[70] Sydserff SG, Borelli AR, Green AR, et al. Effect of nxy-059 on infarct volume after transient or permanent middle cerebral artery occlusion in the rat; studies on dose, plasma concentration and therapeutic time window. Br J Pharmacol 2002;135:103–12.

[71] Lapchak PA, Song D, Wei J, et al. Coadministration of nxy-059 and tenecteplase six hours following embolic strokes in rabbits improves clinical rating scores. Exp Neurol 2004;188:279–85.

[72] Marshall JW, Cummings RM, Bowes LJ, et al. Functional and histological evidence for the protective effect of nxy-059 in a primate model of stroke when given 4 hours after occlusion. Stroke 2003;34: 2228–33.

[73] Marshall JW, Duffin KJ, Green AR, et al. Nxy-059, a free radical–trapping agent, substantially lessens the functional disability resulting from cerebral ischemia in a primate species. Stroke 2001;32:190–8.

[74] Lapchak PA, Araujo DM, Song D, et al. Effects of the spin trap agent disodium- [tert-butylimino)methyl]-benzene-1,3-disulfonate n-oxide (generic nxy-059) on intracerebral hemorrhage in a rabbit large clot embolic stroke model: combination studies with tissue plasminogen activator. Stroke 2002;33:1665–70.

[75] Lees KR, Sharma AK, Barer D, et al. Tolerability and pharmacokinetics of the nitrone nxy-059 in patients with acute stroke. Stroke 2001;32:675–80.

[76] Strid S, Borga O, Edenius C, et al. Pharmacokinetics in renally impaired subjects of nxy-059, a nitrone-based, free-radical trapping agent developed for the treatment of acute stroke. Eur J Clin Pharmacol 2002; 58:409–15.

[77] Baird AE, Warach S. Magnetic resonance imaging of acute stroke. J Cereb Blood Flow Metab 1998;18: 583–609.

[78] Kidwell CS, Alger JR, Saver JL. Beyond mismatch: evolving paradigms in imaging the ischemic penum-

bra with multimodal magnetic resonance imaging. Stroke 2003;34:2729–35.

[79] Schlaug G, Benfield A, Baird AE, et al. The ischemic penumbra: operationally defined by diffusion and perfusion mri. Neurology 1999;53:1528–37.

[80] Sorensen AG, Copen WA, Ostergaard L, et al. Hyper-acute stroke: simultaneous measurement of relative cerebral blood volume, relative cerebral blood flow, and mean tissue transit time. Radiology 1999;210: 519–27.

[81] Schaefer PW, Ozsunar Y, He J, et al. Assessing tissue viability with mr diffusion and perfusion imaging. AJNR Am J Neuroradiol 2003;24:436–43.

[82] Lev MH, Segal AZ, Farkas J, et al. Utility of per-fusion-weighted ct imaging in acute middle cerebral artery stroke treated with intra-arterial thrombolysis: prediction of final infarct volume and clinical out-come. Stroke 2001;32:2021–8.

[83] Wintermark M, Reichhart M, Thiran JP, et al. Prog-nostic accuracy of cerebral blood flow measurement by perfusion computed tomography, at the time of emergency room admission, in acute stroke patients. Ann Neurol 2002;51:417–32.

[84] Wintermark M, Reichhart M, Cuisenaire O, et al. Comparison of admission perfusion computed to-mography and qualitative diffusion- and perfusion-weighted magnetic resonance imaging in acute stroke patients. Stroke 2002;33:2025–31.

[85] Hunter GJ, Hamberg LM, Ponzo JA, et al. Assess-ment of cerebral perfusion and arterial anatomy in hyperacute stroke with three-dimensional functional ct: early clinical results. AJNR Am J Neuroradiol 1998; 19:29–37.

[86] Hacke W, Albers G, Al-Rawi Y, et al. DIAS Study Group. The Desmoteplase in Acute Ischemic Stroke Trial (DIAS): a phase II MRI-based 9-hour window acute thrombolysis trial with intravenous desmote-plase. Stroke 2005;36:66–73.

[87] Singhal AB, Benner T, Roccatagliata L, et al. A pilot study of normobaric oxygen therapy in acute ische-mic stroke. Stroke 2005;36:797–802.

[88] Lin JY, Chung SY, Lin MC, et al. Effects of mag-nesium sulfate on energy metabolites and glutamate in the cortex during focal cerebral ischemia and re-perfusion in the gerbil monitored by a dual-probe microdialysis technique. Life Sci 2002;71:803–11.

[89] Nowak L, Bregestovski P, Ascher P, et al. Magnesium gates glutamate-activated channels in mouse central neurones. Nature 1984;307:462–5.

[90] Chi OZ, Pollak P, Weiss HR. Effects of magnesium sulfate and nifedipine on regional cerebral blood flow during middle cerebral artery ligation in the rat. Arch Int Pharmacodyn Ther 1990;304:196–205.

[91] Izumi Y, Roussel S, Pinard E, et al. Reduction of infarct volume by magnesium after middle cerebral artery occlusion in rats. J Cereb Blood Flow Metab 1991;11:1025–30.

[92] Marinov MB, Harbaugh KS, Hoopes PJ, et al. Neuroprotective effects of preischemia intraarterial

magnesium sulfate in reversible focal cerebral ische-mia. J Neurosurg 1996;85:117–24.

[93] Muir KW, Lees KR. A randomized, double-blind, placebo-controlled pilot trial of intravenous magne-sium sulfate in acute stroke. Stroke 1995;26:1183–8.

[94] Saver JL, Kidwell C, et al. Prehospital neuroprotec-tive therapy for acute stroke: results of the field administration of stroke therapy-magnesium (FAST-MAG) pilot trial. Stroke 2004;35:e106.

[95] Belayev L, Pinard E, Nallet H, et al. Albumin ther-apy of transient focal cerebral ischemia: in vivo analy-sis of dynamic microvascular responses. Stroke 2002; 33:1077–84.

[96] Belayev L, Liu Y, Zhao W, et al. Human albumin therapy of acute ischemic stroke: marked neuropro-tective efficacy at moderate doses and with a broad therapeutic window. Stroke 2001;32:553–60.

[97] Liao JK, Laufs U. Pleiotropic effects of statins. Annu Rev Pharmacol Toxicol 2005;45:89–118.

[98] Amin-Hanjani S, Stagliano NE, Yamada M, et al. Mevastatin, an hmg-coa reductase inhibitor, reduces stroke damage and upregulates endothelial nitric oxide synthase in mice. Stroke 2001;32:980–6.

[99] Laufs U, Gertz K, Huang P, et al. Atorvastatin up-regulates type iii nitric oxide synthase in thrombo-cytes, decreases platelet activation, and protects from cerebral ischemia in normocholesterolemic mice. Stroke 2000;31:2442–9.

[100] Cheung BM, Lauder IJ, Lau CP, et al. Meta-analysis of large randomized controlled trials to evaluate the impact of statins on cardiovascular outcomes. Br J Clin Pharmacol 2004;57:640–51.

[101] Jonsson N, Asplund K. Does pretreatment with stat-ins improve clinical outcome after stroke? A pilot case-referent study. Stroke 2001;32:1112–5.

[102] Greisenegger S, Mullner M, Tentschert S, et al. Ef-fect of pretreatment with statins on the severity of acute ischemic cerebrovascular events. J Neurol Sci 2004;221:5–10.

[103] Marti-Fabregas J, Gomis M, Arboix A, et al. Favor-able outcome of ischemic stroke in patients pretreated with statins. Stroke 2004;35:1117–21.

[104] Yoon SS, Dambrosia J, Chalela J, et al. Rising statin use and effect on ischemic stroke outcome. BMC Med 2004;2:4.

[105] Chen J, Zhang ZG, Li Y, et al. Statins induce angio-genesis, neurogenesis, and synaptogenesis after stroke. Ann Neurol 2003;53:743–51.

[106] Sironi L, Cimino M, Guerrini U, et al. Treatment with statins after induction of focal ischemia in rats reduces the extent of brain damage. Arterioscler Thromb Vasc Biol 2003;23:322–7.

[107] Elkind MS, Flint AC, Sciacca RR, et al. Lipid-lowering agent use at ischemic stroke onset is as-sociated with decreased mortality. Neurology 2005; 65:253–8.

[108] Moonis M, Kane K, Schwiderski U, et al. Hmg-coa reductase inhibitors improve acute ischemic stroke outcome. Stroke 2005;36:1298–300.

[109] Parra A, Kreiter KT, Williams S, et al. Effect of prior statin use on functional outcome and delayed vasospasm after acute aneurysmal subarachnoid hemorrhage: a matched controlled cohort study. Neurosurgery 2005;56:476–84 [discussion: 476–84].

[110] Tseng MY, Czosnyka M, Richards H, et al. Effects of acute treatment with pravastatin on cerebral vasospasm, autoregulation, and delayed ischemic deficits after aneurysmal subarachnoid hemorrhage: a phaseII randomized placebo-controlled trial. Stroke 2005;36: 1627–32.

[111] Gertz K, Laufs U, Lindauer U, et al. Withdrawal of statin treatment abrogates stroke protection in mice. Stroke 2003;34:551–7.

[112] Singhal AB, Topcuoglu MA, Dorer DJ, et al. Ssri and statin use increases the risk for vasospasm after subarachnoid hemorrhage. Neurology 2005;64:1008–13.

[113] Montaner J, Chacon P, Krupinski J, et al. Safety and efficacy of statins in the acute phase of ischemic stroke: the MISTICS trial. Stroke 2004;35:293.

[114] Astrup J, Siesjo BK, Symon L. Thresholds in cerebral ischemia-the ischemic penumbra. Stroke 1981; 12:723–5.

[115] Cardell M, Boris-Moller F, Wieloch T. Hypothermia prevents the ischemia-induced translocation and inhibition of protein kinase c in the rat striatum. J Neurochem 1991;57:1814–7.

[116] Globus MY, Busto R, Lin B, et al. Detection of free radical activity during transient global ischemia and recirculation: effects of intraischemic brain temperature modulation. J Neurochem 1995;65:1250–6.

[117] Krieger DW, Yenari MA. Therapeutic hypothermia for acute ischemic stroke: what do laboratory studies teach us? Stroke 2004;35:1482–9.

[118] Han HS, Karabiyikoglu M, Kelly S, et al. Mild hypothermia inhibits nuclear factor-kappab translocation in experimental stroke. J Cereb Blood Flow Metab 2003;23:589–98.

[119] Wang GJ, Deng HY, Maier CM, et al. Mild hypothermia reduces icam-1 expression, neutrophil infiltration and microglia/monocyte accumulation following experimental stroke. Neuroscience 2002; 114:1081–90.

[120] Han HS, Qiao Y, Karabiyikoglu M, et al. Influence of mild hypothermia on inducible nitric oxide synthase expression and reactive nitrogen production in experimental stroke and inflammation. J Neurosci 2002; 22:3921–8.

[121] Prosser CL. Temperature. In: Prosser CL, editor. Comparative animal physiology. Philadelphia: WB Saunders; 1973. p. 362–428.

[122] Markarian GZ, Lee JH, Stein DJ, et al. Mild hypothermia: Therapeutic window after experimental cerebral ischemia. Neurosurgery 1996;38:542–50 [discussion: 551].

[123] Welsh FA, Harris VA. Postischemic hypothermia fails to reduce ischemic injury in gerbil hippocampus. J Cereb Blood Flow Metab 1991;11:617–20.

[124] Ginsberg MD. Hypothermic neuroprotection in cerebral ischemia. In: Welch KMA, Caplan LR, Reis DJ, et al, editors. Primer on cerebrovascular diseases. San Diego: Academic Press; 1997. p. 272–5.

[125] Corbett D, Hamilton M, Colbourne F. Persistent neuroprotection with prolonged postischemic hypothermia in adult rats subjected to transient middle cerebral artery occlusion. Exp Neurol 2000;163:200–6.

[126] The Hypothermia After Cardiac Arrest Study Group. Mild therapeutic hypothermia to improve the neurologic outcome after cardiac arrest. N Engl J Med 2002;346:549–56.

[127] Bernard SA, Gray TW, Buist MD, et al. Treatment of comatose survivors of out-of-hospital cardiac arrest with induced hypothermia. N Engl J Med 2002; 346:557–63.

[128] Schwab S, Schwarz S, Spranger M, et al. Moderate hypothermia in the treatment of patients with severe middle cerebral artery infarction. Stroke 1998;29: 2461–6.

[129] Krieger DW, De Georgia MA, Abou-Chebl A, et al. Cooling for acute ischemic brain damage (COOL AID): an open pilot study of induced hypothermia in acute ischemic stroke. Stroke 2001;32:1847–54.

[130] Kammersgaard LP, Rasmussen BH, Jorgensen HS, et al. Feasibility and safety of inducing modest hypothermia in awake patients with acute stroke through surface cooling: a case-control study: the Copenhagen Stroke Study. Stroke 2000;31:2251–6.

[131] Hayashi S, Nehls DG, Kieck CF, et al. Beneficial effects of induced hypertension on experimental stroke in awake monkeys. J Neurosurg 1984;60:151–7.

[132] Cole DJ, Matsumura JS, Drummond JC, et al. Focal cerebral ischemia in rats: Effects of induced hypertension, during reperfusion, on cbf. J Cereb Blood Flow Metab 1992;12:64–9.

[133] Fischberg GM, Lozano E, Rajamani K, et al. Stroke precipitated by moderate blood pressure reduction. J Emerg Med 2000;19:339–46.

[134] Kassell NF, Peerless SJ, Durward QJ, et al. Treatment of ischemic deficits from vasospasm with intravascular volume expansion and induced arterial hypertension. Neurosurgery 1982;11:337–43.

[135] Rordorf G, Cramer SC, Efird JT, et al. Pharmacological elevation of blood pressure in acute stroke. Clinical effects and safety. Stroke 1997;28:2133–8.

[136] Rordorf G, Koroshetz WJ, Ezzeddine MA, et al. A pilot study of drug-induced hypertension for treatment of acute stroke. Neurology 2001;56:1210–3.

[137] Hillis AE, Ulatowski JA, Barker PB, et al. A pilot randomized trial of induced blood pressure elevation: effects on function and focal perfusion in acute and subacute stroke. Cerebrovasc Dis 2003; 16:236–46.

[138] Hillis AE, Wityk RJ, Beauchamp NJ, et al. Perfusion-weighted mri as a marker of response to treatment in acute and subacute stroke. Neuroradiology 2004; 46:31–9.

[139] Hillis AE, Barker PB, Beauchamp NJ, et al. Restoring

blood pressure reperfused wernicke's area and improved language. Neurology 2001;56:670–2.

[140] Ingvar HD, Lassen NA. Treatment of focal cerebral ischemia with hyperbaric oxygen. Acta Neurol Scand 1965;41:92–5.

[141] Badr AE, Yin W, Mychaskiw G, et al. Dual effect of hbo on cerebral infarction in MCAO rats. Am J Physiol Regul Integr Comp Physiol 2001;280:R766.

[142] Burt JT, Kapp JP, Smith RR. Hyperbaric oxygen and cerebral infarction in the gerbil. Surg Neurol 1987;28: 265–8.

[143] Lou M, Eschenfelder CC, Herdegen T, et al. Therapeutic window for use of hyperbaric oxygenation in focal transient ischemia in rats. Stroke 2004;35: 578–83.

[144] Veltkamp R, Warner DS, Domoki F, et al. Hyperbaric oxygen decreases infarct size and behavioral deficit after transient focal cerebral ischemia in rats. Brain Res 2000;853:68–73.

[145] Sunami K, Takeda Y, Hashimoto M, et al. Hyperbaric oxygen reduces infarct volume in rats by increasing oxygen supply to the ischemic periphery. Crit Care Med 2000;28:2831–6.

[146] Schabitz WR, Schade H, Heiland S, et al. Neuroprotection by hyperbaric oxygenation after experimental focal cerebral ischemia monitored by mr-imaging. Stroke 2004;35(5):1175–9.

[147] Roos JA, Jackson-Friedman C, Lyden P. Effects of hyperbaric oxygen on neurologic outcome for cerebral ischemia in rats. Acad Emerg Med 1998;5:18–24.

[148] Kawamura S, Yasui N, Shirasawa M, et al. Therapeutic effects of hyperbaric oxygenation on acute focal cerebral ischemia in rats. Surg Neurol 1990;34: 101–6.

[149] Weinstein PR, Anderson GG, Telles DA. Results of hyperbaric oxygen therapy during temporary middle cerebral artery occlusion in unanesthetized cats. Neurosurgery 1987;20:518–24.

[150] Anderson DC, Bottini AG, Jagiella WM, et al. A pilot study of hyperbaric oxygen in the treatment of human stroke. Stroke 1991;22:1137–42.

[151] Nighoghossian N, Trouillas P, Adeleine P, et al. Hyperbaric oxygen in the treatment of acute ischemic stroke. A double-blind pilot study. Stroke 1995;26: 1369–72.

[152] Rusyniak DE, Kirk MA, May JD, et al. Hyperbaric oxygen therapy in acute ischemic stroke: Results of the hyperbaric oxygen in acute ischemic stroke trial pilot study. Stroke 2003;34:571–4.

[153] Veltkamp R, Siebing DA, Heiland S, et al. Hyperbaric oxygen induces rapid protection against focal cerebral ischemia. Brain Res 2005;1037:134–8.

[154] Schabitz WR, Schade H, Heiland S, et al. Neuroprotection by hyperbaric oxygenation after experimental focal cerebral ischemia monitored by mri. Stroke 2004;35:1175–9.

[155] Miljkovic-Lolic M, Silbergleit R, Fiskum G, et al. Neuroprotective effects of hyperbaric oxygen treatment in experimental focal cerebral ischemia are associated with reduced brain leukocyte myeloperoxidase activity. Brain Res 2003;971:90–4.

[156] Flynn EP, Auer RN. Eubaric hyperoxemia and experimental cerebral infarction. Ann Neurol 2002;52: 566–72.

[157] Mori T, Wang X, Jung JC, et al. Mitogen-activated protein kinase inhibition in traumatic brain injury: in vitro and in vivo effects. J Cereb Blood Flow Metab 2002;22:444–52.

[158] Furie KL, Singhal AB, McCarthy C, et al. Stop-stroke study: Utility of early contrast computed tomography in assessing stroke mechanism. Stroke 2004;35:269.

[159] Liu S, Shi H, Liu W, et al. Interstitial po2 in ischemic penumbra and core are differentially affected following transient focal cerebral ischemia in rats. J Cereb Blood Flow Metab 2004;24:343–9.

[160] Singhal AB, Wang X, Sumii T, et al. Effects of normobaric hyperoxia in a rat model of focal cerebral ischemia-reperfusion. J Cereb Blood Flow Metab 2002;22:861–8.

[161] Singhal AB, Dijkhuizen RM, Rosen BR, et al. Normobaric hyperoxia reduces mri diffusion abnormalities and infarct size in experimental stroke. Neurology 2002;58:945–52.

[162] Kim HY, Singhal AB, Lo EH. Normobaric hyperoxia extends the reperfusion window in focal cerebral ischemia. Ann Neurol 2005;57:571–5.

[163] Watson BD, Busto R, Goldberg WJ, et al. Lipid peroxidation in vivo induced by reversible global ischemia in rat brain. J Neurochem 1984;42:268–74.

[164] Mickel HS, Vaishnav YN, Kempski O, et al. Breathing 100% oxygen after global brain ischemia in mongolian gerbils results in increased lipid peroxidation and increased mortality. Stroke 1987;18: 426–30.

[165] Dubinsky JM, Kristal BS, Elizondo-Fournier M. An obligate role for oxygen in the early stages of glutamate-induced, delayed neuronal death. J Neurosci 1995;15:7071–8.

[166] Warach S. New imaging strategies for patient selection for thrombolytic and neuroprotective therapies. Neurology 2001;57:S48–52.

[167] Parsons MW, Barber PA, Chalk J, et al. Diffusion- and perfusion-weighted mri response to thrombolysis in stroke. Ann Neurol 2002;51:28–37.

[168] Kidwell CS, Saver JL, Mattiello J, et al. Thrombolytic reversal of acute human cerebral ischemic injury shown by diffusion/perfusion magnetic resonance imaging. Ann Neurol 2000;47:462–9.

[169] Bernaudin M, Nedelec AS, Divoux D, et al. Normobaric hypoxia induces tolerance to focal permanent cerebral ischemia in association with an increased expression of hypoxia-inducible factor-1 and its target genes, erythropoietin and vegf, in the adult mouse brain. J Cereb Blood Flow Metab 2002; 22:393–403.

[170] Fisher M, Ratan R. New perspectives on developing acute stroke therapy. Ann Neurol 2003;53:10–20.

[171] Wada K, Miyazawa T, Nomura N, et al. Preferential conditions for and possible mechanisms of induction of ischemic tolerance by repeated hyperbaric oxygenation in gerbil hippocampus. Neurosurgery 2001; 49:160–6 [discussion: 166–7].

[172] Menzel M, Doppenberg EM, Zauner A, et al. Increased inspired oxygen concentration as a factor in improved brain tissue oxygenation and tissue lactate levels after severe human head injury. J Neurosurg 1999;91:1–10.

[173] Rockswold SB, Rockswold GL, Vargo JM, et al. Effects of hyperbaric oxygenation therapy on cerebral metabolism and intracranial pressure in severely brain injured patients. J Neurosurg 2001;94:403–11.

[174] Calvert JW, Zhou C, Nanda A, et al. Effect of hyperbaric oxygen on apoptosis in neonatal hypoxia-ischemia rat model. J Appl Physiol 2003;95:2072–80.

[175] Hempel FG, Jobsis FF, LaManna JL, et al. Oxidation of cerebral cytochrome aa3 by oxygen plus carbon dioxide at hyperbaric pressures. J Appl Physiol 1977; 43:873–9.

[176] Duong TQ, Iadecola C, Kim SG. Effect of hyperoxia, hypercapnia, and hypoxia on cerebral interstitial oxygen tension and cerebral blood flow. Magn Reson Med 2001;45:61–70.

[177] Ratai EM, Benner T, Sorensen AG, et al. Therapeutic effects of normobaric hyperoxia in acute stroke: multivoxel mr-spectroscopy and adc correlations on serial imaging. 13th Scientific Meeting of the International Society of Magnetic Resonance in Medicine. Miami, Florida, 2005.

[178] Lyden PD, Jackson-Friedman C, Shin C, et al. Synergistic combinatorial stroke therapy: a quantal bioassay of a gaba agonist and a glutamate antagonist. Exp Neurol 2000;163:477–89.

[179] Onal MZ, Li F, Tatlisumak T, et al. Synergistic effects of citicoline and mk-801 in temporary experimental focal ischemia in rats. Stroke 1997;28: 1060–5.

[180] Barth A, Barth L, Newell DW. Combination therapy with mk-801 and alpha-phenyl-tert-butyl-nitrone enhances protection against ischemic neuronal damage in organotypic hippocampal slice cultures. Exp Neurol 1996;141:330–6.

[181] Du C, Hu R, Csernansky CA, et al. Additive neuroprotective effects of dextrorphan and cycloheximide in rats subjected to transient focal cerebral ischemia. Brain Res 1996;718:233–6.

[182] Ma J, Endres M, Moskowitz MA. Synergistic effects of caspase inhibitors and mk-801 in brain injury after transient focal cerebral ischaemia in mice. Br J Pharmacol 1998;124:756–62.

[183] Barth A, Barth L, Morrison RS, et al. Bfgf enhances the protective effects of mk-801 against ischemic neuronal injury in vitro. Neuroreport 1996;7:1461–4.

[184] Schmid-Elsaesser R, Hungerhuber E, Zausinger S, et al. Neuroprotective efficacy of combination therapy with two different antioxidants in rats subjected to transient focal ischemia. Brain Res 1999;816: 471–9.

[185] Schabitz WR, Li F, Irie K, et al. Synergistic effects of a combination of low-dose basic fibroblast growth factor and citicoline after temporary experimental focal ischemia. Stroke 1999;30:427–31.

[186] Ma J, Qiu J, Hirt L, et al. Synergistic protective effect of caspase inhibitors and bfgf against brain injury induced by transient focal ischaemia. Br J Pharmacol 2001;133:345–50.

[187] Asahi M, Asahi K, Wang X, et al. Reduction of tissue plasminogen activator-induced hemorrhage and brain injury by free radical spin trapping after embolic focal cerebral ischemia in rats. J Cereb Blood Flow Metab 2000;20:452–7.

[188] Meden P, Overgaard K, Sereghy T, et al. Enhancing the efficacy of thrombolysis by ampa receptor blockade with nbqx in a rat embolic stroke model. J Neurol Sci 1993;119:209–16.

[189] Zivin JA, Mazzarella V. Tissue plasminogen activator plus glutamate antagonist improves outcome after embolic stroke. Arch Neurol 1991;48:1235–8.

[190] Sumii T, Lo EH. Involvement of matrix metalloproteinase in thrombolysis-associated hemorrhagic transformation after embolic focal ischemia in rats. Stroke 2002;33:831–6.

[191] Andersen M, Overgaard K, Meden P, et al. Effects of citicoline combined with thrombolytic therapy in a rat embolic stroke model. Stroke 1999;30: 1464–71.

[192] Yang Y, Li Q, Shuaib A. Enhanced neuroprotection and reduced hemorrhagic incidence in focal cerebral ischemia of rat by low dose combination therapy of urokinase and topiramate. Neuropharmacology 2000; 39:881–8.

[193] Bowes MP, Rothlein R, Fagan SC, et al. Monoclonal antibodies preventing leukocyte activation reduce experimental neurologic injury and enhance efficacy of thrombolytic therapy. Neurology 1995;45: 815–9.

[194] Shuaib A, Yang Y, Nakada MT, et al. Glycoprotein iib/iiia antagonist, murine 7e3 f(ab′) 2, and tissue plasminogen activator in focal ischemia: evaluation of efficacy and risk of hemorrhage with combination therapy. J Cereb Blood Flow Metab 2002;22:215–22.

[195] Lyden P, Jacoby M, Schim J, et al. The clomethiazole acute stroke study in tissue-type plasminogen activator-treated stroke (class-t): final results. Neurology 2001;57:1199–205.

[196] Grotta J. Combination therapy stroke trial: recombinant tissue-type plasminogen activator with/without lubeluzole. Cerebrovasc Dis 2001;12:258–63.

ELSEVIER
SAUNDERS

Neuroimag Clin N Am 15 (2005) 721

NEUROIMAGING
CLINICS OF
NORTH AMERICA

Correction in Print

The affiliation of the Guest Editor of "Stroke I" and "Stroke II" (this issue), Michael H. Lev, MD, was published incorrectly in the preface of the prior issue. His correct affiliation appears here below:

Michael H. Lev, MD

Director
Emergency Neuroradiology and
Neurovascular Laboratory
Department of Radiology
Massachusetts General Hospital
Boston, MA, USA

Associate Professor (Radiology)
Harvard Medical School
Boston, MA, USA

ELSEVIER
SAUNDERS

Neuroimag Clin N Am 15 (2005) 723–726

NEUROIMAGING
CLINICS OF
NORTH AMERICA

Index

Note: Page numbers of article titles are in **boldface** type.

Changing Your Address?

Make sure your subscription changes too! When you notify us of your new address, you can help make our job easier by including an exact copy of your Clinics label number with your old address (see illustration below.) This number identifies you to our computer system and will speed the processing of your address change. Please be sure this label number accompanies your old address and your corrected address—you can send an old Clinics label with your number on it or just copy it exactly and send it to the address listed below.

We appreciate your help in our attempt to give you continuous coverage. Thank you.

```
┌─────────────────────────────────────────────────────────┐
│  W. B. Saunders Company                                 │
│                                                         │
│  SHIPPING AND RECEIVING DEPTS.    ┌─────────────────────┐│
│     151 BENIGNO BLVD.             │ SECOND CLASS POSTAGE││
│     BELLMAWR, N.J. 08031          │ PAID AT BELLMAWR, N.J.││
│                                   └─────────────────────┘│
│ ■■■■■■■■■■■■■■■■■■■■■■■■■■■■■■■■■■■■■■■■■■■■■■■■■■■■■■■■■■■ │
│  This is your copy of the                               │
│  _____ CLINICS OF NORTH AMERICA                  │
│ ■■■■■■■■■■■■■■■■■■■■■■■■■■■■■■■■■■■■■■■■■■■■■■■■■■■■■■■■■■■ │
│                                                         │
│  00503570 DOE—J32400        101       NH       8102     │
│                                                         │
│  JOHN C DOE MD                                          │
│  324 SAMSON ST                                          │
│  BERLIN      NH       03570                             │
│                                                         │
│  XP-D11494                                              │
│                                                         │
│                                             JAN ISSUE   │
└─────────────────────────────────────────────────────────┘
```

Your Clinics Label Number

Copy it exactly or send your label
along with your address to:
W.B. Saunders Company, Customer Service
Orlando, FL 32887-4800
Call Toll Free 1-800-654-2452

Please allow four to six weeks for delivery of new subscriptions and for processing address changes.